# DIFFICULT CONCEPTS IN CARDIOLOGY

# DIFFICULT CONCEPTS IN CARDIOLOGY

*Edited by*

*Graham Jackson,* FRCP, FESC
*Consultant Cardiologist*
*Guy's Hospital*
*London, UK*

MARTIN DUNITZ

© Martin Dunitz Ltd 1994

First published in the United Kingdom in 1994 by
Martin Dunitz Ltd
The Livery House
7–9 Pratt Street
London NW1 0AE

A CIP catalogue record for this book is available
from the British Library

ISBN 1-85317-111-5

Composition by Scribe Design, Gillingham, Kent
Printed and bound in Great Britain by The University Press, Cambridge

# CONTENTS

# List of Contributors

**Mr David R Anderson**
Consultant Cardiac Surgeon, Cardiothoracic Unit, Guy's Hospital, London SE1 9RT

**Dr D John Betteridge**
Reader in Medicine and Consultant Physician, Department of Medicine, University College London Medical School, The Middlesex Hospital, London W1N 8AA

**Professor Alasdair Breckenridge**
Professor of Clinical Pharmacology, Department of Pharmacology and Therapeutics, University of Liverpool L69 3BX

**Dr A Yazdani Butt**
Research Fellow, Department of Respiratory Physiology, Papworth Hospital, Cambridge CB3 8RE

**Professor A John Camm**
Professor of Clinical Cardiology and Chairman of Medicine, Department of Cardiological Sciences, St George's Hospital Medical School, London SW17 0RE

**Professor Ronald WF Campbell**
Professor of Cardiology, Academic Cardiology, Freeman Hospital, Newcastle upon Tyne NE7 7DN

**Dr John Chambers**
Senior Lecturer and Honorary Consultant in Cardiology, Department of Cardiology, Guy's Hospital, London SE1 9RT

**Dr Pim J de Feyter**
Director of the Catheterization Laboratory, Thoraxcentrum, Erasmus University, 3000DR Rotterdam, The Netherlands

**Dr Peter PT de Jaegere**
Clinical Director of the Catheterization Laboratory, Thoraxcentrum, Erasmus University, 3000DR Rotterdam, The Netherlands

**Dr David P Foley**
Research Fellow, Thoraxcentrum, Erasmus University, 3000DR Rotterdam, The Netherlands

**Dr Jaswinder S Gill**
Lecturer in Cardiology, Department of Cardiological Sciences, St George's Hospital Medical School, London SW17 0RE

**Dr Ever D Grech**
Clinical Research Fellow, Department of Cardiology, The Cardiothoracic Centre, Liverpool L14 3PE

**Dr Tim W Higenbottam**
Director, Regional Pulmonary Physiology Laboratory, and Consultant Physician, Department of Respiratory Physiology, Papworth Hospital, Cambridge CB3 8RE and Addenbrooke's Hospital, Cambridge CB2 5QQ

**Dr Graham Jackson**
Consultant Cardiologist, Department of Cardiology, Guy's Hospital, London SE1 9RT

**Dr David Keane**
Cardiology Fellow, Department of
Cardiology, Guy's Hospital, London SE1
9RT; Research Fellow, Thoraxcentrum,
Erasmus University, 3000DR Rotterdam,
The Netherlands

**Professor William J McKenna**
Professor of Cardiac Medicine, Department
of Cardiological Sciences, St George's
Hospital Medical School, London SW17
0RE

**Professor Celia M Oakley**
Professor of Clinical Cardiology,
Department of Medicine (Cardiology),
Hammersmith Hospital and the Royal
Postgraduate Medical School, London W12
0NN

**Dr Shakeel A Qureshi**
Consultant Paediatric Cardiologist,
Department of Paediatric Cardiology, Guy's
Hospital, London SE1 9RT

**Dr David R Ramsdale**
Consultant Cardiologist, Department of
Cardiology, The Cardiothoracic Centre,
Liverpool L14 3PE

**Professor Patrick W Serruys**
Professor of Interventional Cardiology,
Erasmus University, Professor of the
Interuniversity Cardiology Institute of The
Netherlands, Director of Research of the
Catheterization Laboratory, Thoraxcentrum,
Erasmus University, 3000DR Rotterdam,
The Netherlands

**Dr Iain A Simpson**
Consultant Cardiologist, Wessex
Cardiothoracic Centre, Southampton
General Hospital, Southampton SO9 4XY

**Dr Alistair KB Slade**
British Heart Foundation Junior Research
Fellow, Department of Cardiological
Sciences, St George's Hospital Medical
School, London SW17 0RE

**Mr Peter R Taylor**
Senior Lecturer in Vascular Surgery, Guy's
Hospital, London SE1 9RT; and Consultant
Vascular Surgeon, Lewisham Hospital,
London SE13 6LH

**Mr Tom Treasure**
Consultant Cardiothoracic Surgeon,
Cardiothoracic Unit, St George's Hospital,
London SW17 0QT

**Dr Andonis G Violaris**
Research Fellow, Thoraxcentrum, Erasmus
University, 3000DR Rotterdam, The
Netherlands

**Professor James J Walker**
Professor of Obstetrics and Gynaecology,
Leeds University, Department of Obstetrics
and Gynaecology, St James's University
Hospital, Leeds LS9 7TF

**Dr Thomas Walley**
Senior Lecturer in Clinical Pharmacology,
Department of Pharmacology and
Therapeutics, University of Liverpool,
Liverpool L69 3BX

# Preface

This book is not a textbook of cardiology and so it is not comprehensive. It is meant to be a stimulating addition to the conventional (and excellent) textbooks currently available. All the authors were given the same challenge of reviewing their subject and translating the grey areas into a firmer decision making process. Finally, we encouraged the personal ending to each chapter entitled 'If I had ...' where individual authors had to imagine they or a close relative had the problem under discussion and decide what they would or would not like to be done.

In this way I hope each of the eighteen chapters will be fun to read purely for interest. Fun may be a strange word to use but I'd like to feel cardiology can be enjoyable whether in agreement or disagreement and the personal input I hope adds a special interest. Each chapter is also fully referenced and the book can therefore be used as an up-to-date source of information.

Our first collection, *Difficult Cardiology* (1990), was well-received and I hope this second collection is of similar value. As before, we cannot cover all areas of contention but we have focused on as many topical issues as possible trying to make entertaining contributions to each subject.

It has been 'fun' editing this book and I have learnt a lot from my fellow authors. I hope others will feel and benefit the same way enjoying the book as they read it.

# Acknowledgements

Grateful thanks are due to my secretary Helen Symeou for co-ordinating the manuscripts; the authors for delivering on time (well almost) and to Robert Peden and Alan Burgess of Martin Dunitz Ltd for their splendid efforts in achieving a rapid publication time.

# Dedication

It is better to be an ordinary patient than a difficult one. This book is dedicated to our difficult patients in the hope we can make more of them ordinary.

# 1

# Drug therapy for patients with angina pectoris

*David Keane and Graham Jackson*

## Introduction

Myocardial ischaemia occurs when an imbalance develops between myocardial oxygen supply and demand. In the presence of a fixed coronary artery stenosis, increases in heart rate, blood pressure and left ventricular wall stress can lead to an imbalance in the supply/demand ratio, resulting in ischaemia. Most coronary stenoses, however, have an arc of normal arterial wall capable of dilatation and constriction. Myocardial oxygen supply may therefore be influenced by alterations in vasomotor tone, with ischaemic episodes resulting from vasoconstriction of such normal segments of stenoses. Episodes of ischaemia may also result from platelet aggregation at sites of coronary stenosis, resulting in transient obstructions to coronary blood flow and reduced oxygen supply.

Anti-anginal therapy should therefore be directed at reduction of myocardial oxygen demand, increase of myocardial oxygen supply and inhibition of platelet aggregation. Furthermore, anti-anginal strategies should be aimed at an improvement in long-term prognosis in addition to the prevention of symptoms.

In addition to sublingual glyceryl trinitrate as required, most patients with stable angina pectoris will require prophylactic anti-anginal medication. Before commencing an anti-anginal agent, however, the following points should be considered.

In obese patients, symptoms may be ameliorated or even disappear with weight reduction.

The importance of stopping smoking should be stressed to all patients with angina, as not only is it a well-established risk factor for coronary artery disease but it has also been shown that smoking may render anti-anginal medication less effective.[1]

The patient should be advised to avoid known triggering activities of his angina where possible, e.g. strenuous effort in very cold, windy weather or after meals. Regular exercise over a prolonged period, however, can reduce the total ischaemic burden[2] and thus reduce the requirement for prophylactic anti-anginal medication. Patients should also be reminded that they may take sublingual nitroglycerin prophylactically prior to undertaking routine triggering activities.

Uncontrolled hypertension in patients with angina should be treated vigorously.

Congestive heart failure may aggravate angina, particularly nocturnal angina. Heart failure increases myocardial oxygen demand by an increase in heart rate, increase in sympathetic tone, cardiac enlargement and reduced cardiac output with reduced coronary bloodflow. Treatment of heart failure with a diuretic, an angiotensin converting enzyme inhibitor or digitalis may relieve angina.

Allowance should be made for possible effects of other cardiovascular medications which the patient may already be taking, e.g. the anti-anginal effect of amiodarone,[3] the negative inotropic effect of other anti-arrhythmic agents and the donation of a sulphydryl group by an angiotensin converting enzyme inhibitor, which may limit nitrate tolerance.

While many pharmacological agents have been shown to improve exercise capacity in angina,[4-6] established prophylactic therapy of angina continues to be limited to three classes of drugs; beta-blockers, nitrates and, more recently, calcium antagonists.[7] While all three classes of drugs share a common end-point, the reduction of myocardial oxygen demand, they have individual mechanisms of action.

## Beta-blockers

Beta-blockers achieve a reduction in myocardial oxygen demand by decreasing heart rate, myocardial contractility and left ventricular afterload with a reduction in blood pressure at rest and on exercise. No major improvement in oxygen supply is seen with this class of medication.

Beta-adrenoceptors are present in the heart, peripheral vasculature, bronchi, pancreas, kidney and liver. Most receptors in the heart are $beta_1$-receptors, and at the other sites $beta_2$-receptors. A third $beta_3$-receptor has recently been identified but its relevance to the drug therapy of angina is undetermined.[8]

Beta-blocker compounds reduce catecholamine-induced formation of cyclic adenosine monophosphate (cAMP) and reduce calcium influx into the myocardial cells. While they may reduce peripheral vasodilatation, there is little evidence that beta-blockers have a clinically significant effect on coronary vasodilatation and they may in fact prevent a paradoxical, exercise-induced constriction seen in coronary stenoses.[9]

Fifteen beta-blockers are currently available and, while they have comparable efficacy, they differ from each other in terms of lipid solubility, $beta_1$-selectivity, intrinsic sympathomimetic activity, alpha-blocking activity and rate of excretion. These added properties may affect the choice of drug in an individual patient. Characteristics of eleven beta-blockers are given in Table 1.1.

Drugs with low lipid solubility cross the blood–brain barrier poorly and may be less likely to cause adverse effects in the central nervous system such as sleep disturbance.

Propanolol blocks both $beta_1$- and $beta_2$-receptors but later drugs like atenolol, bisoprolol and metoprolol are more selective for the $beta_1$-receptor and hence less likely to produce the adverse effects associated with $beta_2$-antagonism, e.g. bronchoconstriction. Selectivity is a relative quality, though, and at higher doses cardioselectivity is reduced. In our experience a limited number of patients with a history of mild obstructive airway disease have tolerated celiprolol, a third-generation beta-blocker, without exacerbation of symptoms or reduction in peak expiratory flow rate. Even at lower doses, however, it is generally not recommended that beta-blocking drugs be administered to patients with a history of obstructive airway disease.

Intrinsic sympathomimetic activity (ISA) or partial agonist activity is seen when, if endogenous sympathetic activity is low, the drug has an ability to cause some stimulation at the beta-receptor, but when endogenous sympathetic activity is high, the drug antagonizes the beta-receptor. Beta-blockers with ISA include celiprolol, acebutolol, oxprenolol, pindolol, carteolol and penbutolol. Beta-blockers with ISA are most useful in the anti-anginal management of patients who have atrial fibrillation, enabling the ventricular rate to be controlled without causing excessive bradycardia at rest. The value of beta-blockers with ISA in the secondary prevention of myocardial infarction is unknown.

| Drug | Optimum dose dynamic half-life (hours) | Beta$_1$ selectivity | Penetrates blood–brain barrier | ISA | Comment |
|------|----------------------------------------|----------------------|-------------------------------|-----|---------|
| Propranolol | 11 | – | ++++ | – | Extensive clinical experience |
| Sotalol | 24 | – | – | – | Class III anti-arrhythmic also |
| Atenolol | 24 | ++ | – | – | Extensive clinical experience |
| Metoprolol | 10–12 | ++ | +++ | – | Extensive clinical experience |
| Bisoprolol | 24 | ++ | ++ | – | Long half-life |
| Nadolol | 39 | – | – | – | Long half-life |
| Labetolol | 8–12 | – | ++++ | + | Alpha-blocker also |
| Acebutolol | 24 | + | ++ | + | Useful in atrial fibrillation |
| Pindolol | 8 | – | ++++ | +++ | Useful in atrial fibrillation |
| Oxprenolol | 13 | – | ++ | ++ | Useful in atrial fibrillation |
| Celiprolol | 24 | ++ | + | +++ | Few adverse effects and beneficial metabolic effects. Limited clinical experience |

– no significant presence
+ degree of effect from + (least) to ++++ (most)

**Table 1.1**
*Characteristics of the commonly used beta-blockers.*

Labetolol antagonizes both alpha- and beta-adrenoreceptors, though it is more potent as a beta-blocker. The alpha-blockade effect may make labetolol particularly useful in patients who develop cold peripheries when taking selective beta-blockers.

## Adverse effects of beta-blockers

Fatigue and cold peripheries are the most common adverse effects of beta-blocking drugs. The drugs are generally contraindicated in obstructive airway disease even with agents that are selective for the beta$_1$-adrenoceptor. Other contraindications to their use are second- and third-degree heart block and moderate to severe heart failure. Recent studies, however, suggest that beta-blockers can have a propitious effect on heart failure,[10,11] although the exact role for beta-blockers in this context has yet to be determined. In addition to beta$_1$- and beta$_2$-blockade, sotalol has some class III activity (potassium channel blockade) and may prolong the QT interval—occasionally this has resulted in torsade de pointes ventricular tachycardia. Unlike selective agents, non-selective beta-blockers may increase platelet aggregation and plasma adrenaline levels.[12]

There is evidence that the sudden withdrawal of beta-blockers in patients with angina may cause an exacerbation of symptoms on account of upregulation of beta-receptors. Withdrawal of beta-blocker therapy should therefore be gradual to permit the number of beta-receptors to fall.[13]

## Nitrates

Nitrates achieve a reduction in myocardial oxygen requirement predominantly by preload reduction with lowering of filling pressure and reduction of intraventricular volume. Nitrates act predominantly as venodilators at low doses. At higher doses, the arterial effects are more marked, and decreased systemic vascular resistance is accompanied by a reduction in blood pressure. The venodilating and arterial dilating effects of nitrates are termed the 'indirect or peripheral' effects, since they relieve ischaemia by reducing determinants of myocardial oxygen demand. The 'direct or central' effects of organic nitrates relieve ischaemia by actions on the coronary vasculature, reversing coronary spasm and increasing intercoronary collateral flow, thereby improving determinants of myocardial oxygen supply.[14] While coronary vasodilatation occurs to a variable extent, the principal mechanism of action of nitrates in chronic stable angina is dilatation of the capacitance vessels.

Endothelium-derived relaxing factor (EDRF), which is generated within the vascular endothelium, is one of the most active endogenous vasodilators, and is involved particularly in the modulation of coronary vascular diameter and flow. In 1987 it was confirmed that the biological effects of EDRF are identical to those of nitric oxide (NO). The intracellular precursor of NO is L-arginine and the enzyme responsible for NO generation is NO synthase. Once produced, NO stimulates guanylate cyclase to produce cyclic guanosine monophosphate (cGMP). The production of EDRF is dependent on an intact endothelium which can become damaged by diseases such as arteriosclerosis, hypertension or diabetes. All the organic nitrates act through a single common mechanism, the release of nitric oxide (NO). Unlike EDRF, however, nitrates do not require intact endothelium in order to become effective.

While the vascular effects of nitrates have been well documented, studies show that, in vivo, nitrates are endowed with platelet-inhibiting and therefore anti-thrombotic properties as well.[15] These anti-aggregating effects are triggered by NO. Nitrates act via a different mechanism than currently used aggregation inhibitors, such as acetylsalicylic acid, and their actions appear additive. The combination of the platelet-inhibiting action with their haemodynamic effects may be important for their anti-ischaemic effectiveness, particularly in preventing vasospastic conditions during unstable angina. Patients with stable angina may also benefit from these effects, since circadian periods of peak ischaemia are frequently associated with increased platelet activity.

Although nitrates can replace the action of EDRF in arteries, the problem of tachyphylaxis (decreased effect with time) which is frequently observed with continuous use of the organic nitrates is not seen with EDRF. The reason for this is not known at present, but the explanation is probably related to the metabolic conversion of organic nitrates to NO, a step not involved in the endogenous production of EDRF. This enzymatic conversion is dependent on the presence of sulphydryl groups, which can become depleted from continuous nitrate exposure. However, this explanation of the phenomenon of tolerance to organic nitrates may be insufficient, since restoration of sulphydryl groups with sulphydryl donors has yet to be demonstrated to be completely effective.

Slow-release formulations of nitrates, maintaining an even 24-h nitrate level, will be subject to tachyphylaxis and should be avoided.[16] Tachyphylaxis to continuous levels of nitrates appears to be a problem in only about a half of patients.[17]

## Nitrate preparations

Glyceryl trinitrate (GTN) has almost 100 per cent first-pass hepatic metabolism and formulations have therefore been developed to enable the trinitrate to bypass the portal system. Even when GTN is administered sublingually, intravenously or topically, it is rapidly converted to inactive metabolites and has a plasma half-life of 1–3 min. Despite this, GTN can be used prophylactically when formulated in a slow-release delivery system and when taken sublingually immediately before physical activity or before situations that involve tension.

The effect of nitrates can be obtained rapidly by sublingual administration, since all organic nitrates are lipid soluble and are easily absorbed from mucous membranes. Sublingual GTN avoids hepatic metabolism, is effective in 2–3 min and may be repeated. GTN lasts up to 30 min sublingually and for more prolonged effect sublingual isosorbide dinitrate may be preferred. GTN loses its potency after 2–3 months, and in view of its volatile properties it should be stored in a fridge in a darkened glass bottle without cotton wool. GTN spray lasts up to 3 years but is more expensive. However, it may be advantageous when the patient's pain is infrequent.

Buccal administration of GTN offers the advantage of immediate release of nitrate, similar to the sublingual route, with a more gradual release over 4 h or so. Buccal preparations would appear to offer a less expensive alternative to intravenous nitrate therapy in the perioperative state or in unstable angina.

Topical (transdermal) nitrates were developed to avoid hepatic metabolism and provide more consistent anti-anginal effects, but unfortunately tolerance rapidly develops. This may be avoided by intermittent administration (12 h on, 12 h off), and in view of a late peak effect (6 h) and long duration, transdermal nitrates may be of value in patients with nocturnal angina. Nitroglycerin ointment has for the most part been replaced by prepacked preparations with adhesive patches. The slightly higher cost is offset by greater convenience to the patient. Application of the nitrate patch over the praecordium may give some patients additional psychological comfort. Except for occasional dermal reactions at the site of application, these preparations are well tolerated. Accelerated absorption may occur if the skin to which the patch is applied is erythematous.

Sublingual or chewable isosorbide dinitrate (ISDN) may be used in place of GTN. Isosorbide dinitrate (ISDN) has a relatively longer plasma half-life ($\sim$36 min) with active hepatic metabolites, isosorbide 2-mononitrate and isosorbide 5-mononitrate. Isosorbide 5-mononitrate appears in higher concentrations than isosorbide 2-mononitrate and is a more potent vasodilator. ISDN is subject to a high degree of hepatic 'first-pass metabolism', which varies considerably between individuals. This may lead to an unpredictable response to treatment, particularly with slow-release preparations.

Only 20–25 per cent of an administered oral dose of ISDN is systemically available. In contrast, isosorbide mononitrate has a high bioavailability and has a comparatively long half-life (4–5 h), making it a more effective and reliable agent for the prophylaxis of angina. On the basis of bioavailability, there may no longer be a need for ISDN in oral preparations.

## Adverse effects of nitrates

When initially prescribed, long-acting nitrates may cause headaches. This side-effect abates if the medications are started at low doses and gradually built up over a few days. Rarely, headaches may be absent initially and appear insidiously after several weeks or months on sustained-action nitrate preparations.

Nitrates can cause postural hypotension, particularly in the elderly. As baroreceptor reflexes are unimpaired when nitrates are used as monotherapy, reduction in arterial pressure is occasionally associated with a reflex tachycardia which is usually mild and not of importance in the exercising patient. Flushing occurs rarely with prophylactic nitrate therapy.

Overall, the organic nitrates are the safest of all anti-anginal drugs and are particularly useful in patients with heart failure where a haemodynamic benefit may be achieved.

## Calcium antagonists

Since the first calcium antagonist was developed in the 1960s, these drugs have proven to be effective in the management of both chronic stable angina and hypertension. The number of calcium antagonists under development continues to increase and calcium antagonists have now become the most commonly prescribed group of cardiovascular drugs.

Calcium antagonists reduce myocardial oxygen demand predominantly by afterload reduction and some (verapamil and diltiazem) reduce heart rate. Furthermore, calcium antagonists may improve myocardial oxygen supply by coronary artery dilatation. The calcium channel blockers inhibit the slow, inward, voltage-sensitive calcium channels in the cell membrane. They have action in (vascular) smooth muscle and nodal tissue and at higher concentrations they may have a negative inotropic effect on the myocardium. Additionally, calcium antagonists may protect tissue during ischaemia and may have effects on red blood cells which influence blood viscosity.[18] Recent evidence suggests that calcium antagonists may retard the atherosclerotic process.

This heterogeneous group of drugs has three subclasses which possess varying degrees of vasoselectivity. Differences between the three subclasses are outlined in Table 1.2 and their principal agents and pharmacological characteristics are given below.

| Drug | Half-life | Bioavailability (%) | Vasoselective | Heart rate | AV conduction |
|------|-----------|---------------------|---------------|------------|---------------|
| Nifedipine | 6–11 h | 43–68 | +++ | ↑↑ | 0 |
| Nicardipine | 8–9 h | 35 | ++++ | ↑↑ | 0 |
| Amlodipine | 35–50 h | 60–65 | ++++ | ↑0 | 0 |
| Diltiazem | 4–6 h | 40 | ++ | ↑↓ | ↓ |
| Verapamil | 3–12 h | 20–35 | + | ↓↓ | ↓↓ |

+ degree of effect from + (least) to ++++ (most)

**Table 1.2**
Calcium antagonists.

## *Dihydropyridines—nifedipine, nicardipine, amlodipine, felodipine, isradipine and nimodipine*

The dihydropyridines vary not only with respect to their overall vasoselectivity but also in their selectivity for specific vascular beds. For instance, nimodipine has little effect on peripheral or coronary vasculature but is a potent vasodilator of cerebral vasculature, while isradipine and nicardipine are potent dilators of both peripheral and coronary vessels.[19]

Nifedipine acts predominantly as a peripheral arterial vasodilator, with no clinically significant effects on electrophysiological tissue. It has good bioavailability, and therapeutic plasma levels are achieved within 20–40 min. This rapid achievement of plasma levels results in frequent vasodilatory side-effects, with reflex tachycardia, flushing and peripheral dilatation with fluid retention and ankle swelling. This reflex tachycardia may occasionally exacerbate symptoms of angina. Slow-release preparations of nifedipine have been developed to achieve a smoother profile and improve compliance.

While, at higher doses, most dihydropyridine calcium antagonists have a mildly negative inotropic effect on the myocardium, cardiac output may increase due to the reduction in afterload. In a study on patients with angina, intravenous or intracoronary administration of nicardipine had no effect or improved left ventricular function,[20] and studies are currently assessing the role of the more vasoselective dihydropyridines in patients with heart failure.

The second-generation dihydropyridines have a higher degree of vasoselectivity and may be associated with improved tolerance and a reduced incidence of adverse effects. Their clinical indications will be further defined by comparative studies of efficacy and safety.

Amlodipine has a long intrinsic half-life, offering full 24-h cover with a once-daily dosage,[21] which should improve compliance. Amlodipine may also have some activity on the benzothiazepine receptor and felodipine may prolong AV conduction.[22]

## *Benzothiazepines—diltiazem*

Diltiazem's pharmacodynamic profile makes it an attractive choice when a calcium antagonist is used as monotherapy. Diltiazem combines a significant negative chronotropic effect with moderate vasodilatation. Diltiazem has a mildly negative dromotropic effect which is usually not clinically significant unless prescribed in combination with a beta-blocker. In a study of 135 patients with angina, first-degree AV block occurred in four patients treated with diltiazem and in six patients treated with diltiazem and hydrochlorothiazide.[23] Diltiazem has a less active metabolite which tends to accumulate with chronic therapy. Diltiazem has a relatively short half-life so that even when slow-release preparations are used a bid dosage is required. A kinetic interaction may occur with digoxin, resulting in increased drug levels. Diltiazem should not be prescribed after infarction to patients with a low ejection fraction or pulmonary congestion,[24] but it may have a limited role following uncomplicated non-q-wave myocardial infarction in patients intolerant of beta-blockers.

## *Phenylalkylamines—verapamil*

Verapamil behaves in many ways like a beta-blocker and presents a useful alternative in patients intolerant of beta-blockers on account of asthma etc. The drug is highly protein-bound and has an active metabolite, norverapamil. Verapamil may exert significant effects on non-vascular smooth muscle which may result in constipation and other gastrointestinal complaints. In addition, verapamil has a significant effect on the SA and AV nodes and, therefore, is relatively contraindicated in sick sinus syndrome or in the presence of AV node disease and in the Wolf–Parkinson–White (WPW) syndrome with antegrade conduction through the accessory pathway. Verapamil may interact with beta-blockers, digoxin, quinidine and disopyramide. Slow-release (once-daily) formulations of verapamil are available which should improve compliance. Verapamil may be used to treat angina following uncomplicated myocardial infarction when left ventricular function is relatively well preserved in patients intolerant of beta-blockers.

## Calcium antagonists and vasoselectivity

In addition to pharmacokinetic properties, vascular selectivity is a key area of difference among the calcium antagonists which may influence drug choice. This is a measure of the relative potency of effect on the vasculature compared with that on the heart. Thus, with a vascular/cardiac selectivity ratio of 1, verapamil affects the heart to the same extent as the peripheral vasculature. Diltiazem, with a selectivity ratio of 5, is only a little different, while nifedipine has a ratio of 15. In contrast, the second-generation calcium antagonists have markedly higher ratios and appear to be free of clinically significant effects on the myocardium at therapeutic dosages.

By virtue of the wide spectrum of clinical effects of calcium antagonists, dihydropyridines may be combined with verapamil or diltiazem to provide effective dual therapy in patients intolerant of beta-blockers.[25] In view of their effect on arterial dilatation, dihydropyridine calcium antagonists should be avoided in obstructive conditions such as aortic stenosis

and hypertrophic obstructive cardiomyopathy. Verapamil, however, may be used to treat angina in patients with hypertrophic obstructive cardiomyopathy who are intolerant of beta-blockers.

## Adverse effects

In general, calcium antagonists are well tolerated, with a low incidence of adverse effects and no unfavourable metabolic effects. Adverse effects vary according to the subclass used. Rapid vasodilatation may cause flushing, headache and oedema, while a more gradual onset of action may reduce some of these side-effects; diltiazem may cause bradycardia; and verapamil may cause bradycardia and rarely AV block. Ankle oedema can occur despite a diuretic and natriuretic effect of dihydropyridine calcium antagonists. Both diltiazem and verapamil may lead to increased levels and toxicity of the anticonvulsant drugs carbamazepine and phenytoin.[26] Calcium antagonists may possibly have an adverse effect on outcome when used as monotherapy in unstable angina.[27]

## Aspirin

Should drug therapy of angina include aspirin? The case for aspirin in secondary prevention post-infarction has been demonstrated by ISIS-2.[28] The benefit of aspirin has also been demonstrated in patients with unstable angina.[29] The risk reduction with aspirin in secondary prevention is around 25 per cent; vascular mortality can be reduced by one-sixth, and non-fatal stroke and myocardial infarction by about a third. While studies have not primarily addressed patients with chronic stable angina, it seems likely that the reduction in cardiovascular mortality associated with aspirin would be extended to those patients with stable angina who have not had a myocardial infarction.

Enteric-coated aspirin was developed to reduce gastric complications. An additional benefit of enteric-coated aspirin over soluble aspirin has been proposed. When aspirin is slowly absorbed, it is entirely deacetylated to salicylate during its passage through the liver and salicylate is not capable of inhibiting prostacyclin production by endothelium in the systemic circulation. Thromboxane synthesis by platelets, however, will be irreversibly blocked during the circulation of platelets through the portal system.[30] The clinical importance of using enteric-coated aspirin remains undetermined and an adequate degree of selective inhibition of thromboxane synthesis can probably be adequately achieved by using low-dose soluble aspirin.

During aspirin therapy, blood pressure should be controlled, to reduce the slightly increased risk of intracranial haemorrhage possibly associated with aspirin.[31]

# Interpretation and design of studies on anti-anginal drug therapy

The subjective and variable nature of angina inherently induces problems with objective assessment. The absence of a standardized approach in trials of anti-anginal medication has rendered direct comparisons of studies difficult. In order to understand the true significance of anti-anginal studies, we need to determine which parameter of exercise testing is the most relevant end-point; total exercise time, time to ischaemia or time to chest pain. Perhaps greater importance should be attached to the performance of anti-anginal medications

in reducing symptomatic and asymptomatic ischaemia on ambulatory electrocardiographic monitoring rather than on exercise testing.[32]

We need to determine whether standard or maximally tolerated dosages of each drug should be used in both monotherapy and combination therapy studies on angina.[33] Preferably, each individual component of combination therapy should be titrated with complete dose–response curves before combination. Furthermore, in view of the different pharmacokinetics of each class of anti-anginal medication, studies on combination therapy should include several time-points over a 24-h period to cover peaks and troughs of each individual drug of the combination under assessment. 'Acute' studies do not assess the possible physiological adjustments that can occur with chronic vasodilator therapy.[34]

The results of previous studies on anti-anginal therapy should not necessarily be applied to newer agents of the same class, particularly when agents of the same class vary considerably in their pharmacodynamics e.g. first- and third-generation beta-blockers or verapamil, and second-generation dihydropyridine calcium antagonists. Moreover, results of studies on drug therapy of chronic stable angina should not be applied to the management of unstable angina.

As yet, the design of published studies does not permit conclusions to be drawn on the relative prognostic benefit of individual anti-anginal agents. Placebo-controlled long-term anti-anginal studies, however, are becoming more difficult to justify.

# Monotherapy

Short-term studies on monotherapy comparing the three classes of anti-anginal drugs with each other have failed to show a consistent advantage of one class over another.[35-39] In principle, however, it is difficult to recommend the long-term use of nitrates as prophylactic monotherapy in view of problems with tachyphylaxis and lack of 24-h cover. Effective, long-term monotherapy of mild to moderate angina can be achieved by use of either a beta-blocker or a calcium antagonist.

Again, while no single beta-blocker has been shown to be clearly superior to other beta-blockers in anti-anginal monotherapy, it is preferable to use a long-acting, cardioselective beta-blocker without ISA[40,41] when possible.

Use of a cardioselective beta-blocker will reduce adverse effects, particularly in patients with a tendency to develop mild bronchospasm or insulin-dependent diabetes mellitus. Cardioselective beta-blockers are less likely to impair glucose release in response to hypoglycaemia. They will, however, mask the tachycardia which diabetic patients may be using as a warning sign. Quality of life is likely to be higher when a cardioselective rather than a non-selective beta-blocker is prescribed which, in turn, will improve compliance. Prescription of a non-selective beta-blocker should nowadays be restricted to specific indications. Such circumstances include the presence of arrhythmias, when sotalol may be effective; when angina is aggravated by thyrotoxicosis, when propanolol may be preferred; and when an agent with ISA is required, although in view of its (mild) cardioselectivity, acebutolol may be used rather than oxprenolol and pindolol.

A beta-blocker with a long half-life will provide more complete 24-h cover. While tachyphylaxis is not seen during beta-blocker therapy, there may in fact be upregulation of beta-receptors and withdrawal of the beta-blocker may result in precipitation of anginal symptoms.[13] For this reason it may be preferable to avoid beta-blocker therapy when poor compliance is suspected. While patients with symptomatic angina comply better than those with silent ischaemia, as little as 1 in 10 patients may be presumed to be perfect compliers, and once-daily drug dosaging results in better compliance than twice- or thrice-daily regimes.

When choosing a calcium antagonist as monotherapy for angina, diltiazem offers peripheral vasodilatation (afterload reduction), coronary dilatation, negative chronotropic effect on the SA node with minimal effect on the AV node and only a mild negative inotropic effect on the myocardium. Verapamil may also be useful monotherapy and in many ways offers the same advantages as a beta-blocker and is available in a once-daily, slow-release preparation. When poor compliance is anticipated despite lengthy discussions with the patient, prescription of amlodipine should be considered in view of its long half-life (36 h).[21] In general, short-acting dihydropyridine calcium antagonists should probably be avoided as monotherapy as occasionally patients may develop a paradoxical increase in angina as a result of a reflex tachycardia or a possible coronary steal phenomenon.

## Combination therapy

The distinctly different mechanisms of action of the three classes of anti-anginal drugs would suggest that their combination may confer additional benefit over monotherapy.

Conceivable advantages of combining anti-anginal medication are as follows:

1 Combination therapy might permit lower doses of each individual medication with lessening of dose-related side-effects.

2 Most episodes of myocardial ischaemia in stable angina pectoris appear to be related to transient reduction in myocardial oxygen supply rather than increase in myocardial

demand,[42] which makes the combination of beta-blockers with nitrates or calcium antagonists appear advantageous.

3 The peripheral, and possible coronary,[43] vasoconstrictor effects of beta-blockers might be overcome by the addition of dihydropyridine calcium antagonists, and in turn the reflex tachycardia seen with some dihydropyridine calcium antagonists may be overcome by the co-prescription of a beta-blocker.

4 The negative inotropic effect of beta-blocker therapy might be offset by the co-prescription of nitrates.[44]

5 The unprotected periods of interval therapy with nitrates might be covered by combination with sustained doses of beta-blockers or calcium antagonists.[16]

Possible disadvantages of combination therapy in angina are as follows:

1 Excessive hypotension may result not only in postural hypotension[45] but also in reduced myocardial perfusion.[46]

2 Symptomatic bradycardia or atrioventricular block from the combined negative chronotropic and dromotropic effects of beta-blockers and certain calcium antagonists (diltiazem and verapamil).

3 Precipitation of heart failure by the combined negative inotropic effects of beta-blockers and calcium antagonists. (While most calcium antagonists have a negative inotropic effect, there is usually no overall fall in cardiac output with the more vaso-selective dihydropyridines due to afterload reduction,[47] reflex tachycardia and improved lusitropy.)

4 Insofar as the ability of calcium antagonists to enhance ventricular relaxation is related to reflex activation of the sympathetic nervous system, this potentially beneficial action may be lost when these drugs are combined with beta-blockers.[48]

5 The particular combination of beta-blockers with verapamil is fraught with a high incidence of adverse events.[49] These relate primarily to the close resemblance in structure of verapamil to catecholamines, enabling verapamil itself to directly antagonize both alpha-adrenergic and beta-adrenergic receptors. In addition, verapamil and beta-blockers may interfere with each other's metabolic degradation, resulting in unexpectedly high plasma levels of both drugs when administered in combination in their usual doses.[50]

6 Compliance becomes more difficult with a greater number of medications. This is of particular concern in patients taking beta-blockers where poor compliance may precipitate an ischaemic episode. Polypharmacy is unfortunately common in patients with ischaemic heart disease, as most are already taking GTN and aspirin and many patients may also be on concomitant medication for hypercholesterolaemia, heart failure or arrhythmias.

## Studies on combination therapy

Of the limited number of studies which have assessed double therapy in stable angina, most but not all have found additional improvement in exercise parameters with double therapy compared to monotherapy.[36,51–53] In studies combining beta-blockers with calcium antagonists, double therapy often prolonged the exercise time to chest pain but failed to improve maximal exercise capacity.[54,55] In studies which titrated the beta-blocker therapy to the maximally tolerated dose prior to adding a calcium antagonist, such a significant improvement occurred with maximizing the beta-blocker dose that little further benefit was detected with double therapy.[54,56,57]

To date, few studies have addressed triple therapy in stable angina.[58] In one such study,[59] the effect of adding a calcium antagonist to maximal nitrate and beta-blocker therapy was assessed in 14 patients. Exercise was initially limited by angina in all 14 patients on double therapy, while after the addition of a calcium antagonist exercise was limited by angina in only five patients on triple therapy. Overall there was a statistically significant increase of 21 per cent in exercise duration on triple therapy.

A second study on combination therapy compared monotherapy, double therapy and triple therapy.[60] Monotherapy consisted of a beta-blocker (slow-release metoprolol at an optimal dose). Double therapy consisted of a beta-blocker combined with a calcium antagonist or a nitrate, while triple therapy involved all three agents. The combinations were compared in 11 patients with stable angina in a randomized, double-blind, crossover design. Patients underwent serial, symptom-limited exercise testing at five intervals over a 24-h period on each treatment combination. Based on ST-segment depression, all combinations of double therapy led to a significant or at least relative increase in effectiveness compared to monotherapy with a beta-blocker. In addition, triple therapy was significantly or relatively more effective than the various double combinations. Of note is the fact that the effectiveness of the above combinations varied considerably according to the timing of the exercise test.

A double-blind, randomized and placebo-controlled study on stable angina assessed the 'acute' effect of adding a calcium antagonist, a nitrate or both to beta-blocker therapy.[34] All patients were on a beta-blocker prior to entering the study which was continued at the same dose without titration. Both nitrate and calcium antagonist increased exercise duration significantly compared to monotherapy with beta-blocker alone. However, when all three drugs were combined together, exercise duration was actually worse in 9 out of 16 patients on triple therapy compared to double therapy with beta-blocker and calcium antagonist. Exercise was stopped more often from leg fatigue and dyspnoea than from chest pain during triple therapy.

A recent study[61] on combination therapy compared mono-, double and triple therapy (all combinations involving a beta blocker) in 18 patients with stable angina in a randomized, double-blind, crossover design. Beta-blocker therapy was titrated to control resting and exercise heart rates prior to entering the study. Each combination of anti-anginal medication was taken for 4 weeks prior to physiological assessment. Most exercise tests were terminated due to chest pain. Both double and triple combination therapies failed to confer a statistically significant improvement over monotherapy in angina attack rates, GTN consumption, duration of symptomless ischaemia on 24-h tape or exercise duration to angina or 1-mm ST depression. Total exercise duration, however, was significantly longer with the combination of beta-blocker and nitrate (double therapy) compared to the combination of beta-blocker and calcium antagonist (double therapy) or beta-blocker alone. Of interest is the fact that the addition of calcium antagonist to the combination of beta-blocker and nitrate therapy (i.e. triple therapy) was associated with a reduction in total exercise duration in 12 out of 18 patients, no change in 1 patient and an improvement in only 5 patients.

These studies on the management of stable angina indicate that only in highly symptomatic patients will the addition of a second anti-anginal agent confer advantage over monotherapy with a beta-blocker at a maximally tolerated dose. The need to titrate beta-blockade to the optimal dosage is emphasized.[62] The addition of a third prophylactic agent will not consistently result in an improvement in either asymptomatic ischaemia or in exercise capacity and may in fact occasionally reduce exercise tolerance. The effect of alteration of patients' medication should be assessed physiologically after each change to confirm benefit and more importantly to exclude deterioration in the patient's functional capacity.

While general policies may preclude individual patients from potential benefit, for patients with stable angina and persistent symptoms on double therapy it may be more expedient to substitute rather than add another agent in the first instance, i.e. 'switch therapy' rather than 'triple therapy'.

## Drug scheduling

Ambulatory electrocardiographic monitoring has clearly demonstrated[63] a circadian pattern in myocardial ischaemic episodes, with peak ischaemic activity in the first two waking hours and a second peak in the early evening. This coincides with diurnal peaks of myocardial infarction, sudden death and strokes. These cardiovascular trends have been attributed to concomitant surges in catecholamine secretion, sympathetic nervous system activity, blood pressure, heart rate, cortisol secretion, reduced fibrinolysis and increased tendency for platelets to aggregate. Scheduling of medical therapy should therefore be adjusted to optimally cover this vulnerable period. This can be achieved by taking a beta-blocker just before going to bed. This may be augmented by a slow-release preparation of isosorbide mononitrate or long-acting calcium antagonist. Persistent early-morning angina may be pre-empted by taking a buccal or sublingual nitrate preparation upon waking in the morning. Dosage and scheduling of drugs should be titrated against symptoms, adverse effects, treadmill test performance and 24-h ischaemic burden.[64]

## Anti-anginal therapy in the elderly

As pain perception during myocardial ischaemic episodes decreases in older age,[65] elderly patients usually require less anti-anginal medication. Particular attention is still required, however, to avoid postural hypotension. Anti-anginal drugs should be started at lower doses than usual and titrated more gradually. Arterial vasodilators which achieve plasma levels rapidly should be avoided. The first dose of sublingual GTN should be taken at the clinic and, as usual, patients should be warned of any likely adverse effects. To an elderly person, quality of life may be more important than any potential prognostic benefit.

## Anti-anginal therapy and metabolic considerations

First-generation beta-blockers (e.g. propranolol) are known to have an adverse effect on the lipid profile by reducing the ratio of HDL to LDL cholesterol. Second-generation beta-blockers (e.g. atenolol, bisoprolol) have a smaller effect on lipids. Celiprolol, one of the new generation of vasodilating beta-blockers, is associated with beneficial metabolic effects.

The clinical significance of adverse effects of beta-blockers on serum lipids is unknown, although it has previously been shown that a 1 per cent rise in serum cholesterol may be associated with a 2 per cent rise in coronary heart disease mortality. For patients with a normal baseline cholesterol the mild effects on lipids associated with the second-generation beta-blockers are likely to be outweighed by an overall reduction in risk of myocardial infarction or sudden death. For patients with hypercholesterolaemia or diabetics with hyper-triglyceridaemia and hypercholesterolaemia it may be preferable to use calcium antagonists and nitrates rather than beta-blockers. Furthermore, beta-blockers are best avoided in patients with diabetes as they interfere with the autonomic and metabolic responses to hypoglycaemia. Choice of anti-anginal medication should be tailored to accommodate the individual patient's clinical and metabolic status.

## Anti-anginal therapy and prognosis

Is it enough for medical therapy of angina to only relieve or prevent symptoms of angina? While angina is the subjective presentation of ischaemia, most episodes of which are silent, repeated episodes of ischaemia may possibly lead to myocardial cell death in the absence of infarction. Therefore, anti-anginal therapy should at least be anti-ischaemic as well as being effective in preventing symptoms. Furthermore, we should not stop at achieving an anti-ischaemic effect; we should aim for regression of coronary artery disease if we are to achieve a significant improvement in long-term prognosis for the patient. Reversal of risk factors for coronary artery disease by non-pharmacological means should be pursued whenever possible, and hypercholesterolaemia, diabetes mellitus and hypertension may require independent drug therapy.

Trials comparing beta-blockers with placebo following myocardial infarction have shown significant reduction in 1-year mortality.[66] The beneficial effect may be due to reduction in ischaemia and arrhythmias. It is unknown if patients with angina, but without myocardial infarction, show similar benefit from beta-blockers, but it is tempting to believe that beta-blockers may confer some protection in these circumstances, particularly in male patients, who have a higher incidence of sudden death.

Calcium antagonists may reduce the rate of progression and possibly cause some regression of early atheroma; however, further study is required in this area.[67] Nifedipine when used as monotherapy does not improve prognosis in unstable angina.[68]

There is little information on the effects of nitrates on prognosis, although pooled data suggest a small benefit in prognosis in acute myocardial infarction. It is possible that the anti-aggregatory effect on platelets associated with nitrate therapy might reduce the likelihood of myocardial infarction.

No drug is known to prevent fissuring of coronary artery plaque. Platelets may play an important role in the development of atheromatous plaque and myocardial infarction and aspirin may prevent platelet aggregation and subsequent thrombus formation.

Heparin has been shown to promote the development of coronary artery collateralization in both animals and man.[69] Development of collaterals might be expected to improve prognosis and further study is required on oral agents which may provide a similar benefit.

While it has been shown that the burden of asymptomatic ischaemia[32] and severity of symptoms[70] predicts survival up to 4 years and all cardiac events up to 5 years, it has not been shown that individual or combined prophylactic medication for stable angina prolongs the survival of patients who have not had a previous myocardial infarction. The necessity of continuing a patient's long-term combination of anti-anginal medications should, therefore, be reviewed periodically. The overall prognosis for patients with chronic stable angina receiving standard medical therapy is relatively good, with an annual mortality ranging from 1.5 to 4.0 per cent, and angina is more likely to be uncomplicated in women.[71]

## *If I had...*

If I developed angina, my primary concern would be to reduce the possibility of myocardial infarction and my secondary aim would be the prevention (rather than the relief) of symptomatic ischaemia. I would take a beta-blocker, GTN spray sl prn and aspirin from day one. I would chew my first tablet of aspirin and thereafter would take enteric-coated aspirin.

To cover the early morning peak period of infarction risk, I would take a beta-blocker with a long half-life last thing before going to bed at night, e.g. atenolol or bisoprolol. If I continued to have early-morning angina I would also take a slow-release preparation of isosorbide mononitrate last thing at night or a buccal nitrate in the morning before getting out of bed.

To cover symptomatic ischaemia throughout the daytime I would take a second dose of beta-blocker if necessary in the morning with or without the addition of isosorbide mononitrate. If I was getting frequent breakthrough symptoms on this regime I would increase the dose of medication and titrate against symptoms, exercise-induced ischaemia and 24-h ischaemic burden on Holter monitoring. If the combination of beta-blocker and nitrate failed to control ischaemia I would continue on the beta-blocker at a maximally tolerated dose and switch from the nitrate to a calcium antagonist. I would take either slow-release diltiazem or amlodipine, depending on my resting heart rate. Again, I would titrate the dose against symptom control and physiological testing.

I would pursue any reversible risk factors vigorously and would exercise daily. Most importantly, on the first day that I developed angina (even if my exercise ECG was only mildly positive) I would book myself for an urgent coronary angiogram!

# References

1 Deanfield J et al, Cigarette smoking and the treatment of angina with propanolol, atenolol and nifedipine, *New Engl J Med* (1984) 310:951.

2 Todd I, Ballantyne D, Effect of exercise training on the total ischaemic burden: an assessment by 24 hour ambulatory electrocardiographic monitoring, *Br Heart J* (1992) 68:56–6.

3 Dabrowski A et al, Effect of amiodarone and disopyramide on the results of electrocardiographic exercise stress testing in patients with coronary disease, *Kardiol Pol* (1990) 33:165–72.

4 Thomassen A et al, Effects of glutamate on exercise tolerance and circulating substrate levels in stable angina pectoris, *Am J Cardiol* (1990) 65:173–8.

5 Sellier P et al, Acute effects of trimetazidine evaluated by exercise testing, *Eur J Clin Pharmacol* (1987) 33:205–7.

6 Guerchicoff S et al, Acute double blind trial of a new anti-anginal drug: molsidomine, *Eur J Clin Pharmacol* (1978) 13:247–50.

7 Quyyumi AA et al, Medical treatment of patients with severe exertional and rest angina: double blind comparison of beta blocker, calcium antagonist, and nitrate, *Br Heart J* (1987) 57:505–11.

8 Emorine LJ et al, Molecular characterisation of the human beta3 adrenergic receptor, *Science* (1989) 245:1118–21.

9 Gaglione et al, Is there coronary vasoconstriction after intracoronary beta-adrenergic blockade in patients with coronary artery disease, *J Am Coll Cardiol* (1987) 10:299–310.

10 Waagstein F et al, Long-term beta-blockade in dilated cardiomyopathy: effects of short- and long-term metoprolol treatment followed by withdrawal and readministration of metoprolol, *Circulation* (1989) 80:551–63.

11 Tuininga YS, Beta-blockers in heart failure—a possible approach to treatment? *Controv Cardiol* (1991) 3:11–13.

12 Winther K et al, Differential effects of timolol and metoprolol on platelet function at rest and during exercise, *Eur J Clin Pharmacol* (1988) 33:587–92.

13 Psaty BM et al, The relative risk of incident coronary artery disease associated with recently stopping the use of beta-blockers, *JAMA* (1990) 263:1653–7.

14 Tonkon M, Haemodynamic profiles of antianginal agents, *Pharmacology* (1987) 7:72S–75S.

15 Stamler JS, Loscalzo J, The antiplatelet effects of organic nitrates and related nitrous compounds in vitro and in vivo and their relevance to cardiovascular disorders, *J Am Coll Cardiol* (1991) 18:1529–36.

16 Parker JO, Nitrate tolerance in angina pectoris, *Cardiovasc Drugs Ther* (1989) 2:823–9.

17 Elkyayam U et al, Incidence of continuous infusion of nitroglycerin in patients with coronary artery disease and heart failure, *Circulation* (1987) 76:577.

18 Ernst E, Matrai A, Diltiazem alters blood rheology, *Pharmatherapeutica* (1988) 5:213–6.

19 Parmley W, New calcium antagonists: relevance of vasoselectivity, *Am Heart J* (1990) 120:1408–13.

20 Rousseau MF et al, Effects of nicardipine on coronary blood flow, left ventricular inotropic state and myocardial metabolism in patients with angina pectoris, *Br J Clin Pharmacol* (1985) 20(suppl 1):147S–57S.

21 Glasser SP, West TW, Clinical safety and efficacy of a once-a-day amlodipine for chronic stable angina pectoris, *Am J Cardiol* (1988) 62:518–22.

22 Been M, Mcfarlane PW, Hillis WS, Electrophysiological effects of felodipine. *Drugs* (1985) 29(suppl 2):476–80.

23 Frishman WH et al, Comparison of hydrochlorothiazide and sustained-release diltiazem for mild to moderate systemic hypertension, *Am J Cardiol* (1987) 59:615–23.

24 Multicentre Diltiazem Postinfarction Trial Research Group, The effect of diltiazem on mortality and reinfarction after myocardial infarction, *New Engl J Med* (1988) 319:385–92.

25 Pucci PD et al, Acute effects on exercise tolerance of felodipine and diltiazem, alone and in combination, in stable effort angina, *Eur Heart J* (1991) 12:55–9.

26 Bahls FH, Ozuna J, Ritchie DE, Interactions between calcium channel blockers and the anticonvulsants carbamazepine and phenytoin, *Neurology* (1991) 41:740–2.

27 Tijssen JG, Lubsen J, Early treatment of unstable angina with nifedipine and metoprolol—the HINT trial, *J Cardiovasc Pharmacol* (1988) 12(suppl 1):S71–7.

28 ISIS-2 (Second International Study of Infarct Survival) Collaborative Group, Randomised trial of intravenous streptokinase, oral aspirin, both, or neither among 17,187 cases of suspected acute myocardial infarction, *Lancet* (1988) ii:349–60.

29 Lewis DH et al, Protective effects of aspirin against acute myocardial infarction and death in men with unstable angina, *New Engl J Med* (1983) 309:396–403.

30 Vermylen J, Should aspirin be used in the primary prevention of myocardial ischaemia? *Controv Cardiol* (1989) 1:6–9.

31 Orme M, Should aspirin be used in the primary prevention of myocardial ischaemia? *Controv Cardiol* (1989) 1:6–9.

32 Yeung AC et al, Effects of asymptomatic ischemia on long-term prognosis in chronic stable coronary disease, *Circulation* (1991) 83:1598–604.

33 Weber JR, Problems associated with clinical evaluation of antianginal medications, *Am J Cardiol* (1985) 56:141–81.

34 Tolins M et al, 'Maximal' drug therapy is not necessarily optimal in chronic angina pectoris, *J Am Coll Cardiol* (1984) 3:1051–7.

35 Stone PH et al, Comparison of propranolol, diltiazem, and nifedipine in the treatment of ambulatory ischemia in patients with stable angina. Differential effects on ambulatory ischemia, exercise performance, and anginal symptoms. The ASIS Study Group, *Circulation* (1990) 82:1962–72.

36 Storstein L, The effect of pindolol and isosorbide dinitrate and their combination on exercise tolerance and ECG changes in angina pectoris, *Acta Med Scand* (1981) 209:357–62.

37 Meyer EC, Makov UE, Palant A, Monotherapy of stable angina pectoris with bopindol in comparison with diltiazem, *Cardiology* (1991) 78:179–84.

38 Barilla F et al, Acute effects of nifedipine versus isosorbide dinitrate on exercise tolerance in patients with isolated coronary artery occlusion and collaterals, *Cardiovasc Drugs Ther* (1990) 4(suppl 5):905–8.

39 Eldridge JE et al, Comparison of nitroglycerin patches and nifedipine, *J Cardiovasc Pharmacol* (1987) 10:315–9.

40 Madger S et al, Comparisons of the effects of pindolol and propanolol on exercise performance in patients with angina pectoris, *Am J Cardiol* (1987) 59:1289–94.

41 Berkenboom GM et al, Comparison of the immediate effects of two beta-blocking drugs: a nonselective and a cardioselective with a modest ISA in exercise induced angina, *Cardiology* (1987) 74:43–8.

42 Chierchia S et al, Role of heart rate in pathophysiology of chronic stable angina, *Lancet* (1984) 2:1353–7.

43 Tilmant PY et al, Detrimental effect of propanolol in patients with coronary arterial spasm countered by combination with diltiazem, *Am J Cardiol* (1983) 52:230–3.

44 Carlens P, Left ventricular pump function in effort angina. Influence of nitroglycerin, propranolol, verapamil, and coronary bypass surgery, *G Ital Cardiol* (1984) 14:809–16.

45 Hyldstrup L, Mogensen NB, Nielsen PE, Orthostatic response before and after nitroglycerin in metoprolol and verapamil treated angina pectoris, *Acta Med Scand* (1983) 214:131–4.

46 Boden WE, Korr KS, Bough EW, Nifedipine-induced hypotension and myocardial ischaemia in refractory angina pectoris, *JAMA* (1985) 253:1131–5.

47 Krikler DM, Calcium antagonists for chronic stable angina pectoris, *Am J Cardiol* (1987) 59:95B–100B.

48 Walsh RA, O'Rourke RA, Direct and indirect effects of calcium entry blocking agents on left

ventricular isovolumic relaxation in conscious dogs, *J Clin Invest* (1985) **75**:1426–34.

49 Findlay IN et al, A double blind placebo controlled comparison of verapamil, atenolol and their combination in patients with chronic stable angina pectoris, *Br Heart J* (1987) **57**:336–43.

50 Packer M, Combined beta-adrenergic and calcium-entry blockade in angina pectoris, *New Engl J Med* (1989) **320**:709–18.

51 Vogler AC et al, Combination therapy with isosorbide dinitrate and verapamil in patients with coronary heart disease and hypertension: effect on blood pressure, ischaemia and left ventricular function, *Z Kardiol* (1989) **78**(suppl 2):183–7.

52 Douard H et al, Anti-ischaemic effects of celiprolol in patients with exercise induced angina pectoris, *Int J Cardiol* (1989) **25**:63–8.

53 Johnston DL et al, Clinical and haemodynamic evaluation of propanolol in combination with verapamil, nifedipine and diltiazem in exertional angina pectoris; a placebo-controlled, double-blind, randomised, cross-over study, *Am J Cardiol* (1985) **55**:680–7.

54 Jenkins RM, Nagle RE, The symptomatic and objective effects of nifedipine in combination with beta-blocker therapy in severe angina pectoris, *Postgrad Med J* (1982) **58**:697–700.

55 Straus WE, Parisi AF, Superiority of combined diltiazem and propanolol therapy for angina pectoris, *Am J Cardiol* (1985) **71**:951–7.

56 Uusitalo A et al, Metoprolol, nifedipine and the combination in stable effort angina pectoris, *Am J Cardiol* (1985) **55**:680–7.

57 Frishman WH et al, Combination propanolol and bepridil therapy in stable angina pectoris, *Am J Cardiol* (1985) **55**:43C–49C.

58 Keane D, Jackson G, Only two drugs in angina, *J Irish Coll Physicians Surg* (1992) **21**:267–70.

59 White HD et al, Addition of nifedipine to maximal nitrate and beta adreno-receptor blocker therapy in coronary artery disease, *Am J Cardiol* (1985) **55**:1303–7.

60 Lehmann G et al, Effectiveness of various combination therapies in patients with coronary heart disease. *Herz* (1990) **15**:399–409.

61 Akhras F, Jackson G, Efficacy of nifedipine and isosorbide mononitrate in combination with atenolol in stable angina, *Lancet* (1991) **338**:1036–9.

62 Jackson G, Atkinson L, Oram S, Reassessment of failed beta blocker treatment in angina pectoris by peak exercise heart rate measurements, *Br Med J* (1975) **3**:616–9.

63 Pepine CJ, Circadian variations in myocardial ischaemia. Implications for management, *JAMA* (1991) **265**:386–90.

64 Egstrup K, The sensitivity of the symptom angina pectoris as a marker of transient myocardial ischaemia in chronic stable angina pectoris, *Acta Med Scand* (1987) **222**:301–6.

65 Miller PF et al, Aging and pain perception in ischaemic heart disease, *Am J Cardiol* (1990) **120**:22–30.

66 The Norwegian Multicentre Study Group, Timolol-induced reduction in mortality and reinfarction in patients surviving acute myocardial infarction, *New Engl J Med* (1981) **304**:801–7.

67 Collins P, Fox K. The pathogenesis of atheroma and the rationale for its treatment, *Eur Heart J* (1992) **13**:560–5.

68 Lubsen J, Tijssen JG, Efficacy of nifedipine and metoprolol in the early treatment of unstable angina in the coronary care unit: findings from the Holland Interuniversity Nifedipine/Metoprolol Trial (HINT), *Am J Cardiol* (1987) **60**:18A–25A.

69 Fujita et al, Improvement of treadmill capacity and collateral circulation as a result of exercise with heparin pretreatment in patients with effort angina, *Circulation* (1988) **77**:1022–9.

70 Hultgren HN, Peduzzi P, Relation of severity of symptoms to prognosis in stable angina pectoris, *Am J Cardiol* (1984) **54**:988–93.

71 Lerner D, Kannel W, Patterns of coronary heart disease morbidity and mortality in the sexes: a 26-year follow-up of the Framingham population, *Am Heart J* (1986) **111**:383–90.

# 2

# Post-angioplasty restenosis: definition, diagnosis and management

*David P Foley and Patrick W Serruys*

## Introduction: what is restenosis?

To embark on the discussion of a vexatious and controversial issue, a clear and unambiguous definition of the substrate is the vital initial step. In view of the vast jungle of literature, which continues to grow, contribute to and compound the controversy surrounding the subject of 'restenosis' following percutaneous transluminal coronary angioplasty, this may not be such a simple first task. Nevertheless, in our view, 'restenosis', in simple terms, refers to the tendency of a blood vessel to renarrow as a consequence of healing processes following the mechanical injury exerted by a procedure or device. Of the currently available percutaneous revascularization devices, this process of response to injury has been most extensively investigated following percutaneous transluminal coronary balloon angioplasty (PTCA) and, as such, is generally considered to consist of four components:

1 Elastic recoil, a natural property of intact vessels in response to stretch. This has only been recently recognized as a 'phenomenon' by computer-assisted quantitative coronary angiography[1] and intravascular ultrasound (IVUS).[2] Data are scarce and somewhat conflicting but, on balance, it appears that recoil occurs immediately following balloon deflation and has a doubtful contribution to the process of late restenosis.[1,3,4]

2 Subintimal platelet deposition, mural thrombus formation, and consequent organization, which may result in 'early restenosis'[5] and may play a role in the development of fibrocellular neointimal hyperplasia.

3 Fibrocellular neointimal hyperplasia, which is widely regarded as the main pathological process by which progressive luminal renarrowing occurs in the months following PTCA,[6,7] and will be described further below.

4 Reaccumulation of 'classical' atherosclerotic plaque.[7]

## Pathological information and hypotheses

Vessel wall injury is frequently extensive as a consequence of coronary balloon angioplasty. Intracoronary angioscopy reveals intimal disruption, to some extent, immediately after successful dilatation, in virtually all cases, while angiography may appear completely normal in two-thirds of cases.[8] These findings are corroborated by autopsy findings of a high incidence of intimal dissection, haemorrhage and thrombus formation, and even severe medial injury, following an angiographically successful procedure, in patients who died within 30 days of PTCA.[9]

The exact nature and time course of biological events occurring as a consequence of vessel wall injury caused by balloon dilatation have been the subject of much speculation. Forrester et al have proposed a paradigm, based on inferential evidence provided by cell biology.[10] In response to intimal disruption, it appears that there is immediate platelet aggregation and adhesion with consequent release of a plethora of substances, including growth factors. Many growth factors, exhibiting a spectrum of potentiating and inhibitory biological effects, have been identified as playing a part in this process, but the complete picture of their complex interaction, at cellular and subcellular level in vivo, remains to be clarified. Suffice it to state that the end result of the cascade of reactions initiated by intimal destruction is conversion of the quiescent contractile smooth muscle cell to its synthetic proliferative phenotype. According to the conventional understanding of the process, this activation is initiated in the media, but within the first few days, migration takes place into the disrupted intima, where the endothelial cells are also furiously proliferating, in an attempt to restore an intact surface. The damaged area may, depending on its size, be resurfaced by a new layer of endothelial cells by day 7. It has been suggested that if the denuded area is <1 cm long, then intimal hyperplasia does not ensue. Therefore, it is likely that there is a critical area of intimal disruption, and perhaps time interval, for endothelial cells to provide a complete covering of the disrupted area, before maximal smooth muscle cell proliferation begins. Thus, if earlier re-endothelialization could be promoted, perhaps the final extent of the process might be usefully controlled or restricted.

Still within the early days, the synthetic smooth muscle cells begin to produce proteoglycan (a bulky, extracellular matrix substance) in abundance. By 2 weeks after injury, some of the synthetic smooth muscle cells already begin to readopt a quiescent, contractile appearance and this pattern progresses, at a rate depending on a number of factors, particularly the extent of injury, and is in parallel with the gradual replacement of proteoglycan in the extracellular matrix by collagen during the succeeding months. Throughout this period, the now characteristic histological appearance of intimal hyperplasia is observed, i.e. proliferating smooth muscle cells in varying concentrations, against a background of a loose matrix largely composed of proteoglycan.[11]

By 6 months, basal conditions of the pre-injury vessel wall are restored, with intact endothelial layer, and predominance of contractile smooth muscle cells in a mainly collagenous matrix. In some cases, where there was extensive injury with chronic persistent endothelial denudation, proliferative cell types may predominate beyond this time and intimal hyperplasia continues. Human post-mortem studies are (fortunately for the future of the procedure as a treatment option!) scarce, and involve small patient numbers; however, findings in lesions where PTCA has been carried out more than 2 years previously appear to be histologically indistinguishable from conventional atherosclerotic plaque.[11]

## An alternative hypothesis based on experimental evidence

An alternative scheme for the early pathological process of restenosis has been proposed by Schwartz et al.[12] Based on extensive experience with a domestic swine model,[13,14] they assign a central role to early mural thrombus formation at the site of injury (already previously well recognized as a key event,[5,11,15,16] which becomes rapidly endothelialized (3–4 days after injury), and is then infiltrated by mononuclear cells, from the luminal surface inward. The degenerating thrombus is subsequently colonized by proliferating alpha-actin staining cells (becoming visible from day 6 onwards), whose origin and exact nature is uncertain (most probably smooth muscle cells or myofibroblasts), again from the luminal surface inward (in the opposite direction to that which is hypothesized in the current conventional model), with concomitant production of extracellular matrix and eventual complete resorption of the thrombus, and the ultimate formation of mature neointima.

## Conflicting and corroborating findings using the same experimental model

Karas et al[17] have also developed an animal model of restenosis, by using balloon dilatation or implantation of a balloon expandable stent, also in normolipaemic domestic swine, but point out that their method of inducing injury is less aggressive than that of Schwartz et al (deliberate device oversizing by 1.2 compared with a factor of approximately 1.5–2.0 in the Mayo Clinic model). They observed marked intimal smooth muscle cell proliferation and an increase in extracellular matrix, destruction of the internal elastic membrane and thinning of the arterial medial layer, both in stented and balloon-dilated segments. Intimal proliferation was more prominent and significantly greater in stented segments, by morphometric analysis, and, in addition, residual luminal area was significantly less in these segments. These histopathological changes were described as being comparable with those observed in human restenosis. Furthermore, reactive inflammatory infiltrates were frequently observed in proximity to the stent filaments, suggesting a foreign body type of reaction. The authors hypothesize that, despite provoking more intimal proliferation, stenting maintains a greater morphometric luminal area than balloon dilatation, through the achievement of a larger lumen, by continued mechanical opposition of elastic recoil. These findings present circumstantial evidence which is in agreement with previous accumulated evidence of the importance of the degree of vessel injury in the development of intimal hyperplasia[5,7,10,11,15,18,19] as well as the more recent demonstration of an actual proportional relationship between the extent of neointimal hyperplasia and the severity of vessel wall injury.[14]

However, the Emory group disagrees with the hypothesis of Schwartz et al,[12] regarding the central role of thrombus in the process of restenosis, on the basis of the rarity of large space-occupying clots in their extensive experience with balloon-injured arteries without stent implantation (as well as the rarity of such clots seen angiographically in clinical practice), and suggest that the induction of excessive arterial injury and the presence of the endoluminal device is responsible for the thrombotic tendency in the Mayo Clinic model, therefore limiting its utility as a screening tool. Thus the role of thrombus formation in the pathological scheme of restenosis remains to be clarified. The possibility of a spectrum of importance for thrombus, from little or none in many cases of PTCA, to considerable relevance in patients following implantation of endoluminal prosthesis or atheroma extraction, must be considered. Increasing clinical use of intracoronary angioscopy,[20] and indeed recently developed intracoronary microscopy,[21] may provide some useful clinical enlightenment in this area.

## Clinical correlations of the pathological process and patient follow-up after PTCA

These histological time patterns of response to arterial injury, observed mainly in the animal model but borne out by the previously mentioned human studies, using tissue specimens obtained at autopsy, and by directional atherectomy, correlate extremely well with the findings of serial angiographic studies depicting restenosis as a ubiquitous, time-related phenomenon, occurring primarily at 1–3 months,[22,23] with some further emergence up to 6 months, and a small percentage of lesions expressing 'late' restenosis at 6–12 months[23] (Figure 2.1). Symptomatic recurrence has been shown to mirror the angiographic evidence,

most patients with symptomatic restenosis manifesting re-emergence of angina by the third month after successful PTCA.[24]

The next logical question is—how to follow up patients after successful PTCA in order to detect restenosis? There is no easy answer to this, since the concept of recurring stenosis may be viewed as angiographic progression of a focal narrowing without implying any functional or clinical consequences, or may be defined by a functional parameter such as coronary flow reserve which can identify a physiologically significant obstruction to bloodflow, or by the presence of reversible ischaemia by a battery of available sophisticated non-invasive diagnostic tests, or by re-emergence of cardiac ischaemic symptoms. Depending on the methodology of assessment and definition criteria used, the incidence of

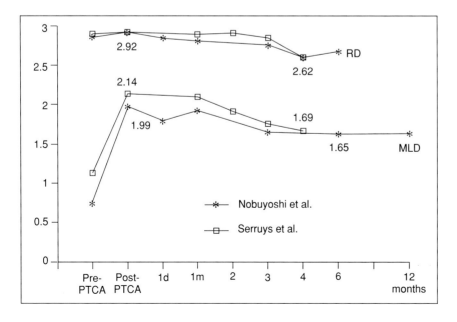

**Figure 2.1**
*Graphic representation of minimal luminal diameter (MLD) and reference diameter (RD) values as reported in the studies of Nobuyoshi et al[23] and Serruys et al,[22] showing virtually identical time trends during 6-month follow-up.*

restenosis will obviously vary widely. For the purposes of scientific studies, it is imperative that the most objective and reproducible methodology be used for data acquisition and description, and that an unambiguous approach be applied, in order to enable valid and meaningful comparisons to be made between studies, to increase available knowledge, and thereby to improve and update approaches and treatments, for the benefit of all practising physicians, and ultimately for patient benefit.

# Symptoms, function, bloodflow or anatomy as criteria for restenosis?

## Symptoms

Although improvement in quality of life (as well as life expectancy) is the goal of any therapeutic modality, it is also the least objective yardstick by which to evaluate the impact of treatment. Symptomatic improvement following an angiographically successful PTCA has been reported to be as low as 70 per cent,[24] and the positive predictive value of symptomatic recurrence for the occurrence of angiographic restenosis ranges from 48 to 92 per cent. In addition, up to 33 per cent of patients who remain asymptomatic following PTCA may exhibit angiographic restenosis.[25] In view of these considerations, the use of symptomatic criteria alone in patient surveillance after PTCA in restenosis prevention trials is not recommended.[26] On the contrary, for clinicians in practice the symptomatic status of the individual patient will be an important determinant as to the need for further investigations and will be discussed further in a later section.

## Disturbance in myocardial perfusion

A wide range of specific tests of myocardial perfusion and viability are available: provocation testing by exercise (bicycle ergometry or treadmill), atrial pacing or pharmacological agents (incremental intravenous infusions of dipyridamole, dopamine, or dobutamine with or without atropine bolus) to detect electrocardiographic changes associated with ischaemia, with, or without, additional imaging techniques, e.g. epicardial or transoesophageal echocardiography, to detect wall motion abnormalities associated with transient myocardial hypoperfusion; radionuclide scanning by single photon emission computed tomography (SPECT) using thallium-201, technetium-99m, teburoxime or isonitrile, to detect reversible perfusion defects, as an indication of reversible myocardial ischaemia. In addition, contrast echocardiography, magnetic resonance imaging and positron emission tomography etc. contribute vital information for evaluation of patients following intervention, as well as at clinical presentation. These tests, singly or in combination, depending on availability and resources, are becoming increasingly useful (perhaps even indispensable) for clinical decision-making in individual patients. Unfortunately, however, widespread and indiscriminate application of these valuable investigational techniques cannot provide the reproducibility and objectivity required to assess the process of luminal renarrowing following PTCA in large patient groups.[25]

## Haemodynamic consequences

Angioplasty-related technology continues to evolve and it is now possible to derive accurate measurement of intracoronary arterial pressure using 0.015-inch fluid-filled guidewire, or

0.018-inch fibre optic wire, and intracoronary bloodflow velocity may be measured by 0.018-inch Doppler wire. Using this technology, a comprehensive assessment of the haemodynamic consequences of non-critical coronary stenoses (the lesions which characteristically create the greatest dilemma regarding the need for intervention) can be readily provided. Theoretical haemodynamic estimates may also be derived using measurements obtained by quantitative angiography, using fluid dynamic equations, such as that described in the past by Gould et al[27] and Kirkeeide et al.[28] At the current time, application of these techniques is still in its relative infancy, is mainly confined to large academic institutions and is still largely research orientated; nevertheless, continual technical improvements and simplifications give hope for more widespread availability and applicability of these techniques in the future. Furthermore, non-invasive approaches, such as ultrafast computed tomography, contrast echocardiography, magnetic resonance imaging and positron emission tomography, are being actively investigated for their ability to measure coronary flow reserve and may well open a whole new perspective for studying coronary pathophysiology.

## Anatomical configuration

This is the degree of luminal narrowing. For the present this aspect is best assessed by conventional contrast angiographic techniques, although IVUS is emerging as an exciting and promising imaging modality[29] and will undoubtedly have a useful application in the future in this area. As yet, although its application is increasing, IVUS is still in the developmental stage and many technical obstacles need to be surmounted, particularly transducer size and flexibility, correlation of images obtained with actual vessel wall morphology

and an objective and reproducible method of quantification of lumen and plaque area, before it can be considered as an alternative to carefully controlled quantitative angiography.[30–32]

## Coronary angiography is still the cornerstone of patient follow-up in clinical PTCA trials

Despite its well-known limitations, the coronary cineangiogram is still the only universally available imaging modality for examination of coronary anatomy, and quantitative angiographic techniques have emerged, in recent years,[30–34,36,37] as the gold standard for the accurate measurement of luminal dimensions from images provided by the basic cineangiogram.

## Difficulties in interpreting outcome of clinical trials due to variability in the definition of angiographic restenosis

One of the most persistent and major obstacles in addressing the restenosis issue is the lack of agreement on an angiographic definition which conveys a measure of change in stenosis severity in the follow-up period after PTCA. As evidence of this lack of concordance, Figure 2.2 shows the differing 'restenosis rates' associated with the use of many (at least 13) different 'definitions'. Most of these are arbitrary categorical cut-off points, although some are based on historical physiological concepts, whereby it was demonstrated, in the past, that the vessel hyperaemic response becomes impaired at a diameter stenosis >50 per cent.[27]

1  A diameter stenosis ≥50 per cent at follow-up.
2  An immediate post-PTCA diameter stenosis <50 per cent that increases to ≥50 per cent at follow-up.
3  As for (2) above, but a diameter stenosis ≥70 per cent at follow-up (NHLBI 2).
4  Loss during follow-up of at least 50 per cent of the initial gain at PTCA (NHLBI 4).
5  A return to within 10 per cent of the pre-PTCA diameter stenosis (NHLBI 3).
6  Loss ≥20 per cent diameter stenosis from post-PTCA to follow-up.
7  Loss ≥30 per cent diameter stenosis from post-PTCA to follow-up (NHLBI 1).
8  A diameter stenosis ≥70 per cent at follow-up.
9  Area stenosis ≥85 per cent at follow-up.
10  Loss ≥1 mm² in stenosis area from post-PTCA to follow-up.
11  Loss ≥0.72 mm in minimal luminal diameter from post-PTCA to follow-up.
12  Loss ≥0.5 mm in minimal luminal diameter from post-PTCA to follow-up.
13  Diameter stenosis >50 per cent at follow-up, if >10 per cent deterioration in diameter stenosis since PTCA in a successfully dilated lesion (defined as diameter stenosis <50 per cent, with a gain of >10 per cent at PTCA).

A number of angiographic definitions of restenosis which have been used in various clinical studies. NHLBI 1, 2, 3 and 4 are criteria for angiographic restenosis, as laid out by the National Heart, Lung, and Blood Institute of the United States.

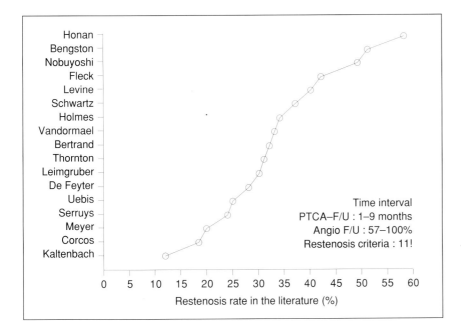

**Figure 2.2**

Non-scientific figure depicting restenosis rates from a selection of published studies with different angiographic follow-up rates (57–100 per cent), follow-up intervals (1–9 months), 11 different restenosis criteria and various angiographic analysis techniques.

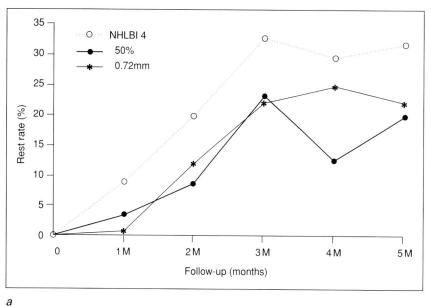
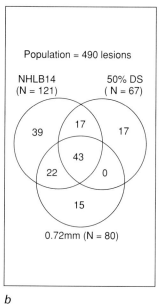

a                                                                                   b

**Figure 2.3**

*(a) Cumulative incidence of restenosis during a 5-month follow-up period, as defined by three different criteria, among a group of 490 successfully dilated lesions. NHLBI 4 = criterion 4 of the National Heart, Lung and Blood Institute of America; loss of >50 per cent of the initial gain at angioplasty. >/50% = >/50 per cent diameter stenosis at follow-up. >/0.72 mm = >/0.72 mm loss in minimal luminal diameter from post-angioplasty to follow-up. (b) Venn diagram showing the distribution of lesions fulfilling the different criteria applied in (a). Note that, of a total of 153 lesions undergoing restenosis according to at least one of the three criteria applied, only 43 fulfil all three. It is appreciated how different definitions of restenosis define separate populations. (Reproduced with permission from Beatt et al.[36])*

The measurement used, however, is percentage diameter stenosis, which is inherently flawed by both the method of its computation (percentage diameter stenosis is calculated by assuming a 'normal' diameter value for the segment of coronary vessel immediately proximal or distal to the area of interest, as the reference diameter; this assumption has been shown to be invalid, particularly in the context of multivessel disease, when there is virtually always diffuse intimal and/or subintimal thickening,[29,38] as well as variable age-related or compensatory ectasia,[38,39] and following interventions when the 'reference diameter' may be altered by the therapeutic procedure[40] and at follow-up when the adjacent apparently normal vessel may become involved in the restenosis process[41–43]), and the inability of a single measurement to accurately describe what is essentially a 'moving target', as has been independently demonstrated by our group[22] and Nobuyoshi et al[23] (Figure 2.1). Applying three different and widely used definitions to a series of 490 lesions in patients treated by PTCA and serially followed up by quantitative coronary angiography, our group[22] demonstrated that: (1) the greatest single determinant of the restenosis rate is the choice of definition (Figure 2.3a); and (2), even if the eventual incidence of restenosis is similar, different definitions identify different patient populations (Figure 2.3b), making risk factor determination impossible. These diversities are almost certainly responsible for most of the confusion surrounding the concept of angiographic restenosis following PTCA.

A further problem which has compounded the situation in the past was the use of visual assessment to analyse cineangiograms in scientific studies. The large inter- and intraobserver variation and lack of correlation with physiological measurements, and pathological and intraoperative findings, are now well recognized,[32] and thus these pre-quantitative angiography studies are impossible to compare with modern quantitative-based studies. The inaccuracy of this methodology in measuring apparently 'small' luminal changes in 'moderate' lesions is magnified by the fact that these small changes may have profound haemodynamic consequences. It has recently been shown[44] that observer variability is independent of experience and that observers trained in visual estimation techniques tend to overestimate the severity of lesions pre-PTCA and underestimate the degree of residual luminal narrowing afterward, possibly because the 'see' area stenosis

and call it diameter stenosis (a percentage diameter stenosis of 74 per cent, in a lesion 6 mm in length and a vessel of 2–6 mm correlates with an area stenosis of 95 per cent[45]).

## Insights into restenosis gleaned through quantitative coronary angiography

Increasing use of quantitative coronary angiography (QCA)[30,31] over the past decade has clearly and definitely demonstrated that absolute measurements such as mean luminal diameter, minimal luminal diameter (MLD) or minimal cross-sectional area of narrowings, provide more reliable and meaningful information than percentage diameter stenosis, with regard to haemodynamic significance of an obstructive coronary lesion.[33,34] The use of QCA must now be considered essential in any scientific study purporting to contribute to current knowledge or understanding in this vital and controversial area.[36,37] Of further and more practical clinical relevance, quantitative coronary measurements (at follow-up after successful PTCA) have, in fact, recently been shown to have useful correlations with exercise-induced angina and exercise electrographic testing.[35]

The pathology of restenosis, as summarized earlier—although still somewhat hypothetical—as well as the angiographic evidence presented separately by ourselves[22] and Nobuyoshi[23] demonstrates that restenosis is, in fact, rather more a continuous (occurring to varying degree in virtually all treated lesions) than 'all or nothing' process (occurring in some but not others). In addition, our group has subsequently shown that the change in minimal luminal diameter values during follow-up post-PTCA follows a near-Gaussian distribution[41,45] and others have reported the same phenomenon in patients treated by directional atherectomy and stent implantation.[46] These corroborative findings collectively demonstrate the limitations of applying categorical angiographic definitions to studying the immediate and long-term outcome of intervention in large patient groups or clinical trials. Since it is also apparent that there is no specific threshold for loss in minimal luminal diameter above which physiological or clinical significance is reached, it is much more meaningful and realistic, therefore, to study the effect of a pharmacological agent, or intervention using a continuous statistical approach,[47] where all patients treated in a common manner are considered as a single group. Thus, the mean (quantitatively measured) loss in minimal luminal diameter during follow-up will best reflect the restenosis process for that group, and this is the measure of greatest interest in restenosis prevention trials.[26,48,49] In addition to providing more relevant and informative results, the analysis and application of continuous variables requires many fewer patients in the treatment groups to be compared.[47] We consider it misleading, therefore, to discuss the issue of restenosis in terms of 'incidence' or 'restenosis rate', and can verily state that restenosis is, indeed, still a rapidly evolving concept.

## Pharmacological attempts to prevent restenosis— information gained from multicentre trials

Many different pharmacological interventions, including antiplatelet agents, thromboxane $A_2$ antagonists, calcium channel blockers, antimitotic agents, angiotensin converting enzyme inhibitors, steroids, anticoagulants and fish-oil,

have been used in prospective randomized trials to prevent restenosis, with no convincing success.[50] Considerable difficulty is encountered in making valid comparisons between studies, the four salient problems being: (1) inadequate population size; (2) inadequate angiographic follow-up; (3) non-standardized angiographic follow-up interval; and (4) use of arbitrary definitions of 'restenosis'.[36,50] It is therefore difficult to draw any meaningful conclusions from this morass of data, other than that there is still no clear or conclusive evidence that any pharmacological agent can control or inhibit the restenosis process. Lack of meaningful dialogue between the main protagonists involved in pushing back the frontiers of knowledge would appear to be an important contributory cause of continued discrepancies in the methodological approach to scientific studies.

At the core laboratory in Rotterdam, we have now accumulated, through the cooperative efforts of institutions throughout Europe and North America, a large databank of quantitative angiographic, procedural and clinical information on patients undergoing various transluminal coronary interventions with comprehensive follow-up. To date, among 1452 patients who underwent coronary balloon angioplasty in two European multicentre restenosis prevention trials,[48,49] a number of adjunctive reports have been compiled. Multivariate analysis, using clinical, procedural and quantitative angiographic data, has been carried out for each of these trials, with luminal loss as the 'outcome'.

In the multivariate model of the CARPORT trial,[51] diabetes mellitus and duration of angina (<2.3 months) as well as luminal gain (in minimal luminal diameter, measured in millimetres) at angioplasty, pre-PTCA minimal luminal diameter lesion length (>6.8 mm) and presence of angiographically visible thrombus post-PTCA were found to be independently predictive of luminal loss during follow-up after PTCA. Restriction of independent variables to quantitative angiographic parameters revealed the gain in lumen at intervention adjusted for the vessel size ('relative gain') to be the greatest determinant of late luminal renarrowing, and lesion length was also retained in the model.[4]

Multivariate analysis applied to clinical, angiographic and procedural data collected during the MERCATOR trial as independent predictors of luminal renarrowing (loss in minimal luminal diameter during follow-up)[52] revealed relative gain as the strongest associated factor, with minimal luminal diameter after angioplasty (partly included in the relative gain, which is calculated as: (MLD post – MLD pre)/vessel size), and non-right coronary artery dilatation. This latter association was not confirmed by examination of the two groups together, for the purpose of investigating restenosis throughout the coronary tree, where no significant differences in relative loss (luminal loss normalized for the vessel size) or restenosis rate (percentage diameter stenosis ≥50 per cent at follow-up) were evident between segments or vessels.[53] No clinical or procedural characteristics were found to be independently associated with a greater loss in lumen during follow-up in the multivariate model, although in univariate analysis duration of angina (<86 days) was associated with more luminal loss, and borderline association was found for total balloon inflation duration (>240 s), maximum inflation pressure (>9 atm), lesion located in the LAD, lesion calcification and balloon/artery ratio (>1.2). In a separate study, the presence of an angiographically visible but non-flow-limiting dissection, after an otherwise successful balloon angioplasty (so-called 'therapeutic dissection'), was demonstrated *not* to be associated with relative luminal loss during follow-up, or 'restenosis rate'.[54]

The overall predictability of luminal loss by these multivariate models was poor, which is not all that surprising in view of many previous reports of a diversity of clinical (male gender, unstable angina, diabetes, hypercholesterolaemia and other lipid abnormalities, current smoking, recent-onset angina, severity of angina, coexistence of multivessel disease, post-infarction angina and hypertension) as well as a wide variety of lesion- and procedure-related factors associated with the occurrence of restenosis,[47] as defined by a spectrum of angiographic definitions (Table 2.1), making comparison of findings impossible.

Reading between the lines of all these data, it is apparent that restenosis after balloon angioplasty, and indeed after other interventions, is a multifactorial phenomenon. Nevertheless, it is clear that a fundamental direct relationship has been demonstrated between injury imparted at intervention and the degree of subsequent intimal hyperplasia,[5,7,10,11,14,15,17–19] thus indicating restenosis as the inevitable healing response of the coronary artery (or bypass graft) to the traumatic therapeutic procedure.[11,55] Quantitative angiographic studies have recently demonstrated a corresponding phenomenon, through the examination of the relationship between luminal changes after intervention and during follow-up, normalized for the individual vessel size, in patients treated by directional atherectomy or stent implantation as well as by balloon angioplasty[37,56,57] (Figure 2.4). These findings represent further elaboration on the previously described results of the multivariate analyses in patients treated by balloon angioplasty. The Beth Israel group have reported similar findings using absolute luminal changes after intervention and during follow-up in patients treated by directional atherectomy or

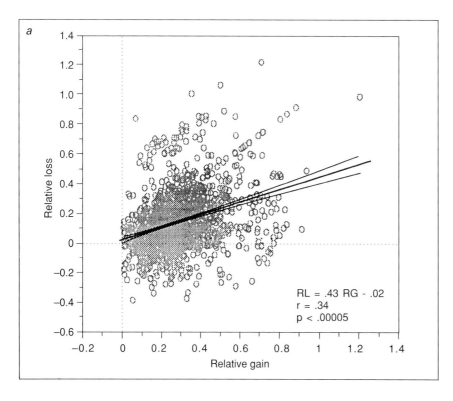

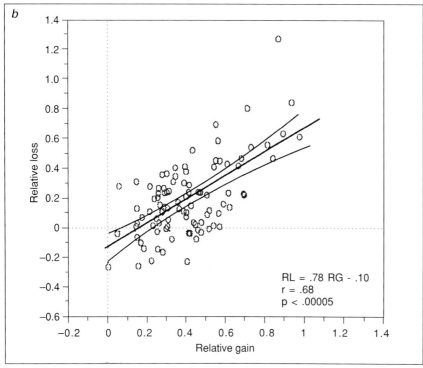

**Figure 2.4**

*(a–d) Graphic display of the linear regression relationship, including 95 per cent confidence intervals for the regression lines (data points are omitted) between relative gain (gain in minimal luminal diameter at intervention normalized for the vessel size) on the x-axes and relative loss (loss in minimal luminal diameter during follow-up, normalized for the vessel size) on the y-axes for four separate patient groups, treated for native coronary artery disease by different 'devices'. Two observations emerge: (1) A clear linear relationship exists between relative loss (representing intimal hyperplasia) and relative*

*gain (representing an index of vessel wall injury at intervention) for each of the four devices. This may represent angiographic manifestation of the injury/hyperplasia phenomenon (the restenosis process). (2) Definite differences in the relative gain/relative loss relationship are notable between the 'devices' which may reflect inherent characteristics of each, with regard to the particular injury/hyperplasia relationship provoked. However, since demographic disparities between the patient groups may also play an important and yet unquantified role, these differences must be interpreted cautiously.[56]*

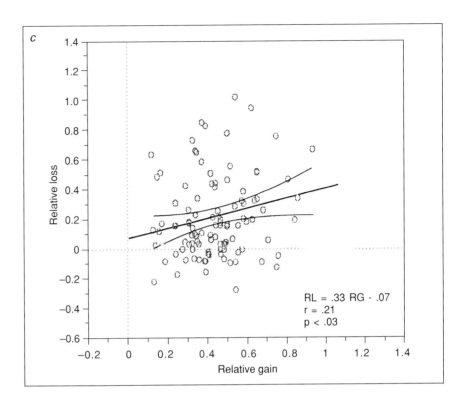

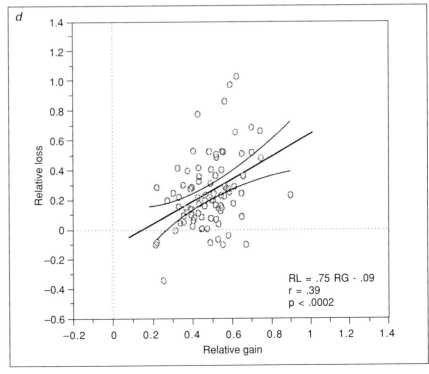

stent implantation.[46] Our proposal is that interventional devices and treatment strategies may be most usefully evaluated and compared by examining the relative gain–relative loss relationship as the quantitative angiographic manifestation of the injury–hyperplasia phenomenon.[37] To further improve our understanding of this persistently elusive and vexatious limitation of percutaneous interventions, justifiably termed the 'Achilles heel', further and extensive studies addressing the effect of various relevant suspected 'risk factors', such as anginal status, diabetes, hypercholesterolaemia/hyperlipidaemia, cigarette smoking, multivessel disease, lesion location, lesion length, presence of thrombus pre- or post-intervention, lesion symmetry, and type of device used, on the relative gain–relative loss relationship will be necessary.

## Restenosis—management strategy

The management of restenosis presents no greater difficulty than that of the primary presenting coronary lesion. The clinical presentation is, generally, a gradual recurrence of the same type of anginal symptoms, to a variable degree and with variable rapidity of onset and progression, as were present prior to the particular therapy in question.[24] One of the salient features of symptomatic ischaemic heart disease is, of course, the consistency of the symptoms in each individual patient, although the descriptions of angina differ widely between patients.

Our suggestion to the practising family doctor, general physician or non-interventional cardiologist, confronted with patients who have undergone angioplasty or other percutaneous revascularization procedure, is, in general, to be guided by clinical status. The freely exercising asymptomatic patient requires no further routine tests, except in the situation where he or she is involved in a scientific study, in which case other additional examinations may have already been ordained as part of a protocol, examining the benefit of a new pharmacological agent or treatment modality. Alternatively, sedentary or exercise-limited patients, diabetics, or other patients already previously identified as experiencing silent myocardial ischaemia, may require assessment by special techniques, as outlined previously (provocation testing etc.).

The first question to ask the patient who returns to the primary care physician complaining of 'chest pain' is—is it the same as, or different from, the type of discomfort experienced before revascularization? If the answer is a definite 'no'!, then, assuming that the original symptomatology was genuine angina pectoris, this presenting complaint certainly is not angina. Where there is a lingering doubt concerning vague symptoms reported by a patient, discretion is always the better part of valour, and it is advised to err on the side of caution, by taking a serious view of the symptoms, and carrying out a simple 12-lead exercise treadmill (or bicycle ergometer) test, or, alternatively, referring to the cardiologist. Ideally, exercise testing should be 'maximal' rather than 'symptom limited', as the latter may not resolve the question being asked, which is whether or not the patient is experiencing myocardial ischaemia. The increasing armoury of adjunctive non-invasive tests of myocardial perfusion and viability yield improvingly accurate and precise assessments,[58,59] when appropriately applied. Such application may be most reliably managed by the experienced specialist cardiologist, so early and appropriate referral of patients with suspicious symptoms may be the best option, to avoid unnecessary or unsuitable investigation, particularly in these days of rising health care costs and restriction of public health services and budgets. The specialist cardiologist, calling on extensive clinical experience, may consider the symptoms to be non-cardiac, and reassure the patient with a simple explanation of the clinical situation, or, alternatively, may decide that further investigation is indeed warranted. (Incidentally, the interventional cardiologist has a tremendous opportunity, during the interventional procedure, at the time of balloon inflation, to give the patient, who is experiencing anginal pain, an opportunity to use that experience in the future to discriminate between true angina and non-cardiac chest pains.) In cases where angina does recur, the elapsed time from apparently successful PTCA to re-emergence of symptoms has been reported to be clinically useful in identifying the most probable cause:[24]

1 Within one month—incomplete revascularization due to additional, underestimated or untreated coronary artery disease and/or incomplete dilatation should be suspected.
2 One to six months— 'restenosis', as already described, is the likely culprit.
3 After six months—atheroma progression should be considered.

Opinions will differ as to the next step involved in solving the problem. One view is to proceed immediately to angiography, to demonstrate the anatomical scenario, and rapidly answer the ultimate question as to whether or not there is significant restenosis, or indeed new coronary disease of sufficient degree to explain symptomatic recurrence, or to confirm that there is no significant coronary artery obstruction (with the consequent reassurance that there is no imminent myocardial threat), and, therefore, demonstrate that the symptoms are extremely unlikely to be due to myocardial ischaemia. The other approach is to carry out non-invasive diagnostic investigations, as already described. Proponents of the former view will argue that angiography will be eventually required if these tests are positive, in order to delineate the extent of obstructive coronary disease and plan further treatment, and will also be required if the tests are negative or inconclusive (assuming appropriate indication for investigation in the first place), since all of the non-invasive tests are subject to false negativity to some degree. Perhaps newer techniques will emerge which can reliably confirm or deny the presence of significant coronary narrowings non-invasively, but as yet no such techniques are available.

Most authorities would probably agree that in the context of general clinical practice, outside of scientific studies, routine angiographic restudy, in the absence of worrying symptoms, is not warranted. Similarly, potentially misleading non-invasive diagnostic tests, as outlined already, are not indicated on a 'blanket basis'.

Having established that significant recurrence of stenosis, sufficient to cause anginal symptoms and/or myocardial ischaemia, has taken place, the decision regarding the further treatment will depend on a number of patient- and lesion-related factors, many of which have been already mentioned, since there is now a wide range of potential therapeutic options.

## New treatment options

Recently there has been an explosion of new treatment modalities—most notably, atherectomy (directional, extractional or rotational), intracoronary stent implantation and laser devices—which were originally conceived and designed to prevent restenosis, and which are now also applied to therapy of primary obstructive coronary (or graft) disease. Unfortunately, all of these treatment modalities subject the vessel wall to a traumatic insult of variable intensity, and therefore are associated with similar consequences, in terms of restenosis, as balloon dilatation.[37] Nevertheless, their unique and different modes of action introduce the concept of a 'niche' for each of these techniques according to various characteristics of target coronary obstructions.[60,61]

The first of the *atherectomy* devices to be used in human coronary arteries was the Simpson directional atherectomy catheter, which 'shaves' the surface of the plaque and collects the debris within. The device consists basically of a cylindrical tube with a longitudinal opening on one side, through which an enclosed cup-shaped cutter can excise the atheromatous plaque. In general this device is recommended for larger arteries, ≥3 mm in diameter, although the mean vessel size in the recent CAVEAT study was less than this.[62] Recent studies suggest a particular role for this device in the removal of eccentric proximal stenosis and lesions containing thrombus, as well as in the treatment of restenotic lesions.[63] The second atheroma-debulking device, the rotablator, was developed by Auth,[64] and consists of a high-speed rotating metal burr in sizes ranging from 1.25 mm up to 4.5 mm in diameter (for use in peripheral arteries). The distal half of the burr is embedded with fine diamond abrasive particles (approximately 40 µm in size) and rotates at very high speed (up to 175 000 rev/min). Because the majority of the plaque particles are less than 10 µm in size, they are allowed to travel downstream to move through the capillary system and to eventually be trapped in the reticuloendothelial system of the liver and lungs. A particular role for the rotablator may be in small arteries with long, eccentric or calcified lesions or in the recanalization of totally occluded vessels. The third atherectomy device is the transluminal extraction catheter (TEC), developed by Stack.[65] The TEC is essentially a flexible torque tube that tracks over a flexible steerable guidewire under fluoroscopic control to the target lesion in the coronary artery. Once properly positioned, a conical cutter starts to rotate at 750 rev/min, while suction is applied through openings of the cuttery windows, to cause the plaque fragments to be extracted through the catheter and out of the patient.

*Lasers* have been applied to the problem of coronary obstructions for a number of years,[66] with initially poor results because the complex laser–tissue interaction was not appropriately harnessed, until the development of the excimer laser, which emits pulsed ultraviolet light at very high energy levels to ablate tissue at the point of contact.[67] The limitation of the laser is that the orifice it creates is the size of the outer diameter of the catheter, the largest of which is 2.4 mm, and therefore this treatment modality is more appropriate for small to medium-sized vessels and additional PTCA is required in the majority of cases (up to 90 per cent) to provide a satisfactory angiographic result.[68] Recent evidence suggests that the laser may be particularly appropriate for lesions which are long and irregular, calcified lesions and lesions located at the ostia of the main coronary arteries,[68] which cannot realistically be treated with any notable success by conventional balloon angioplasty.

*Intracoronary stenting* was first carried out in humans in 1986,[69] initially to deal with acute occlusion following PTCA, but subsequently to prevent recurrent late restenosis in patients who had previous PTCA, and is now a primary treatment option. There are a number of different types of stent currently under clinical investigation. Because of the scaffolding and anti-recoil effects of endoluminal stents, residual lumen following stent implantation may reach the dimensions of the adjacent apparently normal arterial segments;[70,71] hence the claim that by maximizing the initial gain in lumen, the 'restenosis rate' (when defined as diameter stenosis ≥50 per cent) may be reduced[46] compared with other devices. Previous reports were not as encouraging,[73] although more aggressive and improved anticoagulation control has considerably reduced the frequency of acute and subacute stent thrombosis.[70] Despite the increasingly encouraging acute and long-term clinical results with stent implantation, it must not be forgotten that reduction in 'restenosis rate' does not equate with prevention of the process of restenosis, as is clear from earlier sections of this chapter. Indeed, our group has previously advised a cautionary approach in what is still a largely experimental area.[73]

Critical evaluation of our own experience to date with the newer intracoronary interventions using the comparative technique of matching (comparing the effect of interventions in lesions of the same severity, at the same sites, and in arteries of the same size) reveals that the immediate angiographic outcome is 'better' with atherectomy and stenting than with PTCA,[74] but this improvement in luminal diameter is not maintained at follow-up for atherectomy;[75] however, although also associated with a greater loss in luminal diameter during follow-up, stenting yields a significantly larger vessel lumen (MLD) than PTCA at follow-up, due to the vastly superior initial result.[76] This observation needs to be tested and validated in randomized prospective clinical trials, which are, in fact, in progress in Europe and the USA.

The other available treatment options are, of course, repeat balloon angioplasty, medical therapy or *coronary artery bypass grafting (CABG)*. *Laser balloon angioplasty*[77] or 'hot-balloon' will be abandoned as a treatment possibility because of the unacceptably high restenosis rates which appear to be directly related to the amount of thermal energy used.

# Therapeutic decision-making

The choice of therapy for the individual will depend on many considerations, not the least of which is the centre in which the patient is being treated. Interventionalists at tertiary referral institutions, equipped with all the above treatment modalities, will be in a position to offer the patient the best available modality for his or her particular problem, according to their own experience and the latest information. It may often be largely a choice for the individual patient and referring physician to make, in the light of recommendations made by the interventionalist, since there is as yet no clear-cut objective evidence on the long-term benefits of any of the new treatments, including PTCA, when compared with CABG.

In the 'multiple choice' situation, where CABG, PTCA, atherectomy, laser and stenting are all available, the decision regarding therapy will depend on the following factors:

1 *Age*. Young patients will prefer a non-surgical treatment which can be repeated in the future if necessary, and, at the other end of the spectrum, very elderly patients may not be fit for surgery, so a percutaneous revascularization technique is also preferable.

2 *Clinical condition of the patient*. If a high surgical risk because of extensive myocardial impairment or coexistent non-cardiac disease, then, regardless of other factors, a non-surgical approach may be preferable.

3 *Single or multivessel disease*. In the former situation a non-surgical option is always considered first and then factor (4) becomes central. Traditionally, multivessel disease is considered an indication for surgery but may now also be treated by percutaneous revascularization with comparable immediate and long-term success; however, randomized trials have only been in progress since 1987, so objective long-term results are, as yet, unavailable.

4 *Lesion morphology.* As already pointed out, different lesion characteristics may be more appropriately treated by different modalities.

5 *Access to the lesion.* Tortuous or occluded iliofemoral or coronary arteries may prevent the introduction of bulky or rigid catheters.

6 *Likely compliance of the patient with additional therapy or follow-up investigations.* Rigorous anticoagulant regimes are used in patients being treated by implantation of some intracoronary stents, various pharmacological agents are constantly under investigation for their ability to prevent restenosis, and most clinical trials require angiographic follow-up.

7 *The existence of randomized clinical trials,* comparing various treatment modalities, at the institution, in which case a patient meeting the carefully devised and extremely strict entry criteria, and giving informed consent, may be assigned to a particular treatment modality completely at random. Obviously this last factor applies only to special centres and exists only because of the continued lack of certainty regarding the ultimate clinical niche for all these treatment options.

This embarrassment of riches may, in itself, present an excessive dilemma, and the patient (and physician) in a primary institution, with the relatively simpler options of medical or surgical therapy or conventional PTCA, may, ultimately, be better off.

# The future—'niches', and the 'magic bullet'—cause for optimism?

At this moment in time there is no ideal intracoronary treatment. All available modalities are attended by similar general early success and complication 'rates',[60] and cannot improve on those generally now offered by PTCA. Restenosis continues to occupy pride of place as the 'Achilles Heel'. The recently highlighted value of laser therapy at plaque erosion in particular circumstances (such as chronic occlusions, calcified, long, irregular or ostial coronary lesions) and of directional atherectomy in concentric 'restenotic' lesions and 'complex lesions appearing to contain thrombus' (especially in saphenous vein grafts) has unveiled perhaps a new concept in interventional cardiology—a 'niche' for each of the treatment modalities.[60,78] This would imply only minimal overlap between recommendations of appropriateness for a particular modality and therefore rationalization of approach and consequent increase in the number of patients previously labelled as having 'unsuitable anatomy' (currently about 50 per cent)[60] in whom a non-surgical intervention might offer a reasonable alternative to medical therapy or CABG.

There are, undoubtedly, patients in whom these treatments are doomed to failure, and it is of utmost importance to make every effort to identify these patients using information already collected in prospective studies.

Restenosis is the 'buzz word' of this era and, as such, is the focus of considerable attention throughout the world of invasive cardiology, in the quest for what has been termed the 'magic bullet'. New devices for percutaneous revascularization have not actually provided us with the 'magic bullet' but each appears, nevertheless, to have carved a 'niche' for itself in the treatment of obstructive coronary disease. It appears that the 'magic bullet' will take the form of a combination of a device which can forge great luminal increase and a pharmaco-biological agent,[80,81] to control either the aggressive early proliferation of smooth muscle cells which takes place after endothelial injury, or their effusive production of matrix substances, or to modulate the phenotype of the proliferating cells from synthetic to contractile (non-secretory), or indeed to effect the early restoration of an intact endothelial surface so as to restrict cell proliferation. Steady progress is clearly being made in this area[79–81], and maybe, by the end of the century, the dream of a 'magic bullet' will finally become a reality.

# If I had . . .

My reaction depends on what I mean by 'restenosis'—I shall interpret it as implying, merely, symptomatic recurrence following an initially clinically successful balloon angioplasty, for a single non-left main stem coronary lesion. (If this was a significant left main stem lesion, I would be inclined to lean towards having bypass graft surgery, including, of course, an internal mammary artery graft to my LAD.)

Assuming I can correctly interpret my symptoms, I would consider re-emergence of exercise-induced chest discomfort as indicating significant degree of arterial narrowing. If my symptoms recurred within the first few weeks and were only exercise related, I would first want to undergo a treadmill exercise test, to assess my functional capacity, as some indication of ischaemic threat (preferably associated with either echocardiography or thallium-SPECT, to give an impression of the amount of myocardium in jeopardy). If I performed reasonably well on exercise—say, into stage 3 (6–9 min) of the standard Bruce protocol—and had completely reversible thallium or wall motion abnormalities, which did not constitute more than 25 per cent of my myocardium, then I would start taking a long-acting beta-blocker and prophylactic sublingual or buccal nitrates and bide my time. My reasoning for

this preference is that early re-intervention (<3 months) has been reasonably convincingly demonstrated, by a number of investigators over the years, to be attended by a greater need for further re-intervention than when re-intervention is carried out later (>3 months). The cut-off of 3 months may appear rather arbitrary, but it does correlate with the serial clinical angiographic studies, which demonstrate very little further deterioration in lumen after 3 months, and also with experimental pathological inferences. In the early weeks after angioplasty (when the healing process is at its height, the neointima is still immature and no 'scar' has yet been formed), perhaps repeat injury has a multiplied or magnified effect and the resultant healing response is even more intense and prolonged. Therefore I would want to delay any decision to re-intervene (by whatever means) for as long as possible after the first angioplasty. If I had NYHA class III or IV or unstable angina, a poor exercise test performance or >30 per cent myocardium at risk, then I would want to have repeat angiography, as soon as possible, to decide what type of re-intervention to undergo (i.e. I have no doubt that I would need, and would wish to undergo, fairly urgent revascularization).

Assuming I undergo angiography (either sooner or later, depending on the information outlined above) and significant renarrowing has occurred, as long as the lesion was suitable for PTCA, I would undergo repeat PTCA. Of course, early and aggressive symptomatic recurrence/unstable angina may be associated with intracoronary thrombosis, so I would not object to having intracoronary angioscopy. If thrombus was thus demonstrated, I would opt initially for aggressive antithrombotic and antiplatelet therapy intravenously and perhaps even intracoronary thrombolysis, if a significant volume of red thrombus were present, as well as bedrest and aggressive 'medical' therapy (aspirin + intravenous nitrates + beta-blockade ± calcium antagonists (± anxiolytics!)) and 'aggressive' observation. If I 'cooled off' on this therapy, I would like to gradually mobilize and have an exercise test after a couple of days of symptom-free mobility, then be guided by the outcome of this, as above. On the other hand, if I had a critical eccentric lesion, with super-imposed thrombus, I would opt for directional atherectomy or TEC (depending on the particular expertise of my physician), especially if the artery was >3 mm and the lesion was reasonably accessible. I would like to have full intravenous anticoagulation for at least a few days after such intervention (and I would not mind taking oral anticoagulants for a few weeks either), against a background of intracoronary thrombus.

I would not consider having stent implantation at this stage of my disease (first symptomatic recurrence after balloon angioplasty) as I am not keen on the idea of having a foreign body in my body, if I have an alternative. Maybe if biodegradable or 'temporary' stents show some success in the future, I would be more amenable to such therapy. In the context of the bailout situation, I would certainly accept a stent, ideally Palmaz–Schatz, although in the given situation I suspect the particular model would be the least of my worries!

At this stage in the continuing evolution of interventional cardiology, I would not be keen on undergoing laser therapy, as I believe the restenosis process to be particularly aggressive following this procedure. If I had a heavily calcified or long lesion or an ostial lesion, I think I would prefer to have rotablator, although Professor Karsch might be able to persuade me otherwise, should I fall ill in the vicinity of Tübingen.

Under which circumstances would I consider undergoing bypass graft surgery? Having served some time as a cardiothoracic surgical resident, I must confess to being a little reluctant to having my chest 'opened'. Even in the context of three-vessel disease, with restenosis of one or more lesions (apart from in the 'bailout' scenario), I would not yet opt for surgery, preferring instead to exhaust the percutaneous possibilities, as described above for the single lesion. However, if I were 60–70 years old, I reckon full revascularization by a well-performed CABG should get me well beyond my allotted '3 score and 10'.

What about adjunctive medical therapy? Apart from the obligatory prophylactic daily aspirin, there is none currently available which I would take on a regular basis, to prevent further restenosis (studies in progress may challenge this statement), although I might take a chance on fish oil, since I do not eat fish (merely because of a lifelong personal distaste) and my mother always told me that cod liver oil would be good for me—one should always take heed of one's mother!

# References

1 Rensing BJ et al, Quantitative angiographic assessment of elastic recoil after percutaneous transluminal coronary angioplasty, *Am J Cardiol* (1990) **66**:1039–44.

2 Isner JM et al, Combination balloon-ultrasound imaging catheter for percutaneous transluminal angioplasty. Validation of imaging, analysis of recoil, and identification of plaque fracture, *Circulation* (1991); **84**:739–54.

3 Hanet C et al, Influence of balloon size and stenosis morphology on immediate and delayed elastic recoil after percutaneous transluminal coronary angioplasty, *J Am Coll Cardiol* (1991) **18**:506–11.

4 Rensing BJ et al, Quantitative angiographic risk factors of luminal narrowing after coronary balloon angioplasty using balloon measurements to reflect stretch and elastic recoil at the dilatation site, *Am J Cardiol* (1992) **69**:584–91.

5 Steele PM et al, Balloon angioplasty: natural history of the pathophysiological response to injury in the pig model, *Circ Res* (1985) **57**:105–12.

6 Austin GE et al, Intimal proliferation of smooth muscle cells as an explanation for recurrent coronary artery stenosis after percutaneous transluminal coronary angioplasty, *J Am Coll Cardiol* (1985) **6**:369–75.

7 Waller BF et al, Morphologic observations late after coronary balloon angioplasty: mechanisms of acute injury and relationship to restenosis, *Radiology* (1990) **174**:961–7.

8 Uchida Y et al, Angioscopic observation of the coronary luminal changes induced by coronary angioplasty, *Am Heart J* (1989) **117**:769–76.

9 Potkin BN, Roberts WC, Effects of coronary angioplasty on atherosclerotic plaques and relation of plaque composition and arterial size to outcome, *Am J Cardiol* (1988) **62**: 41–50.

10 Forrester JS et al, A paradigm for restenosis based on cell biology: clues for development of new preventive therapies, *J Am Coll Cardiol* (1991) **17**:758–69.

11 Nobuyoshi M et al, Restenosis after percutaneous transluminal coronary angioplasty: pathologic observations in 20 patients, *J Am Coll Cardiol* (1991) **17**:433–9.

12 Schwartz RS, Holmes DR, Topol EJ, The restenosis paradigm revisited: an alternative proposal for cellular mechanisms, *J Am Coll Cardiol* (1992) **20**:1284–93.

13 Schwartz RS et al, Restenosis after balloon angioplasty. A practical proliferative model in porcine coronary arteries, *Circulation* (1991) **82**:2190–200.

14 Schwartz RS et al, Restenosis and the proportional neointimal response to coronary artery injury: results in a porcine model, *J Am Coll Cardiol* (1992) **19**:267–74.

15 Chesebro JH et al, Restenosis after arterial angioplasty: a haemorrheologic response to injury, *Am J Cardiol* (1987) **60**:10B–16B.

16 Ip JH et al, The role of platelets, thrombin and hyperplasia in restenosis after coronary angioplasty, *J Am Coll Cardiol* (1991) **17**:77B–88B.

17 Karas SP et al, Coronary intimal proliferation after balloon injury and stenting in swine: an animal model of restenosis, *J Am Coll Cardiol* (1992) **20**:467–74.

18 Ip JH et al, Syndromes of accelerated atherosclerosis: role of vascular injury and smooth muscle cell proliferation, *J Am Coll Cardiol* (1990) **15**:1667–87.

19 Barbeau GR et al, Rupture of internal elastic lamina is essential for restenosis following balloon angioplasty, *Circulation* (1991) **84**:II–603 (abstr.).

20 den Heijer P et al, Serial angioscopy during the first hour after successful PTCA. *Circulation* (1992) **86**:I–458 (abstr.).

21 Uchida Y et al, Observation of luminal changes in human coronary artery by an intravascular microscope, *Circulation* (1992) **86**:I–503 (abstr.).

22 Serruys PW et al, Incidence of restenosis after successful angioplasty: a time related phenomenon: a quantitative angiographic

study in 342 consecutive patients at 1, 2, 3 and 4 months, *Circulation* (1988) **77**:361–71.

23 Nobuyoshi M et al, Restenosis after successful percutaneous transluminal coronary angioplasty: serial angiographic follow-up of 299 patients, *J Am Coll Cardiol* (1988) **12**:616–23.

24 Gruentzig AR, Meier B, Percutaneous transluminal coronary angioplasty. The first five years and the future, *Int J Cardiol* (1983) **2**:319–23.

25 Califf RM et al, Restenosis: the clinical issues. In: Topol EJ, ed. *Textbook of interventional cardiology.* (W.B. Saunders: Philadelphia 1990) 363–94.

26 Popma JJ, Califf RM, Topol EJ, Clinical trials of restenosis following angioplasty, *Circulation* (1991) **84**:1426–37.

27 Gould KL, Lipscomb K, Hamilton GW, Physiological basis for assessing critical coronary stenosis: instantaneous flow response and regional distribution during coronary hyperaemia as measures of coronary flow reserve, *Am J Cardiol* (1974) **33**:87–97.

28 Kirkeeide RL, Gould KL, Parsel L, Assessment of coronary stenoses by myocardial perfusion imaging during pharmacologic coronary vasodilation. Validation of coronary flow reserve as a single integrated functional measure of stenosis severity reflecting all its geometric dimensions, *J Am Coll Cardiol* (1986) **7**:103–13.

29 Nissen SE et al, Intravascular ultrasound assessment of lumen size and wall morphology in normal subjects and patients with coronary artery disease, *Circulation* (1991) **84**:1087–99.

30 Brown BG et al, Quantitative coronary angiography. Estimation of dimensions, haemodynamic resistance and atheroma mass of coronary artery lesions using the arteriogram and digital computation, *Circulation* (1977) **53**:329–37.

31 Reiber JHC et al, A cardiac image analysis system. Objective quantitative processing of angiocardiograms, *Proc Comp Cardiol* (1978) 239–42.

32 Reiber JHC, Serruys PW, Quantitative coronary angiography. In: Marcus ML et al, eds. *Cardiac imaging, a companion to Braunwalds heart disease* (Saunders: New York 1991) 211–80.

33 Zijlstra F et al, Does quantitative assessment of coronary artery dimensions predict the physiological significance of a coronary stenosis? *Circulation* (1987) **75**:1154–61.

34 Harrison DG et al, The value of lesion cross-sectional area determined by quantitative coronary angiography in assessing the physiologic significance of proximal left anterior descending coronary arterial stenoses, *Circulation* (1984) **69**:1111–19.

35 Rensing BJ et al, Which angiographic parameter best describes functional status 6 months after successful single vessel coronary balloon angioplasty, *J Am Coll Cardiol* (1993) **21**:317–24.

36 Beatt KJ, Serruys PW, Hugenholtz PG, Restenosis after coronary angioplasty: new standards for clinical studies, *J Am Coll Cardiol* (1990) **15**:491–8.

37 Serruys PW, Foley DP, de Feyter PJ, Restenosis after coronary angioplasty: a proposal of new comparative approaches based on quantitative angiography, *Br Heart J* (1992) **68**:417–24.

38 Arnett EN et al, Coronary artery narrowing in coronary heart disease: comparison of cineangiographic and necropsy findings, *Ann Int Med* (1979) **91**:350–6.

39 Glagov S et al, Compensatory enlargement of human atherosclerotic coronary arteries, *New Engl J Med* (1987) **316**:1371–75.

40 Foley DP et al, Is there a need for angiography after 24 hours to assess the result of coronary balloon angioplasty in clinical studies, *Circulation* (1992) **86**:I–785 (abstr.).

41 Beatt KJ et al, Change in diameter of coronary artery segments adjacent to stenosis after percutaneous transluminal coronary angioplasty: failure of percent diameter stenosis measurement to reflect morphologic changes induced by balloon dilation, *J Am Coll Cardiol* (1988) **12**:315–23.

42 Smucker ML et al, 'Whole artery restenosis' after coronary atherectomy: a quantitative angiographic study, AHA 64th scientific sessions, *Circulation* (1991) **84**:0322 (abstr.).

43 Foley DP et al for the MERCATOR group, Restenotic lesions after PTCA are morphologically different from the original stenosis—a quantitative angiographic study, *Circulation* (1992) **86**:I–596 (abstr.).

44 Fleming RM et al, Patterns in visual interpretation of coronary angiograms as detected by

quantitative coronary angiography, *J Am Coll Cardiol* (1991) **18**:945–51.

45  Rensing BJ et al, Luminal narrowing after percutaneous transluminal coronary balloon angioplasty follows a near Gaussian distribution. A quantitative angiographic study in 1445 successfully dilated lesions, *J Am Coll Cardiol* (1992) **19**:939–45.

46  Kuntz RE et al, Novel approach to the analysis of restenosis after the use of three new coronary devices, *J Am Coll Cardiol* (1992) **19**:1493—99.

47  Serruys PW et al, Restenosis following coronary angioplasty. In: Meier B, ed. *Interventional cardiology* (Hogrefe and Huber: Toronto, Lewiston, NY, Bern, Gottingen, Stuttgart 1990) 79–115.

48  Serruys PW et al, Prevention of restenosis after percutaneous transluminal coronary angioplasty with thromboxane A2 receptor blockade. A randomized, double-blind, placebo controlled trial, *Circulation* (1991) **84**:1568–81.

49  The Mercator Study Group, Does the new angiotensin converting enzyme inhibitor cilazapril prevent restenosis after percutaneous transluminal coronary angioplasty? The results of the Mercator study: a multicentre randomized double-blind placebo-controlled trial, *Circulation* (1992) **86**:100–11.

50  Hermans WRM et al, Prevention of restenosis after percutaneous transluminal coronary angioplasty (PTCA): the search for a 'magic bullet', *Am Heart J* (1991) **122**:171–87.

51  Rensing BJ et al on behalf of the CARPORT study group, Luminal narrowing after coronary angioplasty. Clinical, procedural and lesion factors related to long term angiographic outcome, *Eur Heart J* (1992) **13**(abstract supplement):P1460.

52  Serruys PW et al on behalf of the MERCATOR study group, Are clinical, angiographic or procedural variables predictive of luminal renarrowing after successful coronary balloon angioplasty, *Circulation* (1992) **86**:I-849 (abstr.).

53  Hermans WR et al, Postangioplasty restenosis rate between segments of the major coronary arteries, *Am J Cardiol* (1992) **69**:194–200.

54  Hermans WRM et al on behalf of the MERCATOR study group, Therapeutic dissec-

tion after successful coronary angioplasty: no effect on restenosis nor on clinical outcome nor in 693 patients, *J Am Coll Cardiol* (1992) **20**:767–80.

55  Myler RK et al, There is no such thing as 'restenosis', *J Inv Cardiol* (1992) **4**:282–90.

56  Foley DP et al, Is 'bigger' really 'better'? A quantitative angiographic study of immediate and long term outcome following balloon angioplasty, directional atherectomy and stent implantation, *Circulation* (1992) **86**:I-530 (abstr.).

57  Foley DP et al, The influence of vessel size on restenosis following percutaneous coronary interventions, *Circulation* (1992) **86**:I-255 (abstr.).

58  Fioretti PM et al, Exercise echocardiography versus thallium-201 SPECT for assessing patients before and after PTCA, *Eur Heart J* (1992) **13**:213–19.

59  de Silva R et al, Preoperative prediction of the outcome of coronary revascularization using positron emission tomography, *Circulation* (1992) **86**:1738–42.

60  Forrester JS, Eigler N, Litvack F, Interventional cardiology: the decade ahead, *Circulation* (1991) **84**:942–4.

61  Leon MB et al, Strategies for coronary revascularization using different atherectomy devices: a NACI registry report, *J Am Coll Cardiol* (1992) **19**:731–1.

62  The CAVEAT Investigators, United States and Europe, The coronary angioplasty versus excision atherectomy trial preliminary results, *Circulation* (1992) **86**:I-1491 (abstr.).

63  Ellis SG et al, Relation of stenosis morphology and clinical presentation to the procedural results of directional coronary atherectomy, *Circulation* (1991) **84**:644–53.

64  Ahn SS, Auth D, Marcus DR, Removal of focal atheromatous lesions by angioscopically guided high speed rotary atherectomy, *J Vasc Surg* (1988) **7**:292–300.

65  Stack RS et al, Advances in cardiovascular technologies: interventional cardiac catheterization at Duke Medical Centre, *Am J Cardiol* (1988) **62**:1F–44F.

66  Abela GS et al, Laser angioplasty with angioscopic guidance in humans, *J Am Coll Cardiol* (1986) **8**:184–92.

67  Karsch KR et al, Percutaneous coronary excimer laser angioplasty: initial clinical results, *Lancet* (1989) **2**:647–50.

68  Bittl JA, Sanborn TA, Excimer laser-facilitated coronary angioplasty: relative risk analysis of acute and follow-up results in 200 patients, *Circulation* (1992) **86**:71–80.

69  Sigwart U et al, Intravascular stents to prevent occlusion and restenosis after transluminal angioplasty, *N Eng J Med* (1987) **316**:701–6.

70  Carroza JP Jr et al, Angiographic and clinical outcome of intracoronary stenting: immediate and long term results from a single-center experience, *J Am Coll Cardiol* (1992) **20**:328–37.

71  Colombo A et al, Coronary stenting: single institution experience with the initial 100 cases using the Palmaz-Shatz stent, *Cath Cardiovasc Diagn* (1992) **26**:171–6.

72  Serruys PW et al, Angiographic follow-up after placement of a self-expanding coronary artery stent, *N Eng J Med* (1991) **324**:13–17.

73  Foley DP et al, Stenting of the coronary arteries, the ideal revascularization technique: dream, reality, mystery or myth? In: Sigwart U, Frank GI, eds. *Intravascular Stents* (Springer-Verlag: Berlin, Heidelberg 1992) 101–33.

74  Umans VA et al, Comparative quantitative angiographic analysis of directional coronary atherectomy and balloon angioplasty: a new methodologic approach, *Am J Cardiol* (1991) **68**:1556–63.

75  Umans VA et al, Restenosis after directional coronary atherectomy and balloon angioplasty: comparative analysis based on matched lesions, *J Am Coll Cardiol* (1993) **21**:1382–90.

76  de Jaegere P et al, Stent versus balloon angioplasty; matching based on QCA, a surrogate for randomized studies, *Am Heart J* (1993) **125**:310–19.

77  Spears JR et al, Percutaneous coronary laser balloon angioplasty: preliminary results of a multicenter trial, *J Am Coll Cardiol* (1989) **13**(suppl A):61A (abstr.).

78  Topol EJ, Promises and pitfalls of new devices for coronary artery disease, *Circulation* (1991) **83**:689–94.

79  Epstein SE et al, Cytotoxic effects of a recombinant chimeric toxin on rapidly proliferating vascular smooth muscle cells, *Circulation* (1991) **84**:778–87.

80  Nabel EG, Plautz G, Nabel GJ, Gene transfer into vascular cells, *J Am Coll Cardiol* (1991) **17**:189B–94B.

81  Speir E, Epstein SE, Inhibition of smooth muscle cell proliferation by an antisense oligonucleotide targeting the messenger RNA encoding proliferating cell nuclear antigen, *Circulation* (1992) **86**:538–47.

# 3

## Angioplasty or surgery in the over-70s?

*Peter PT de Jaegere, Andonis G Violaris, PJ de Feyter and*
*Patrick W Serruys*

## Introduction

As the social and medical advances of this century have translated into improved longevity, the number of people over 70 in our society has increased in both absolute and relative numbers. We now have an aging population which is increasing at twice the rate of the general population and which promises to constitute 20–25 per cent of the total population by the first half of the next century.[1] Furthermore, the sector of the population which is increasing most rapidly is the oldest, the over-85s. Coronary artery disease is particularly prevalent in this population, with more than 15 per cent of the over-70s and 20 per cent of the over-80s manifesting evidence of coronary heart disease.[2] It is thus responsible for substantial morbidity and mortality in this age group.

Recent advances in technology have increased our ability to diagnose and treat a wide spectrum of coronary artery disease. It is now technically feasible to perform multivessel angioplasty at little risk and with minimal inconvenience to the patient. As the numbers of elderly increase and both their and their doctor's expectations grow, the demand for specialist cardiology services and cardiac surgery will increase. The cost of providing such services will increase substantially over the next few years and, as our resources are limited, may significantly compromise our ability to offer adequate medical care to everyone. Already in our institution the number of coronary angioplasties performed in patients over the age of 70 has increased from 3 per cent in 1981 to over 19 per cent of the total population in 1991. In the USA, over a third of cardiac catheterizations and coronary bypass operations are performed in the elderly.[3,4] We know that, technically, both coronary angioplasty and bypass surgery can be performed in the elderly with reasonable safety. The question is, should it be done just because it is technically feasible?

In this chapter we review the available evidence on the use of revascularization procedures in the elderly and compare and contrast the results of coronary angioplasty with those of coronary artery bypass grafting. We then propose a management strategy, based on the currently available evidence, which results in clinical decision-making based on a risk–benefit analysis for each individual patient rather than on the technical feasibility or otherwise of coronary angioplasty or surgery. We believe this is better, both for the individual patient, and for the community as a whole.

# The over-70s—are they any different?

It is easy to divide the population on the basis of age and take 70 as an arbitrary cut-off point to define the elderly. This arbitrary cut-off point may be inappropriate, however, as there are marked differences within this elderly group and a distinction needs to be made between the chronological and physiological age of an individual patient. Physiological aging is a continuous process which proceeds at quite different rates amongst individuals, depending on the interplay of internal factors such as genetic disposition and external factors such as overall quality of life (living habits and conditions) and chronic medical conditions.[5] The physiological age of the patient is determined by the activity of the patient before the limitations of severe angina occurred, the mental status of the patient, the motivation of the patient to go back to an active life and the freedom from severe associated disease processes such as chronic renal failure or cerebrovascular disease. The difference between chronological and physiological age is important, as in most studies it is the adequacy of left ventricular function and concomitant disease that is the main determinant of survival after revascularization rather than the chronological age of the patient. Thus each doctor should be able to use his own judgement as to who is and who is not physiologically over 70 and hence elderly.

Unfortunately, most of the literature that addresses the question of revascularization in the elderly fails to take this into account and assumes an arbitrary age threshold of 65–70 as defining the elderly. This results in a marked heterogeneity in the study populations, with wide differences in age, clinical and angiographic variables, all of which may have an appreciable influence on both clinical outcome and long-term prognosis. The heterogeneity in age is particularly important as although in a younger population an age difference of 15 years makes little physiological difference, in the over-70s it makes a substantial difference. It is therefore only possible to extrapolate the results of these studies to individual patients in a very general way.

# Treatment objectives—are they any different?

The lifestyle, life expectancy and response to treatment of patients over 70 are different from those of the average population. Thus our treatment needs to be tailored to their particular requirements and needs.

What then are the aims of treatment in the over-70s? Are we aiming to simply alleviate symptoms and improve the quality of life or are we also aiming to prolong life, reduce cardiac events and improve long-term prognosis? Unlike the younger population, where we are continuously striving to improve prognosis and reduce cardiac events as well as alleviate symptoms, the elderly have a more limited long-term prognosis and often value continued independence and quality of life more than an extra year or two of life. Symptom relief is therefore a more appropriate end-point for this group. Because of this we should be using the path least likely to cause complications. Initial management should therefore be with medical therapy.

The drugs used to treat the elderly are the same as those used to treat the younger population. The response of the over-70s to drug therapy is, however, different because of altered pharmacodynamics and concomitant disease processes.[6,7] Drug therapy must therefore be individualized to avoid adverse reactions.

Drugs should be started at the lowest dose available and increased slowly until an adequate therapeutic effect is achieved. Medical treatment is sometimes insufficient, however, either as a result of the altered pharmacodynamics or as a result of intolerance, and, when symptoms remain limiting, referral for revascularization is indicated.

# Which elderly patients should be referred for revascularization?

The decision as to who should be referred for revascularization should be based on a careful evaluation of the clinical setting and assessment of the risk–benefit ratio. This would involve a full, detailed assessment of the patient's cardiac symptoms and their response to medical therapy, quality of life in general, overall clinical and mental state as well as other concomitant diseases. If the patient's quality of life is compromised, with substantial restrictions of activity, further investigation is warranted. Otherwise, active elderly patients with symptoms refractory to medical therapy or who do not tolerate drug therapy and who accept the risks of cardiac catheterization and subsequent revascularization should then be formally assessed by cardiac catheterization.

Until the introduction of coronary angioplasty in 1977,[8] the only option for revascularization was coronary artery bypass surgery, which itself was in the early stages of development. With the introduction of coronary angioplasty and the subsequent refinements of the technique and the equipment used, balloon angioplasty has opened a whole new approach to revascularization and expanded its indications.

# Coronary angioplasty

## Acute results

Most data regarding the acute success rate and incidence of major complications of balloon angioplasty in the elderly are from retrospective analyses[9-23] (Table 3.1). The immediate angiographic success rate varies between 78 and 93 per cent. Although the complication rate in the over-70s is reasonably low at 0–2.2 per cent death, 0.8–5.1% per cent myocardial infarction and 0.9–9.0 per cent emergency bypass grafting, this rises significantly in the over-80s, with mortality rates of up to 10 per cent[23] and emergency bypass rates of up to 7 per cent.[13,23] There are wide variations between studies, however, perhaps reflecting selection bias. Certainly in at least one large study the incidence of critical complications did not clearly increase with age.

Although the studies cited above have different patient profiles, indications for coronary angioplasty, and definitions of success and complications, it is fair to say that balloon angioplasty can be performed with a high immediate success rate of up to 96 per cent. Furthermore, these acute results compare favourably with the overall National, Heart, Lung and Blood Institute (NHLBI) PTCA registry data.[24] Except for the higher incidence of major complications such as death and myocardial infarction, PTCA can thus be performed with comparable success in the elderly.

## Long-term results

Successful coronary angioplasty results in substantial clinical improvement. Jeroudi and colleagues have shown that over 87 per cent of patients older than 80 were subjectively improved, 33 per cent were physically more

| Patient age (years) | Study | No. patients | Angiographic success (%) | Clinical success (%) | Complications | | |
|---|---|---|---|---|---|---|---|
| | | | | | Death | Acute myocardial infarction | CABG |
| ≥70 | Dorros et al[9] | 109 | 89 | 83 | 1.8 | 2.8 | 0.9 |
| | Holt et al[10] | 54 | – | 80 | 0.0 | 1.8 | 5.6 |
| | Simpfendorfer et al[11] | 124 | – | 90 | 0.0 | 0.8 | 4.0 |
| | | 212 | – | 93 | 0.9 | 0.9 | 2.8 |
| | Thompson et al[12] | 233 | – | 82 | 2.2 | 4.3 | 9.0 |
| | Bedotto et al[13] | 517a | – | 96 | 1.7 | 1.7 | 0.9 |
| | Buffet et al[14] | 99 | – | 84 | 1.0 | 5.1 | 2.0 |
| | Forman et al[15] | 270 | 88 | – | 2.0 | 5.0 | 4.0 |
| | de Jaegere et al[16] | 166 | 85 | 86 | 2.1 | 2.7 | 3.4 |
| ≥75 | Kelsey et al[17] | 92 | 80 | 72 | 3.3 | 8.7 | 5.4 |
| | Thompson et al[12] | 193 | – | 93 | 6.2 | 6.7 | 3.0 |
| | Bedotto et al[13] | 295a | – | 97 | 1.6 | 1.0 | 0.6 |
| | Buffet et al[14] | 86 | – | 79 | 3.5 | 10.4 | 0.0 |
| ≥80 | Kern et al[18] | 21 | 78 | 67 | 19.0 | – | 14.0 |
| | Rich et al[19] | 22 | 89 | 86 | 0.0 | 14.0 | 0.0 |
| | Jeroudi et al[20] | 54 | 93 | 91 | 4.0 | 4.0 | 0.0 |
| | Rizo-Patron et al[21] | 53 | – | 83 | 1.8 | 5.5 | 7.5 |
| | Bedotto et al[13] | 111a | – | 91 | 6.3 | 2.7 | 0.0 |
| | Myler et al[22] | 74 | – | 80 | 1.4 | 0.0 | 4.1 |
| | Jackman et al[23] | 31 | 90 | – | 6.5 | 6.5 | 10.0 |
| | Buffet et al[14] | 30 | – | 73 | 0.0 | 10.0 | 0.0 |
| | Forman et al[15] | 67 | 84 | – | 6.0 | 5.0 | 2.0 |

**Table 3.1**
*Angiographic and clinical success rate and complications of balloon angioplasty in patients 70 years of age and older.*

active and 55 per cent required less medication after angioplasty.[20] Jeroudi's findings also agree with the observation in most studies that more than 75 per cent of patients are free of angina or are clinically improved after angioplasty.

This initial clinical improvement appears to be well maintained during follow-up. Event-free survival (free of myocardial infarction and bypass surgery) exceeds 80 per cent at 1 year and 70 per cent at 4 years.[12,20,22,23] Although

Thompson and colleagues found that event-free survival was considerably lower in patients over 75,[12] Myler and colleagues report event-free survival rates of 89 per cent at 1 year and 82 per cent at 4 years in patients over 80.[22] The incidence of late myocardial infarction is less than 5 per cent and is similar to the infarction rate in the general angioplasty population.[9–12,14–16,19–21] The need for bypass surgery ranges from 3 to 14 per cent in patients over 70[9–12,14–16] and from 6 to 10 per cent in patients over 80.[20,21] This contrasts with the need for repeat balloon angioplasty, which is performed in 14–22 per cent of patients over 70 and in 4–35 per cent of patients over 80.[9–12,14–17,14–23] The higher frequency of repeat PTCA may be explained by referral bias, which may be influenced by the preference of the patient, family or physician for a less invasive procedure.

The impact of coronary angioplasty on the long-term prognosis is not clear and no randomized studies have been performed to assess this. The 1- and 4-year survival rates, however, have been reported to be 91–95 per cent in patients over 70[11] and 80–93 per cent in patients over 80.[20,22] This high rate of overall long-term survival compares favourably with the calculated survival of the general elderly population. In the Netherlands the calculated 4-year survival for the elderly population over 70 is 84 per cent for males and 93 per cent for females, and 64 and 77 per cent for male and female octogenarians respectively.

## Thorax-centre experience

Between January 1983 and September 1988 we performed coronary angioplasty in 166 patients over 70 years old representing 8 per cent of the total coronary angioplasty population ($n = 2002$) during the same time.[16] The median age of the patients was 73 with an age range of 70–84. Indications for coronary angioplasty were unstable angina in 81 patients (49 per cent), stable angina in 76 patients (46 per cent) and acute myocardial infarction in 9 patients (5 per cent). Angioplasty was performed on a total of 226 lesions (one lesion in 117 patients (70 per cent), two or more lesions in 49 patients (30 per cent). Revascularization was complete in 101 patients (61 per cent) and partial in 65 patients (39 per cent).

Of the 226 stenoses attempted, 192 were successfully dilated. The overall primary angiographic success rate of 85 per cent was reflected in a primary clinical success rate of 86 per cent. In 14 patients (8 per cent) the angioplasty did not significantly reduce the diameter stenosis but there were no complications. Ten patients (6 per cent) had a total of 15 major procedure-related complications, and four (2 per cent) died as a result of these. Acute myocardial infarction was seen in four patients, of whom one died and two were referred for emergency bypass surgery. Another four patients underwent urgent bypass surgery; of these, one died of a perioperative myocardial infarction. Two other patients had ventricular fibrillation and subsequently died.

Patients were followed up for a median of 21 months (range 0.5–66). Sixteen patients (10 per cent) died and eight (5 per cent) had sustained a non-fatal myocardial infarction during follow-up. Of the rest, 21 (13 per cent) had undergone repeat dilatation and 17 (10 per cent) elective bypass surgery. The estimated survival at 4 years (mean (SD)) was 89(4) per cent whilst the event-free survival at 4 years was 61(8) per cent (Figure 3.1). Multivariate logistic analysis revealed that the extent of vessel disease and not the completeness of revascularization was the only independent predictive factor for event-free survival: the event-free survival rate was 81(10) per cent at

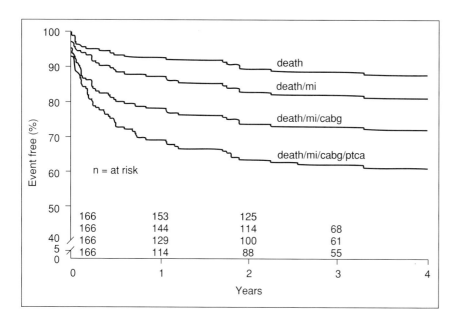

**Figure 3.1**
*Thorax-centre experience. Overall long-term cumulative survival and event-free survival curves after balloon angioplasty according to the Kaplan–Meier method for patients aged >70.*

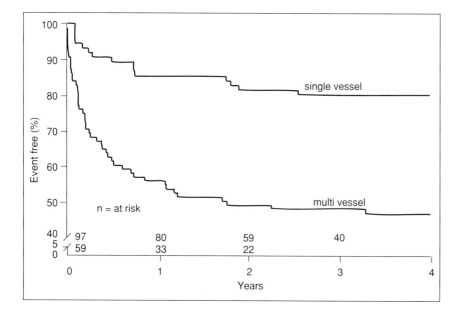

**Figure 3.2**
*Thorax-centre experience. Event-free survival after balloon angioplasty according to the Kaplan–Meier method for patients aged >70 with single- and multi-vessel disease.*

4 years for patients with single-vessel disease compared with 45(12) per cent for patients with multivessel disease (Figure 3.2).

Thus coronary angioplasty, both single- and multivessel, is a safe and effective treatment for obstructive coronary disease in the over-70s.

# Coronary artery bypass grafting

## Acute results

Because no randomized studies have been published to date on CABG in the elderly, most data regarding the success, operative mortality and morbidity of the procedure come from retrospective studies[25-44] (Table 3.2). In spite of the different patient populations, widespread age distribution and different operative techniques in different centres, a number of points emerge.

Firstly, because of refinements in anaesthesia, myocardial preservation and operative techniques, the operative mortality for the procedure has fallen substantially in this age group over recent years. When Elayda and colleagues examined the operative mortality in 1275 patients over 70 operated on for CABG alone from 1970 to 1981 they found that the operative mortality fell from 13.9 per cent in the 1970–1975 cohort to 4.7 per cent in the 1976–1981 cohort, despite the two groups having similar baseline characteristics.[29] More recent studies suggest that the operative mortality in large centres is around 6–9 per cent.[33-35] It still remains, however, much higher than in the younger population and appears to increase substantially with increasing age after 70,[28,34] reaching rates of up to 41 per cent in the over-80s.[44] This may be as a consequence of the greater frequency of risk factors with increasing age, particularly the much higher incidence of unstable and post-infarction angina in the over-80s, both of which are associated with increased mortality in younger age groups.[32,41] These increased risk factors are probably also responsible for the very high mortality rates associates with emergency surgery: 35 per cent compared with 14.9 per cent for urgent cases and 3.6 per cent for elective operations.[40] Performing additional procedures such as valve replacements or left ventricular aneurysmectomy at the time of CABG further increases the mortality rate.[35,42] Other variables predictive of perioperative mortality are similar to those of the younger population and include severe left ventricular dysfunction and associated medical diseases.[32,35,39]

Although the actual mortality rate in the over-70s may not be high, because of concomitant disease, extracorporeal support during the operation and slow healing of the thoracotomy wound, bypass surgery in this age group is associated with significant perioperative morbidity of up to 65 per cent secondary to both cardiac and non-cardiac complications, particularly neurological.[25-45] These are much more common than in the younger population, perhaps because of cerebral atherosclerosis, which results in a reduced ability to withstand hypotension, hypoperfusion and extracorporeal circulation. Furthermore, they are particularly devastating in this age group, resulting in perhaps additional burdens on the, also elderly, partner. Variables predictive of perioperative morbidity include concomitant disease such as diabetes mellitus, cerebral and peripheral vascular disease, renal impairment and chronic obstructive pulmonary disease.[32,35,39] The increased incidence of major postoperative complications results in a slower recovery with substantially longer hospital stays and increases the financial cost of the procedure in this age group.[32]

| Patient age (years) | Study | No. patients | Mean age (range) | Mortality (%) | Morbidity (total) (%) | Actuarial survival (%) (months) |
|---|---|---|---|---|---|---|
| ≥70 | Berry et al[25] | 65 | 72.4 | 3 | 37 | 94 (12) |
| | Hochberg et al[26] | 75 | 72.3 | 12 | 33 | 96 (22) |
| | Faro et al[27] | 105 | 72.5 (70–81) | 10.5 | 33 (cardiac) 44 (non-cardiac) | 94 (–) |
| | Gersh et al[28] | 241 | (70–75) | 6.6 | – | – |
| | Elayda et al[29] | 1275 | (70–90) | 5.8 | – | 80 (30) |
| | Gersh et al[30] | 200 | (70–75) | – | – | 77 (–) |
| | Ennabli et al[31] | 102 | 72 (70–78) | 7.0 | 39 | – |
| | Horneffer et al[32] | 228 | 73.3 | 9.3 | 37 (cardiac) 31 (non-cardiac) | – |
| | Acinapura et al[33] | 685 | 74.2 (70–85) | 8 | 8 (cardiac) 17 (non-cardiac) | 85 (72) |
| | Grondin et al[34] | 88 | 74.6 | 6 | – | – |
| | Carey et al[35] | 332 | 74.2 | 9.9 | 38.5 | 69 (60) |
| ≥75 | Gersh et al[28] | 42 | (75–84) | 9.5 | – | – |
| | Rahimtoola et al[36] | 178 | (75–84) | 2.8 | – | – |
| | Saldanha et al[37] | 59 | 76 (75–80) | 2.7 | – | – |
| | Rich et al[38] | 60 | 77.6 (75–86) | 3.3 | 65 | – |
| | Loop et al[39] | 467 | – | 4.7 | 17 | 53 (106) |
| | Horvath et al[40] | 222 | 77 (75–85) | 10.8 | 37 | 75 (48) |
| ≥80 | Montague et al[41] | 16 | (80–87) | 12.5 | – | – |
| | Tsai et al[42] | 33 | (80–89) | 6.1 | – | – |
| | Naunheim et al[43] | 16 | 82 (80–88) | 12.5 | 56 | 82 (24) |
| | Edmunds et al[44] | 41 | (80–97) | 24 | – | – |
| | Myler et al[22] | 49 | 83 (80–89) | 10 | 38 | 82.5 (24) |

**Table 3.2**
Success rate, complications and follow-up of isolated coronary artery bypass grafting in patients 70 years of age and older.

Nevertheless, following CABG a significant immediate improvement in clinical status is achieved in more than 90 per cent of patients, most of whom are functionally in NYHA class I or II.

## Long-term results

The improvement in symptoms is maintained over the long term with up to 67 per cent of survivors continuing to be in NYHA class 1 at

5 years. This falls, however, to 55 per cent by 7 years, perhaps reflecting late graft failure or progression of native atherosclerosis.[36] The overall 5-year survival is comparable to that of the normal population adjusted for age. Surgery does not seem to confer additional benefit compared to medical therapy in those patients with relatively good left ventricular function and no left main stem coronary artery disease, but does seem to improve the 6-year survival in those patients with extensive disease and left ventricular dysfunction despite the high perioperative mortality.[30] Whether this is a true reflection of benefit from surgery or whether it reflects selection bias in therapy, crossover problems or the significant differences in the large number of baseline characteristics between the two groups is not, however, clear.

## Coronary angioplasty versus coronary artery bypass grafting—should we strive for complete revascularization?

Coronary angioplasty is less invasive than coronary artery surgery and by avoiding thoracotomy and extracorporeal support offers the potential for myocardial revascularization with a faster recovery and lower morbidity, resulting in shorter hospitalization times and lower costs than bypass surgery. Furthermore, the acute success is maintained in a high proportion of patients. Intuitively it is therefore an attractive proposition for the over-70s. Unfortunately, however, the elderly patient is likely to have advanced disease with rigid, tortuous vessels, calcified lesions and poor left ventricular function. The elderly patient is also more likely to be female and to present with unstable angina. These angiographic and clinical characteristics are likely to make PTCA technically more difficult to perform and only a minority of patients are likely to achieve complete revascularization from balloon angioplasty.

The question then posed is whether complete revascularization is necessary or not. Should we strive for complete revascularization with PTCA and, if this cannot be achieved, refer the patients for CABG, or should we settle for incomplete revascularization? Does complete revascularization improve the short- and long-term outcomes after coronary angioplasty? These are important questions to answer, as multivessel angioplasty carries a significantly higher morbidity and mortality than single-vessel angioplasty.

That remaining stenoses are not always functionally significant has been demonstrated by a number of reports which have shown that a strategy of incomplete revascularization can provide immediate clinical benefit.[46-59] Thomas and colleagues, for example, reported that although 67 per cent of patients had incomplete revascularization, post-angioplasty exercise test performed within 2 months of the procedure showed an ischaemic response in only 34 per cent of patients with incomplete revascularization versus 19 per cent in patients with complete revascularization.[54] The functional performance was comparable in both groups. Thus the majority of patients with incomplete revascularization do not have evidence of residual ischaemia and only a minority of patients with remaining severe ischaemic symptoms unresponsive to pharmacological treatment need an additional revascularization procedure.[46-58]

If clinical outcome is not adversely affected by incomplete revascularization, is long-term prognosis affected? Earlier results from surgery have shown that completeness of revascularization appears to have an important influence

| Author | No. patients | CR (%) | IR (%) | F/U (month) | Death CR (%) | Death IR (%) | AMI CR (%) | AMI IR (%) | Re-PTCA CR (%) | Re-PTCA IR (%) | CABG CR (%) | CABG IR (%) | Symptom free CR (%) | Symptom free IR (%) |
|---|---|---|---|---|---|---|---|---|---|---|---|---|---|---|
| Thomas et al[58] | 92 | 20 | 80 | 12 | 0 | 0 | 0 | 1 | 11 | 12 | 5 | 1 | 63 | 63 |
| Deligonul et al[59] | 470 | 32 | 68 | 27 | 5 | 5.5 | 2.5 | 3.5 | 14 | 13 | 7 | 16 | 80 | 80 |
| Reeder et al[50] | 286 | 44 | 56 | 26 | 3 | 5 | 7.1 | 9.4 | 20 | 9 | 9 | 17 | 69 | 68 |
| Samson et al[51] | 134 | 59 | 41 | 33 | 4 | 11 | 2 | 9 | 4 | 6 | 5 | 19 | 58 | 48 |

Abbreviations:
CR = complete revascularization
IR = incomplete revascularization
F/U = follow-up
AMI = acute myocardial infarction
PTCA = percutaneous transluminal coronary angioplasty
CABG = coronary artery bypass graft

**Table 3.3**
*Long-term follow-up after successful angioplasty of patients with complete and incomplete revascularization.*

on long-term outcome of patients with multi-vessel disease who have undergone coronary artery bypass surgery.[60–62] Complete revascularization was associated with an increased survival rate and more freedom from symptoms during a follow-up period ranging from 16 to 46 months. This difference tended to disappear after a follow-up period of 10 years.[63] However, this does not necessarily mean that the degree of revascularization achieved with PTCA should be similar to that achieved by surgery, for two major reasons. First, angioplasty is easily repeatable and there is therefore no compelling need to treat all lesions in a single procedure. Secondly, moderate stenoses of 40–60 per cent, often bypassed at surgery, are not usually considered for angioplasty because of the risk of developing a recurrent stenosis more severe than the initial lesion.[64]

Intuitively, complete revascularization makes the most sense: few residual stenoses should mean a better long-term outcome. Several earlier reports in both the general population and in the over-70s have shown, as might be expected, that incomplete revascularization after PTCA was associated with a worse outcome in terms of recurrent anginal symptoms and repeat revascularization procedures compared with complete revascularization (Table 3.3). These studies, however, are all flawed by their design methodologies. The patients analysed were not randomly assigned to a specific treatment group and therefore the observed difference in outcome may be explained by differences in baseline characteristics. In fact two studies have clearly identified substantial differences in baseline characteristics between both groups.[46,50] After adjusting for these variables, no difference was found in the risks of death, myocardial infarction, need for revascularization procedures or presence of angina between the groups.[48,50] This is borne out by our own experience. We have demonstrated in our cohort of the over-70s that after adjustment for other baseline differences the only independent predictor of event-free survival is the extent of disease and not the completeness or otherwise of revascularization.[16] Thus the terms complete and incomplete revascularization do not fully describe the clinical problem and incomplete revascularization does not necessarily imply undertreatment. From a practical clinical viewpoint it seems more appropriate to think in terms of adequate and inadequate revascularization. Adequate revascularization should include dilatation of all significant lesions supplying viable myocardium; this can be achieved by either complete or incomplete revascularization. Inadequate revascularization implies that one or more significant lesions supplying large areas of viable myocardium have not been dilated.

## *Coronary angioplasty versus coronary artery bypass grafting—complementary techniques?*

Given the advantages of angioplasty and the risks of bypass surgery outlined above, the elderly patient with single- or multivessel disease in whom all lesions are suitable for balloon angioplasty or in whom adequate, if incomplete, revascularization is justifiable and feasible should be referred for angioplasty. Bypass surgery may be more appropriate for those patients in whom complete revascularization is necessary or who are high-risk PTCA candidates (e.g. those who have a single remaining vessel or who require angioplasty of a vessel that supplies a remaining normal segment of the left ventricle).

# Suggested management strategies

Based on the evidence provided above, it is possible to define a treatment strategy for the management of the over-70s which we believe is scientifically sound, best for the patient and also best for the population as a whole. The strategy is based on relief of symptoms and with this in mind involves a cascade in which the least invasive procedure compatible with a normal lifestyle is recommended at each stage.

## Unstable angina

There is no universally accepted definition of unstable angina, although the term is used to broadly cover a wide spectrum of clinical syndromes ranging from stable angina to acute myocardial infarction.[65] This, together with the variable underlying anatomy and pathophysiological mechanisms involved, makes it difficult to evaluate the impact of different therapeutic modalities on outcome and to suggest strategies for management. This is particularly true in the over-70s, where few specific data are available on revascularization in this situation. In terms of prognosis and therefore for the overall management of patients we have tended to divide patients into three categories similar to the three categories suggested by Braunwald,[65] and broadly reflecting their prognosis.

### Progressive angina (Braunwald IB)

These are patients with new-onset angina of a progressive nature or with chronic angina who experience increased frequency or severity of angina but no rest pain. This subgroup of patients appears to have a more benign course and may only require pharmacological intervention to treat recurrent ischaemia or to prevent progression to myocardial infarction or cardiac death.[66–68]

### Angina at rest (Braunwald IIB, IIIB)

These are patients with repeated episodes of angina at rest. This subgroup also appears to have a worse prognosis, with a high incidence of myocardial infarction and mortality, which in a younger age group requires more aggressive intervention.[69–71]

### Early post-infarction angina (Braunwald IIC, IIIC)

These are patients with early (within 30 days) post-infarction angina at rest with ST-segment or T-wave changes or with angina pectoris induced by light exercise. They also appear to have a high incidence of recurrent myocardial infarction and mortality, suggesting that they may also benefit from more aggressive interventions.[72–74]

## Proposed management of patients with unstable angina

Randomized studies aimed at establishing the merits of current pharmacological treatment, bypass surgery and coronary angioplasty in the management of patients with the various categories of unstable angina are lacking, both in the younger group and in the over-70s. Until further information becomes available, we would suggest the following practical approach. Patients with progressive angina generally have a benign prognosis. They should therefore be treated with aspirin, nitrates, beta-blockers or calcium antagonists, and reassessed in outpatients. Their subsequent treatment follows the pattern outlined below under stable angina pectoris. Because the prognosis for angina at rest and early post-infarction angina is less benign, their treatment should be more aggressive.

Patients should be hospitalized and receive prompt management with stepwise intensification of pharmacological therapy in an attempt

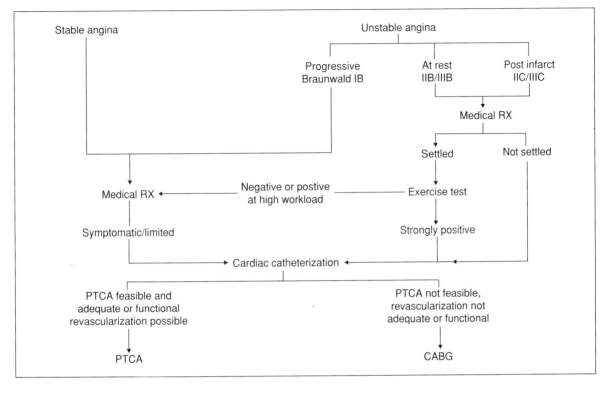

**Figure 3.3**
*Flow chart illustrating suggested management
for patients over 70 years of age with suspected
coronary artery disease.*

to achieve stability (Figure 3.3). This is usually effective in the majority of cases. Patients who settle should be discharged and reviewed in outpatients shortly afterwards. Their subsequent management should follow that of stable patients, with one exception. They should have an exercise test as an outpatient, on therapy, and we believe that if this is strongly positive at an early stage they should be referred for revascularization. If patients do not settle and ischaemic episodes continue despite maximal medical therapy, early angiography is indicated.

The subsequent management is dependent on the underlying coronary anatomy. Coronary angioplasty is indicated if a stenosis, technically suitable for dilatation, is found to be responsible for the unstable state. The decision in favour of coronary angioplasty in patients with single-vessel disease is easy to make. In patients with multivessel disease in which a culprit lesion can be identified, target lesion angioplasty is indicated. In the case of left main stem disease, severe three-vessel disease, unfavourable anatomy for angioplasty or where angioplasty carries a high risk such as in the case of a single remaining vessel supplying viable myocardium, CABG should be considered.

## Stable angina

If the patient has stable angina an accurate history should be taken, focusing on the severity of the symptoms and how restricted the patient is by these. A full clinical examination and baseline investigations then need to be performed to exclude any underlying cause for the angina such as valvular heart disease, as well as any other concomitant disease such as anaemia which may be aggravating the problem.

The patient should be commenced on regular anti-anginal therapy, bearing in mind the altered pharmacodynamics, and then reassessed 2 weeks later. If symptoms persist, the anti-anginal medication should be maximized and if the patient remains limited despite maximal therapy he or she should be referred for cardiac catheterization and revascularization.

The choice between angioplasty and surgery is made by an evaluation of the factors which will determine the immediate success, risk of major complications and long-term outcome of revascularization, namely the coronary anatomy and left ventricular function.

In the case of single-vessel disease, angioplasty is the treatment of choice. In the case of two- and three-vessel disease, angioplasty is the treatment of choice only if adequate functional rather than complete revascularization can be performed.

Bypass surgery is more appropriate for those patients with left main stem disease and severe three-vessel disease with impaired left ventricular function. It is also indicated for those patients in whom complete revascularization is indicated or who are high-risk PTCA candidates (e.g. those who have a single remaining vessel or who require angioplasty of a vessel that supplies a remaining normal segment of left ventricle).

## Conclusions

The increasing number of elderly people in our population and their greater expectation in terms of what cardiology and cardiac surgery can offer is likely to place great strain on our resources over the next few years. As the morbidity and mortality of revascularization techniques increases with age, these procedures should be reserved for patients who were previously fit and active but are now symptomatic despite adequate medical therapy. Age *per se*, however, should not be a bar to revascularization if the patient fits the above criteria, as the older patient may benefit as much from revascularization as the younger patient. Given the high immediate success rate, low incidence of complications and gratifying long-term results, coronary angioplasty is an appropriate initial approach provided that adequate functional revascularization can be attained. If this cannot be attained or the anatomy is unsuitable, coronary artery bypass surgery should be considered.

## If I had...

If I was over 70 and had coronary artery disease I would initially manage myself conservatively by adjusting my lifestyle and maximizing my medical therapy. If, despite these simple changes, I was still symptomatic or restricted in my activities, I would refer myself for further investigation and coronary angiography.

My subsequent decisions regarding revascularization would be based on my coronary anatomy and the state of my left ventricular function. If I had significant single-vessel disease amenable to coronary angioplasty I would like this to be performed. If I had multivessel disease but there was an obvious target lesion responsible for my symptoms, either angiographically or on functional testing for ischaemia, I would again opt for coronary angioplasty to the target lesion. If I had multivessel disease and there was

no obvious culprit lesion I would again opt for multivessel angioplasty, as a staged procedure, if adequate functional revascularization was feasible, but would choose the operator carefully.

If I had left main disease or coronary angioplasty was unable to offer me adequate functional revascularization I would undergo coronary artery bypass grafting, provided I had no other concomitant disease that would greatly increase the risks of the operation. I would choose my surgeon, anaesthetist and perfusionist carefully. If I had concomitant disease as well as severe coronary disease I would seriously reassess my lifestyle and consider continued medical therapy.

# References

1 Satler LF et al, Coronary artery disease in the elderly, *Am J Cardiol* (1989) **63**:245–8.

2 Chaitman BR et al, Angiographic prevalence of high-risk coronary artery disease in patient subsets (CASS), *Circulation* (1981) **64**:360–7.

3 Kashyap M, Cardiovascular disease in the elderly: current considerations, *Am J Cardiol* (1989) **63**:3H–4H.

4 Stason WB, Sanders CA, Smith HC, Cardiovascular care of the elderly: economic considerations, *J Am Coll Cardiol* (1987) **10**:18A–21A.

5 Rogers WB, von Dohlen TW, Frank MJ, Management of coronary heart disease in the elderly, *Clin Cardiol* (1991) **14**:635–42.

6 Greenblatt DJ, Sellers EM, Shader RI, Drug disposition in old age, *N Engl J Med* (1982) **306**:1081–8.

7 Sjoqvist F, Alvan G, Aging and drug disposition–metabolism, *J Chronic Dis* (1983) **36**:31–7.

8 Gruntzig AR, Senning A, Siegenthaler WE, Nonoperative dilatation of coronary artery stenosis: percutaneous transluminal coronary angioplasty, *N Engl J Med* (1979) **301**:61–8.

9 Dorros G, Janke L, Percutaneous transluminal coronary angioplasty in patients over the age of 70 years, *Cath Cardiovasc Diagn* (1986) **12**:223–9.

10 Holt GW et al, Results of percutaneous transluminal coronary angioplasty for unstable angina in patients 70 years of age and older, *Am J Cardiol* (1988) **61**:994–7.

11 Simpfendorfer C et al, Early and long-term results of percutaneous transluminal coronary angioplasty in patients 70 years of age and older with angina pectoris, *Am J Cardiol* (1988) **62**:959–61.

12 Thompson RC et al, Percutaneous transluminal coronary angioplasty in the elderly: early and long-term results, *J Am Coll Cardiol* (1991) **17**:1245–50.

13 Bedotto JB et al, Results of multivessel percutaneous transluminal coronary angioplasty in persons aged 65 years and older, *Am J Cardiol* (1991) **67**:1051–5.

14 Buffet P et al, L'angioplastie transluminale coronaire après 70 ans. Analyse multivariée des paramètres influençant les résultats immédiats et prognostic à long terme, *Arch Mal Coeur* (1992) **85**:287–93.

15 Forman DE et al, PTCA in the elderly: the 'young-old' versus the 'old-old', *J Am Geriatr Soc* (1992) **40**:19–22.

16 de Jaegere P et al, Immediate and long term results of percutaneous coronary angioplasty in patients aged 70 and over, *Br Heart J* (1992) **67**:138–43.

17 Kelsey SF, Miller DP, Holubkov R, and the investigators from the NHLBI PTCA Registry, Results of percutaneous transluminal coronary angioplasty in patients ≥ 65 years of age (from the 1985 to 1986 National Heart, Lung, and Blood Institute's Coronary Angioplasty Registry, *Am J Cardiol* (1990) **66**:1033–8.

18 Kern MJ et al, Percutaneous transluminal coronary angioplasty in octogenarians, *Am J Cardiol* (1988) **61**:457–8.

19 Rich JJ et al, Percutaneous transluminal coronary angioplasty in patients 80 years of age and older, *Am J Cardiol* (1990) **65**:675–6.

20 Jeroudi OM et al, Percutaneous transluminal coronary angioplasty in octogenarians, *Ann Int Med* (1990) **113**:423–8.

21 Rizo-Patron C et al, Percutaneous transluminal coronary angioplasty in octogenarians with unstable coronary syndromes, *Am J Cardiol* (1990) **66**:857–8.

22 Myler RK et al, Coronary angioplasty in octogenarians: comparison to coronary bypass surgery, *Cathet Cardiovasc Diagn* (1991) **23**:3–9.

23 Jackman JD et al, Percutaneous transluminal coronary angioplasty in octogenarians as an effective therapy for angina pectoris, *Am J Cardiol* (1991) **68**:116–19.

24 Detre K et al, One year follow up results of the 1985–86 National Heart, Lung and Blood

Institute's percutaneous transluminal coronary angioplasty registry, *Circulation* (1989) **80**:421–8.

25  Berry BE et al, Coronary artery bypass operations in septuagenarians, *Ann Thorac Surg* (1981) **31**:310–13.

26  Hochberg MS et al, Isolated coronary artery bypass grafting in patients seventy years of age and older: early and late results, *J Thorac Cardiovasc Surg* (1982) **84**:219–23.

27  Faro RS et al, Coronary revascularization in septuagenarians, *J Thorac Cardiovasc Surg* (1983) **86**:616–20.

28  Gersh BJ et al, Coronary arteriography and coronary bypass surgery: morbidity and mortality in patients aged 65 years or older. A report from the Coronary Artery Surgery Study, *Circulation* (1983) **67**:483–91.

29  Elayda MS et al, Coronary revascularisation in the elderly patient, *J Am Coll Cardiol* (1983) **3**:1398–402.

30  Gersh BJ et al, Comparison of coronary artery bypass surgery and medical therapy in patients 65 years of age or older. A nonrandomized study from the Coronary Artery Surgery Study (CASS) registry, *N Engl J Med* (1985) **313**:217–24.

31  Ennabli K, Pelletier LC, Morbidity and mortality of coronary artery surgery after the age of 70 years, *Ann Thorac Surg* (1986) **42**:197–200.

32  Horneffer PJ et al, The effect of age on outcome after coronary bypass surgery, *Circulation* (1987) **76**(suppl V): V6–V12.

33  Acinapura AJ et al, Coronary artery bypass in septuagenarians. Analysis of mortality and morbidity, *Circulation* (1988) **78**:1179–84.

34  Grondin CM et al, Cardiac surgery in septuagenarians: is there a difference in mortality and morbidity? *J Thorac Cardiovasc Surg* (1989) **98**:908–14.

35  Carey JS, Cukingnan RA, Singer LKM, Quality of life after myocardial revascularization, *J Thorac Cardiovasc Surg* (1992) **103**:108–15.

36  Rahimtoola SH, Grunkemeier GL, Starr A, Ten year survival after coronary bypass surgery for angina in patients aged 65 years and older, *Circulation* (1986) **74**:509–17.

37  Saldanha RF et al, Myocardial revascularization in patients over seventy five years, *J Cardiovasc Surg* (1988) **29**:624–8.

38  Rich MW et al, Morbidity and mortality of coronary artery bypass surgery in patients 75 years of age or older, *Ann Thorac Surg* (1988) **46**:638–44.

39  Loop FD et al, Coronary artery bypass graft surgery in the elderly, *Cleve Clin J Med* (1988) **55**:23–34.

40  Horvath KA et al, Favorable results of coronary bypass grafting in patients older than 75 years, *J Thorac Cardiovasc Surg* (1990) **99**:92–6.

41  Montague NT III et al, Morbidity and mortality of coronary bypass grafting in patients 70 years of age and older, *Ann Thorac Surg* (1985) **39**:552–7.

42  Tsai TP et al, Cardiac surgery in the octogenarian, *J Thorac Cardiovasc Surg* (1986) **91**:924–8.

43  Naunheim KS et al, Coronary artery bypass surgery in patients aged 80 years or older, *Am J Cardiol* (1987) **59**:804–7.

44  Edmunds LH Jr et al, Open-heart surgery in octogenarians, *N Engl J Med* (1988) **319**:131–6.

45  Kowalchuk GJ, Siu SC, Lewis SM, Coronary artery disease in the octogenarian: angiographic spectrum and suitability for revascularization, *Am J Cardiol* (1990) **66**:1319–23.

46  Bell MR et al, Percutaneous transluminal angioplasty in patients with multivessel coronary disease: how important is complete revascularization for cardiac event-free survival? *J Am Coll Cardiol* (1990) **16**:553–62.

47  O'Keefe JH et al, Multivessel coronary angioplasty from 1980 to 1989: procedural results and long-term outcome, *J Am Coll Cardiol* (1990) **16**:1097–102.

48  Mabin TA et al, Follow-up clinical results in patients undergoing percutaneous transluminal coronary angioplasty, *Circulation* (1985) **71**:754–60.

49  Vandormael MG et al, Immediate and short-term benefit of multilesion coronary angioplasty: influence of degree of revascularization, *J Am Coll Cardiol* (1985) **6**:983–91.

50  Reeder GS et al, Degree of revascularization in patients with multivessel coronary disease: a report from the National Heart, Lung, and Blood Institute Percutaneous Transluminal

Coronary Angioplasty Registry, *Circulation* (1988) **77**:638–44.

51 Samson M et al, Successful multiple segment coronary angioplasty: effect of completeness of revascularization in single-vessel multilesion and multivessels, *Am Heart J* (1990) **120**:1–12.

52 Holmes DR et al, Co-investigators of the NHLBI-PTCA Registry. Comparison of complications during PTCA from 1977 to 1981 and from 1985 to 1986, *J Am Coll Cardiol* (1988) **12**:1149–55.

53 Bourassa MG et al, Complete revascularization in patients with multivessel coronary disease: an uncommon PTCA outcome, *J Am Coll Cardiol* (1991) **17** (suppl A): 113A (abstr).

54 Thomas ES, Most AS, Williams DO, Objective assessment of coronary angioplasty for multivessel disease: results of exercise testing, *J Am Coll Cardiol* (1988) **11**:217–22.

55 Deligonul U et al, Prognostic value of exercise stress testing after successful coronary angioplasty: importance of the degree of revascularization, *Am Heart J* (1989) **117**:509–14.

56 de Feyter PJ et al, Coronary angioplasty of the unstable angina related vessel in patients with multivessel disease, *Eur Heart J* (1986) **7**:460–7.

57 Vandormael MG et al, Multilesion coronary angioplasty: clinical and angiographic follow-up, *J Am Coll Cardiol* (1987) **10**:246–52.

58 Thomas ES, Most AS, Williams DO, Coronary angioplasty for patients with multivessel coronary artery disease: follow-up clinical status, *Am Heart J* (1988) **115**:8–13.

59 Deligonul U et al, Coronary angioplasty: a therapeutic option for symptomatic patients with two and three vessel coronary disease, *J Am Coll Cardiol* (1988) **11**:1173–9.

60 Jones EL et al, Importance of complete revascularization in performance of the coronary bypass operation, *Am J Cardiol* (1983) **51**:7–12.

61 Cukingnam RA et al, Influence of complete coronary revascularization on relief of angina, *J Thorac Cardiovasc Surg* (1980) **79**:188–93.

62 Tyras DH et al, Long-term results of myocardial revascularization, *Am J Cardiol* (1979) **44**:1290–6.

63 Schaff HV et al, Survival and functional status after coronary artery bypass grafting: results 10 to 12 years after surgery in 500 patients, *Circulation* (1983) **68**(suppl II):II-200–II-204.

64 Ischinger T et al, Should coronary arteries with less than 60% diameter stenosis be treated by angioplasty? *Circulation* (1983) **68**:148–54.

65 Braunwald E, Unstable angina. A classification, *Circulation* (1989) **80**:410–14.

66 Harris PH et al, Survival in medically treated coronary artery disease, *Circulation* (1979) **60**:1259–69.

67 Roberts KB et al, The prognosis for patients with new onset angina who have undergone cardiac catheterization, *Circulation* (1983) **68**:970–8.

68 Mulcahy R, Natural history and prognosis of unstable angina, *Am Heart J* (1985) **109**:753–9.

69 Olson HG et al, The high-risk angina patients, *Circulation* (1981) **64**:674–84.

70 Quyang P et al, Variables predictive of successful medical therapy in patients with unstable angina pectoris: selection by multivariate analysis from clinical, electrocardiographic and angiographic variables, *Circulation* (1984) **70**:376–84.

71 Report of the Holland Interuniversity Nifedipine/Metoprolol Trial (HINT) Research group. Early treatment of unstable angina in the coronary care unit. A randomised, double blind, placebo controlled comparison of recurrent ischaemia in patients treated with nifedipine or metoprolol or both, *Br Heart J* (1987) **56**:400–13.

72 Schuster EH, Bulkley BH, Early postinfarction angina: ischemia at a distance and ischemia in the infarct zone, *N Engl J Med* (1981) **305**:110–15.

73 Fioretti P, Brower RW, Balakumaran K, Early post-infarction angina. Incidence and prognostic relevance, *Eur Heart J* (1986) **7** (suppl c):73–7.

74 Gibson RS et al, The prevalence and clinical significance of residual myocardial ischemia 2 weeks after uncomplicated non Q wave infarction: a prospective natural history study, *Circulation* (1986) **73**:1186–98.

# 4

## The role of PTCA in acute myocardial infarction

*Ever D Grech and David R Ramsdale*

## Introduction

Many studies have demonstrated that, following acute myocardial infarction, early coronary artery recanalization reduces infarction size and improves survival,[1] greatest benefits are seen in patients treated soon after the onset of symptoms.[2]

Percutaneous transluminal coronary angioplasty (PTCA) in acute myocardial infarction may be performed at various time intervals after the initial event, and may be combined with thrombolytic therapy. This chapter reviews data on the wider role of PTCA in acute myocardial infarction with emphasis on primary PTCA, and summarizes current opinion.

## History

In 1980, De Wood et al[3] first reported angiographic evidence of a high incidence of totally occluded or critically stenosed infarction-related arteries in the early hours of acute myocardial infarction. Such findings prompted the use of intracoronary and later intravenous streptokinase therapy. After successful thrombolytic therapy a high-grade residual lesion was frequently observed and led Meyer et al[4] to use PTCA after intracoronary streptokinase during the same sitting. This combination treatment was advocated as a means of avoiding reocclusion and recurrent ischaemia. The rationale for dealing with the flow-limiting potential of the residual plaque following thrombolysis has led to many studies which have examined the need to proceed to PTCA at various times.

The technique of primary therapy in acute infarction, introduced in 1983,[5] avoided the need for thrombolytic therapy and its haemorrhagic complications. Primary PTCA causes mechanical disruption of the occlusive thrombus and the underlying stenosis which results in a rapid restoration of coronary flow. A few centres in the USA perform this technique routinely but for logistical reasons this is uncommon practice in both the USA and the UK.

In the last few years many groups of workers have been examining more closely the value (or otherwise) of PTCA performed at various time intervals after thrombolytic therapy in acute myocardial infarction, as well as the advantages and disadvantages of primary PTCA alone. It is the purpose of this chapter to attempt to clarify the data available so far and we must therefore begin with a clear definition of the terminology in current usage.

## Definitions

An understanding of the terminology of the various forms of PTCA is important in the interpretation of clinical studies.

**Sequential PTCA** is performed after thrombolysis. This category includes the following:

1  *Immediate PTCA* where the patient is taken to the catheter laboratory soon after completion of the thrombolysis with the intention of performing PTCA (Figure 4.1).
2  *Rescue* or *salvage PTCA*, which is performed when thrombolysis has apparently failed to recanalize the infarct-related artery after 60–120 min (Figure 4.2).
3  *Routine* or *deferred PTCA*, which refers to those undergoing PTCA 1–7 days post-thrombolysis.
4  *Elective PTCA*, which refers to those requiring PTCA for treatment of angina or provocable ischaemia more than 1 week post-thrombolysis.

**Primary (or direct) PTCA** is performed without antecedent thrombolytic therapy and was introduced by Hartzler in 1983[5] (Figures 4.3 and 4.4).

## *Immediate PTCA (Figure 4.1)*

The combination of the inevitable procedural delay associated with primary PTCA and the promising results of intravenous thrombolytic therapy led to the anticipation that PTCA immediately *after* thrombolytic therapy (immediate PTCA) would improve the initial advantage of thrombolytic reperfusion. Three major randomized trials (TAMI,[6] ECSG[7] and TIMI-2A[8]) using intravenous tissue plasminogen activator (t-PA) with or without additional

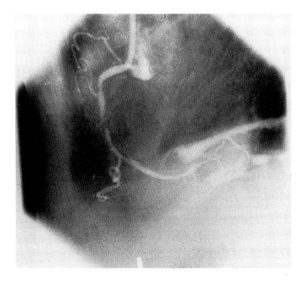 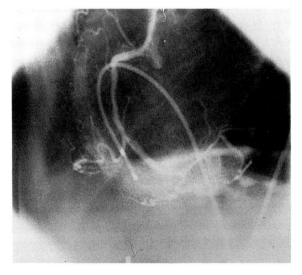

**Figure 4.1**
(Left) Right coronary arteriogram in a 48-year-old man who had received intravenous t-PA 2 h earlier for acute inferior myocardial infarction. The artery is patent but a high-grade stenosis persists.

(Right) The same artery following successful immediate PTCA.

PTCA have been undertaken. The study designs differed significantly.

In the TAMI study, all patients received intravenous t-PA, followed by emergency coronary angiography. Patients were randomized to immediate, or deferred PTCA at 7 days, only if the infarction-related artery was patent with a high-grade residual stenosis suitable for PTCA. In contrast, with the ECSG and the TIMI-2A trials, patients were randomized without prior knowledge of the coronary anatomy. In the ECSG study, immediate angiography and PTCA was compared with angiography before discharge (10–20 days later). In the TIMI-2A trial, 50 per cent of patients were randomized to immediate angiography and PTCA if suitable and 50 per cent to angiography and PTCA, if appropriate, 18–48 h after admission.

Thus the TAMI trial selected patients who had successfully thrombolysed before randomization, whereas the other studies randomly assigned all patients, testing the combined strategy of timing of coronary angiography and angioplasty. Despite these differences, all showed similar results, with little demonstrable improvement in left ventricular function with PTCA. In addition, the immediate PTCA group had a higher mortality and complication rate (more bleeding complications as well as a higher rate of emergency coronary artery bypass graft (CABG) and vessel reocclusion). Overall, these trials support the view that in clinically stable patients following successful pharmacological coronary recanalization nothing is to be gained by immediate PTCA.

## *Rescue/salvage PTCA (Figure 4.2)*

This strategy developed as a consequence of the results of the immediate PTCA trials. A series of seven studies[9–15] have studied the value of PTCA in recanalizing the 25–40 per cent of patients with a persistently occluded artery despite thrombolytic therapy. Although technical success rates were high (71–92 per cent), there is little evidence to support a significant improvement in left ventricular function. Furthermore, reocclusion rates were high (4–29 per cent),[9,11] and mortality rates varied considerably (0–17 per cent).[11,13] A considerably lower mortality rate has been reported in patients undergoing successful rescue PTCA than those in whom PTCA was unsuccessful.[16] A further study[17] showed that patients who had PTCA to the right coronary artery group fared worse in terms of in-hospital mortality, cardiac arrest, hypotension and serious arrhythmias than those undergoing PTCA to the left coronary artery. The mechanism of this discrepancy remains unclear.

In summary, the available data on rescue angioplasty are inadequate. In an editorial review, Ellis et al[18] have focused on the correct role of rescue angioplasty and concluded that randomized trials were needed to replace disparate clinical opinions.

## *Deferred/elective PTCA*

The rationale of the deferred strategy is that the residual coronary artery stenosis after thrombolysis needs to be addressed if recurrent ischaemic events are to be avoided. Initial studies suggested that such a strategy may be beneficial.[6,19] As a result, two large trials, the TIMI-2[20] and SWIFT[21] studies, evaluated the relative benefit of performing prophylactic PTCA within 3 days of infarction or if spontaneous or provocable ischaemia occurred. Both these studies demonstrated that routine early intervention following thrombolysis conferred no benefit and was unnecessary. A further

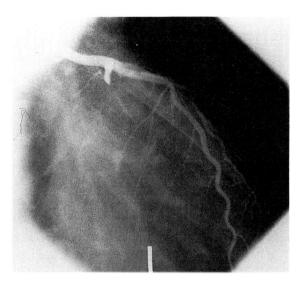 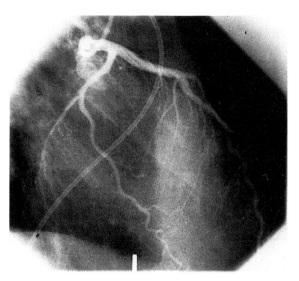

**Figure 4.2**
(Left) A totally occluded left circumflex artery in a 55-year-old man with persistent inferior ST segment elevation and chest pain 2 h after receiving intravenous streptokinase.

(Right) The same artery following successful recanalization by rescue PTCA.

randomized trial by the TOPS study group[22] assessed late PTCA (between 4 and 14 days post-infarction), and again no functional or clinical benefit was evident. At present, one arm of the LIFT (Late Intervention Following Thrombolysis)[23] study is investigating the potential benefit of PTCA at a much later interval of 1–2 months post-infarction.

Subgroup analysis of 1-year follow-up data from the TIMI-2 trial[24] suggested that mortality was lower in patients with a previous history of infarction randomized to PTCA or CABG than in those treated conservatively.

# Primary PTCA
*(Figures 4.3 and 4.4)*

Coronary artery recanalization by primary PTCA using a guidewire and balloon catheter has several advantages over conventional thrombolytic therapy. First, patency rates in the order of 90 per cent are obtained.[25,26] This is significantly higher than the optimal patency rate of 55 per cent with intravenous streptokinase,[27] the commonest thrombolytic agent in use in the UK. Restoration of antegrade coronary bloodflow and normalization of the

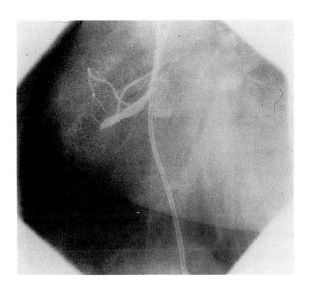 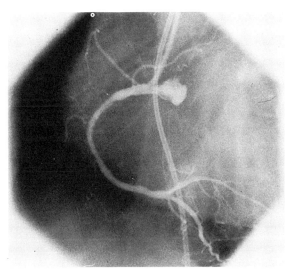

**Figure 4.3**
(Left) A totally occluded right coronary artery in a 64-year-old woman with an acute inferior myocardial infarction.

(Right) The same artery reopened by primary PTCA, 2 h after the onset of chest pain. Note that the residual plaque-related stenosis has been alleviated, resulting in a widely patent artery and brisk antegrade flow.

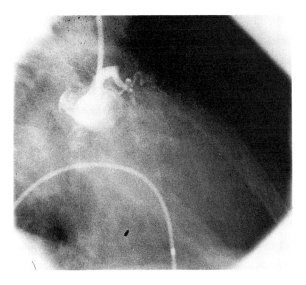 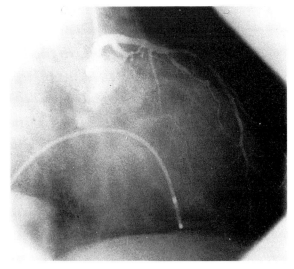

**Figure 4.4**
(Left) Left coronary arteriogram in a 49-year-old woman with a 90-min history of acute anterior myocardial infarction and cardiogenic shock. Both the left anterior descending and left circumflex arteries are occluded.

(Right) Following reopening of the left anterior descending artery by primary PTCA there was a dramatic haemodynamic improvement in left ventricular function. It proved impossible to recanalize the left circumflex artery, which was considered to be chronically occluded.

electrocardiogram is not only more rapid but is also more predictable. Moreover, since systemic fibrinolysis is avoided, the likelihood of bleeding complications as well as intra-plaque and intra-myocardial haemorrhage is reduced.[28]

In their early prospective randomized study of 56 patients, O'Neill et al[29] found that primary PTCA patients were less likely to experience post-infarction angina and to have exercise-induced ischaemia, and were likely to have better regional and global left ventricular function than those receiving intracoronary streptokinase. These observations were attributed to a reduction in peri-infarction ischaemia as a consequence of the alleviation of the residual luminal stenosis by angioplasty. Fung et al[30] reported similar findings. More recently, three larger prospective randomized studies from the Netherlands[31] and the USA[32,33] have compared primary PTCA with intravenous streptokinase or t-PA. PTCA resulted in high patency rates (93–98 per cent), improved left ventricular ejection fractions,[31] fewer bleeding complications and less recurrent myocardial ischaemia and re-infarction than with thrombolysis. Several weeks after infarction, primary PTCA patients were less likely to have a residual coronary stenosis in the infarction-related artery.

Although the importance of a patent infarction-related artery and preservation of left ventricular function after primary PTCA have been confirmed by Brodie et al,[34] who have demonstrated that these determined both short- and long-term survival, data examining these parameters are sparse and conflicting. In their recent prospective randomized study involving 395 patients, Grines et al[32] reported a significantly lower mortality or reinfarction in the primary PTCA than the thrombolytic group during both the in-hospital period (2 and 10.4 per cent respectively) and at 6 months (8.5 and

16.8 per cent respectively). However, in a case-matched study, Martin et al[35] reported similar hospital and 1-year mortality in the two groups.

A number of retrospective studies have been carried out to determine the impact of primary PTCA on myocardial function and to identify subsets of patients who are most likely to benefit.[25,36–38] In a study involving 250 patients, Kahn et al[38] achieved excellent patency rates in excess of 90 per cent, an in-hospital reocclusion rate of less than 10 per cent and an acceptable hospital mortality of 5 per cent. Infarction patients ineligible for thrombolytic therapy, and those with LAD artery occlusions who were at highest risk of cardiogenic shock and death, were particularly likely to benefit from primary PTCA. The most impressive results are seen in patients with single-vessel disease, when a recanalization rate of 99 per cent, an in-hospital death rate of 1 per cent and an urgent CABG rate of <0.5 per cent can be expected.[39]

Primary PTCA has also been shown to be of great value in patients with previous CABG[39] and in the elderly,[41] and can be performed in patients with hypotension and cardiogenic shock. This latter condition, which has an approximate incidence of 10 per cent,[42] is associated with a grave prognosis despite thrombolytic therapy due to the low frequency of recanalization.[43] Primary PTCA has been found to offer a survival advantage in this group of patients[44–46] (Figure 4.4). In our limited experience, however, it would seem to offer little to those with established cardiogenic shock, late (>6 h) after extensive infarction.

In addition to the expense of performing primary PTCA in preference to intravenous streptokinase therapy, there are several other drawbacks. Clearly the procedure can only be performed when cardiac catheterization facilities, staff and experienced operators are available. A 24-hour on-call team and an open, available laboratory are necessary if coronary recanalization by PTCA is to be more rapid than by thrombolysis. Herein lie the major logistical difficulties in the UK. In our centre, where catheter laboratory staff are on call from home, the average time from admission to reopening of the infarction-related artery by PTCA may be in the order of 60 min.

Concern about the potential increased cost of primary PTCA has been examined by two studies[33,47] which have found that although the expense involved in the interventional equipment was considerably greater than with thrombolytic therapy, this was offset by a significantly shorter in-hospital period, fewer readmissions and reduced follow-up costs. However, both these studies, carried out in the USA, used t-PA as the thrombolytic agent. This is much more expensive than streptokinase and therefore in the UK (where streptokinase is the commonest thrombolytic agent in use) this would negate the reduction in overall cost attributed to PTCA.

The risks and complications associated with cardiac catheterization and PTCA are greater than those seen in elective PTCA for chronic angina. Reperfusion arrhythmias are not infrequently observed, although they are usually transient and often do not demand anti-arrhythmic drug therapy. However, a sustained episode of arrhythmia, such as a ventricular tachycardia, may cause profoundly adverse haemodynamic effects.[48] Coronary artery reocclusion can occur in up to 13 per cent, and in-hospital mortality may be as high as 7.2 per cent[49] in unselected groups of patients. Unless cases are carefully selected, many patients who are unsuitable for PTCA may undergo angiography. However, this does not preclude them from receiving thrombolytic therapy as an alternative, and angiography may help to improve their risk stratification and identify appropriate patients who require emergency coronary artery bypass surgery.

Although not contraindicated, patients with previous myocardial infarction(s), a long history of angina, previous CABG and proven multivessel or diffuse coronary disease are often technically unattractive prospects for primary PTCA. However, even here direct PTCA may be shown to have a greater benefit than thrombolytic therapy if undue time delays to treatment can be avoided.

## *Conclusions*

PTCA may be performed at various time intervals after acute infarction, and may be combined with thrombolytic therapy. Although there continue to be unresolved issues about optimal treatment strategies with sequential PTCA, primary PTCA may offer patients an alternative to thrombolytic therapy and may be a superior mode of recanalization.

In an editorial comment in 1990, Meier[50] concluded that primary PTCA had been 'buried alive' and that it was time to 'get the shovel'. However, further large randomized studies must show clear cost and clinical benefits over thrombolytic therapy before a cardiologist would entertain setting up a 24-hour primary PTCA programme in a regional centre. Furthermore, this would require a huge increase in resources, facilities and expertise nationally which, in these financially stringent times, may not be available.

For now, at least, the most widely available therapeutic strategy likely to restore antegrade coronary artery flow following thrombotic occlusion continues to be intravenous thrombolytic therapy. However, where logistics allow and facilities are available, primary PTCA should ideally be preferred for those patients likely to benefit the most. Ideal patients include those who are aged less than 60 years old, present within 4 h of the onset

*Key points.*

- PTCA may be performed at various time intervals after acute infarction, and may be combined with thrombolytic therapy.
- An understanding of the terminology of the various forms of PTCA is important in the interpretation of clinical studies.
- There continue to be unresolved issues about optimal treatment strategies with sequential PTCA.
- However, primary PTCA may offer patients an alternative to thrombolytic therapy and may be a superior mode of recanalization.
- Certain subsets of patients are more likely to benefit from primary PTCA.
- As well as being logistically demanding and requiring experienced operators, primary PTCA is expensive. More evidence of cost and clinical benefits is needed.

of chest pain associated with acute ST-segment elevation, have no previous acute infarction or a long history of angina, and have no contraindication to PTCA. Patients with anterior infarction or contraindication to thrombolytic therapy may be particularly suitable.

## *If I had...*

If I had an acute myocardial infarction—and the facilities and expertise were available for coronary arteriography and primary PTCA—I would wish to undergo primary PTCA to reopen the occluded coronary artery promptly. I also would like to have intracoronary thrombolysis if residual intracoronary thrombus was visible angiographically. I would have intravenous heparin for 48 h, daily oral aspirin and

a beta-blocker long term. The coronary arteriographic findings would also determine whether I should have emergency CABG surgery instead, or deferred PTCA or CABG surgery for prognostic reasons.

If I had an acute myocardial infarction—and the above facilities and expertise were not available or a delay of more than 2 h in receiving primary PTCA was likely—then I would prefer to be admitted directly to a coronary care unit and receive an intravenous thrombolytic agent such as streptokinase or r-TPA. I would also wish to receive oral aspirin without delay and a beta-blocker if I had no evidence of acute heart failure. If my ECG showed no resolution of ST-segment elevation within 90 min, I would wish to be transferred as an emergency to a centre experienced in primary/immediate PTCA for coronary arteriography and rescue PTCA.

If I had an acute myocardial infarction and cardiogenic shock, I would like my family and priest nearby, but my experienced interventional cardiologist nearer still to take me to the catheter laboratory for coronary angiography, whilst supporting me with intravenous inotropes and an intra-aortic balloon pump. If my left anterior descending, left circumflex or dominant right coronary artery could be reopened by direct PTCA, then I would consider this to be ideal. If, however, I had a left main stem stenosis or severe three-vessel coronary disease, I would like emergency CABG surgery with a LIMA to my large left anterior descending artery.

# References

1 Van de Werf F, Arnold AER, Intravenous tissue plasminogen activator and size of infarct, left ventricular function and survival in acute myocardial infarction, *Br. Med J* (1988) **297**:1374–9.

2 ISIS-2 Collaborative Group, Randomised trial of intravenous streptokinase, oral aspirin, both or neither among 17,187 cases of suspected acute myocardial infarction: ISIS-2, *Lancet* (1988) **2**:349–60.

3 De Wood MA et al, Prevalence of total coronary occlusion during the early hours of transmural myocardial infarction, *N Engl J Med* (1980) **303**:897–902.

4 Meyer J et al, Sequential intervention procedures after intracoronary thrombolysis; balloon dilatation, bypass surgery and medical treatment, *Int J Cardiol* (1985) **7**:281–93.

5 Hartzler GO et al, Percutaneous transluminal coronary angioplasty with and without thrombolytic therapy for treatment of acute myocardial infarction, *Am Heart J* (1983) **106**:965–73.

6 Topol EJ et al, A randomized trial of immediate versus delayed elective angioplasty after intravenous tissue plasminogen activator in acute myocardial infarction, *N Engl J Med* (1987) **317**:581–8.

7 Simoons ML et al, Thrombolysis with tissue plasminogen activator in acute myocardial infarction: no additional benefit from immediate percutaneous coronary angioplasty, *Lancet* (1988) **1**:197–203.

8 TIMI Research Group, Immediate vs delayed catheterization and angioplasty following thrombolytic therapy for acute myocardial infarction, *JAMA* (1988) **260**:2849–58.

9 Califf RM et al, Characteristics and outcome of patients in whom reperfusion with intravenous tissue-type plasminogen activator fails; results of the Thrombolysis and Angioplasty in Acute Myocardial Infarction (TAMI) I trial, *Circulation* (1988) **77**:1090–9.

10 Fung AY et al, Value of percutaneous transluminal coronary angioplasty after unsuccessful intravenous streptokinase therapy in acute myocardial infarction, *Am J Cardiol* (1986) **58**:686–91.

11 Topol EJ et al, Coronary arterial thrombolysis with combined infusion of recombinant tissue-type plasminogen activator and urokinase in patients with acute myocardial infarction, *Circulation* (1988) **77**:1100–7.

12 Baim DS et al, PTCA 'salvage' for thrombolytic failures—implications from the TIMI II-A, *Circulation* (1988) **78** (suppl II): 112 (abstr.).

13 O'Connor CM et al, Rescue coronary angioplasty after failure of intravenous streptokinase in acute myocardial infarction: in-hospital and long-term outcomes, *J Invas Cardiol* (1989) **1**:85–95.

14 Grines CL et al, Efficacy, safety and cost effectiveness of a new thrombolytic regimen for acute myocardial infarction using half dose t-PA with full dose streptokinase, *Circulation* (1988) **78-II**:304 (abstr.).

15 Holmes DR et al, 'Rescue' percutaneous transluminal coronary angioplasty after failed thrombolytic therapy—4 year follow-up, *J Am Coll Cardiol* (1989) **13**:193A (abstr.).

16 Ellis SG et al, Implications for patient triage from survival and left ventricular functional recovery analyses in 500 patients treated with coronary angioplasty for acute myocardial infarction, *J Am Coll Cardiol* (1989) **13**:1251–9.

17 Gacioch GM, Topol EJ, Sudden, paradoxical clinical deterioration during angioplasty of the right coronary artery in acute myocardial infarction, *J Am Coll Cardiol* (1989) **14**:1202–9.

18 Ellis SG et al, Present status of rescue coronary angioplasty: current polarization of opinion and randomized trials, *J Am Coll Cardiol* (1992) **19**:681–6.

19 Guerci AD, Gerstenblith G, Brinkler JA, A randomized trial of intravenous tissue plasminogen activator for acute myocardial infarction with subsequent randomization to elective coronary angioplasty, *N Engl J Med* (1987) **317**:1613–8.

20  TIMI Study Group, Comparison of invasive and conservative strategies after treatment with intravenous tissue plasminogen activator in acute myocardial infarction, *N Engl J Med* (1989) **320**:618–27.

21  SWIFT trial of delayed elective intervention v conservative treatment after thrombolysis with anistreplase in acute myocardial infarction. SWIFT (Should We Intervene Following Thrombolysis?) Trial Study Group, *Br Med J* (1991) **302**:555–60.

22  Ellis SG et al, Randomized trial of late elective angioplasty versus conservative management for patients with residual stenoses after thrombolytic therapy of acute myocardial infarction, *Circulation* (1992) **86**:1400–6.

23  Roberts RH, Glenn SP, Balcon R, Should we catheterize patients who are asymptomatic following thrombolysis? Data from the LIFT study registry, *Br Heart J* (1993) **69**:P44 (abstr.).

24  Williams DO et al, One-year results of the Thrombolysis in Myocardial Infarction investigation (TIMI) Phase II Trial, *Circulation* (1992) **85**:533–42.

25  Hartzler GO, Rutherford BD, McConahay DR, Percutaneous transluminal coronary angioplasty: application for acute myocardial infarction, *Am J Cardiol* (1984) **53**:117C–21C.

26  Kahn JK et al, Results of primary angioplasty for acute myocardial infarction in patients with multivessel coronary artery disease, *J Am Coll Cardiol* (1990) **16**:1089–96.

27  Verstraete M, Bernard R, Bury M, Randomised trial of intravenous recombinant tissue-type plasminogen activator versus intravenous streptokinase in acute myocardial infarction, *Lancet* (1985) **1**:842–7.

28  Colavita PG et al, The spectrum of pathology associated with percutaneous transluminal coronary angioplasty during acute myocardial infarction, *J Am Coll Cardiol* (1986) **8**:855–60.

29  O'Neill W et al, A prospective randomized clinical trial of intracoronary streptokinase versus coronary angioplasty for acute myocardial infarction, *N Engl J Med* (1986) **314**:812–8.

30  Fung AY et al, Prevention of subsequent exercise-induced periinfarct ischemia by emergency coronary angioplasty in acute myocardial infarction: comparison with intracoronary streptokinase, *J Am Coll Cardiol* (1986) **8**:496–503.

31  Zijlstra F et al, A comparison of immediate coronary angioplasty with intravenous streptokinase in acute myocardial infarction, *N Engl J Med* (1993) **328**:680–4.

32  Grines CL et al, A comparison of immediate angioplasty with thrombolytic therapy for acute myocardial infarction, *N Engl J Med* (1993) **328**:673–9.

33  Gibbons RJ et al, Immediate angioplasty compared with the administration of a thrombolytic agent followed by conservative treatment for myocardial infarction, *N Engl J Med* (1993) **328**:685–91.

34  Brodie BR et al, Importance of a patent infarct-related artery for hospital and late survival after direct coronary angioplasty for acute myocardial infarction, *Am J Cardiol* (1992) **69**:1113–9.

35  Martin JS et al, Immediate and one year outcome following direct angioplasty versus thrombolytic therapy for acute myocardial infarction, *J Am Coll Cardiol* (1993) **21**:331A (abstr.).

36  Vacek JL et al, Direct angioplasty versus initial thrombolytic therapy for acute myocardial infarction: long-term follow-up and changes in practice pattern, *Am Heart J* (1992) **124**:1141–8.

37  O'Keefe JH Jr et al, Myocardial salvage with direct coronary angioplasty for acute infarction, *Am Heart J* (1992) **123**:1–6.

38  Kahn JK et al, Catheterization laboratory events and hospital outcome with direct angioplasty for acute myocardial infarction, *Circulation* (1990) **82**:1910–5.

39  Stone GW et al, Direct coronary angioplasty in acute myocardial infarction: outcome in patients with single vessel disease, *J Am Coll Cardiol* (1990) **15**:534–43.

40  Kahn JK et al, Usefulness of angioplasty during acute myocardial infarction in patients with prior coronary artery bypass grafting, *Am J Cardiol* (1990) **65**:698–702.

41  Lee TC et al, Emergency percutaneous transluminal coronary angioplasty for acute myocardial infarction in patients 70 years of age and older, *Am J Cardiol* (1990) **66**:663–7.

42  Kuhn LA, The treatment of cardiogenic shock. Part I. The nature of cardiogenic shock, *Am Heart J* (1967) **74**:578–81.

43  Rentrop P et al, Selective intracoronary thrombolysis in acute myocardial infarction and unstable angina pectoris, *Circulation* (1981) **63**:307–16.

44  Lee L et al, Multicenter registry of angioplasty therapy of cardiogenic shock: initial and long-term survival, *J Am Coll Cardiol* (1991) **17**:599–603.

45  Karalis DG, Parris TM, Coronary angioplasty in cardiogenic shock: a bridge to coronary artery surgery, *J Invas Cardiol* (1989) **1**:231–7.

46  Hibbard MD et al, Percutaneous transluminal coronary angioplasty in patients with cardio-genic shock, *J Am Coll Cardiol* (1992) **19**:639–46.

47  Eckleberg T et al, Cost comparison of primary angioplasty versus thrombolytic therapy for acute myocardial infarction, *J Am Coll Cardiol* (1993) **21**:347A (abstr.).

48  Grech ED, Ramsdale DR, Reperfusion arrhythmia, *Lancet* (1993) **341**:1667–8.

49  Topol EJ, Mechanical interventions for acute myocardial infarction. In: Topol EJ, ed. *Textbook of interventional cardiology* (W.B. Saunders Company: Philadelphia 1990) 269–99.

50  Meier B, Balloon angioplasty for acute myocardial infarction. Was it buried alive? *Circulation* (1990) **82**:2243–5.

# 5

## Cardiac surgery for complications of myocardial infarction

*David Anderson*

Following acute occlusion of a major coronary artery the myocardium undergoes necrosis with subsequent softening and weakening of the muscle. This predisposes to structural failure which may express itself in one of four different ways. The most common is for the affected area to gradually heal and form a scar, which will be akinetic, or, in more severe instances, stretch in response to ventricular systole and therefore move paradoxically. As a result there may be no apparent clinical change but a proportion of patients will experience a greater or lesser degree of left ventricular failure, depending on the severity of the infarction, the size of the aneurysm, and the degree of paradoxical motion. In some cases scar formation may not have time to develop before the weakened myocardium ruptures under the stresses of left ventricular systole.

## Rupture

Three forms of rupture may occur. The most common is left ventricular free wall rupture, which is found as the cause of death in up to 10 per cent of patients dying post-myocardial infarction.[1,2] Next most common is rupture of the interventricular septum, responsible for approximately 2 per cent of deaths post-myocardial infarction. The least common, as a

post-mortem finding, is rupture of the head of a papillary muscle, producing mitral incompetence. The incidence of rupture may be increasing since the introduction of coronary care units.[1] Alternatively, it is the detection rate which has improved.

## Predisposing factors to rupture

Precisely why there is rupture of the myocardium following an infarction in some cases and not others is not clearly understood. A number of factors have been implicated and principal among them is post-infarction hypertension.[3–5] It is an observation often associated with rupture of the ventricular septum that the infarction was otherwise silent up until the time that the septum ruptured, precipitating clinical presentation.[6] The fact that the infarction had been otherwise silent meant that the patient continued normal activities instead of having been rested, as would have been the case were they admitted to hospital and the diagnosis confirmed. This would involve rises in blood pressure, which logically must increase the stresses on the walls of the left ventricle. In keeping with the theory of hypertension leading to increased stress on the ventricular wall, it has been shown that hearts which suffered rupture post-infarction had a tendency for thinning and expansion of the infarction zone as compared to unruptured infarctions.[7] It has also been suggested that the incidence of post-infarction rupture is higher among patients in mental institutions. These patients often do not announce their symptoms or, even when diagnosed, follow advice and rest. The incidence of rupture is also higher in older women than one would expect given the number of infarctions which occur in the female population.[5,8,9] Patients who have longstanding hypertension and consequent ventricular hypertrophy seem less likely to suffer rupture than those with normal-thickness ventricles.[5] This again is logical, since even though the ventricle is necrotic, the greater thickness is probably better able to withstand the stresses of ventricular systole. Finally, patients who have had previous infarctions are less likely to suffer rupture following a subsequent infarction than those experiencing their first infarction.[1,5,6,8] There may be two explanations for this. First, the fibrosis and scarring following the initial infarction may provide some strength in the ventricular wall. Second, the occurrence of the second infarction may weaken the pumping power of the ventricle to such an extent that it is incapable of generating the pressures necessary to cause rupture. The relatively recent introduction of thrombolytic therapy, which is intended to salvage myocardium which might otherwise infarct, seems to have led to an increase in the incidence of rupture.[10] This difference is not observed in another large study.[1] The explanation for the effect of thrombolytic therapy may be that the rupture tending to occur would probably lead to thrombus formation within the tearing myocardium. If that thrombus was then lysed by thrombolytic therapy, this could well increase the chances of external rupture. Whatever its cause, rupture of the myocardium is a treatable condition if the diagnosis can be quickly established and appropriate surgical

intervention carried out. In a series of 68 patients operated on for acute ventricular septal defect, none had significant symptoms of cardiac failure prior to the occurrence of a rupture.[6] This suggests, therefore, that the ventricle is quite capable of supporting the circulation adequately, and that clinical deterioration following rupture is due to haemodynamic changes rather than a further deterioration in left ventricular function. Of course, undiagnosed or untreated ruptures will have a knock-on effect on cardiac function, which may subsequently become chronically depressed, greatly increasing the risks of surgical intervention. It is obvious, therefore, that if these patients are in otherwise good cardiovascular condition prior to the occurrence of rupture, the earlier diagnosis is made and treatment instituted, the better chance there is of a successful outcome.

## Left ventricular free wall rupture

This is by far the most common form of cardiac rupture, accounting for approximately 10 per cent of fatal myocardial infarctions. The first report seems to have been by William Harvey in 1647.[11] Clinically, the diagnosis is often not made since the occurrence of rupture of the free wall results in immediate cardiac tamponade and a rapid demise of the patient. Pathologically, there seem to be two forms of rupture. The first, occurring within 24 h of the onset of pain, develops as a tear at the margin of viable and infarcted myocardium. The cause may be a combination of two forces, the first the pressure generated during cardiac systole and second the shearing forces resulting from contractile tissue operating next to an akinetic area.[12] The second form occurs a few days later, classically between the fourth and seventh day following the onset of pain. Here the infarction is expanded, bulging outwards as an aneurysm with thinning of the wall. There is obvious evidence of infarction, both macroscopically and microscopically. The point of rupture is usually at the apex of the bulge and the mechanism is probably quite simply an inability of the necrotic myocardium to contain the pressure of ventricular systole.[7] The pathway through the myocardium may not be direct, instead following planes between the layers of myocardium.[13] In some instances, therefore, rupture is not catastrophic and rather takes the form of a gradual leakage through the myocardium and a slow build-up of tamponade. In these cases clinical diagnosis and appropriate treatment may be possible.

The common clinical presentation is of a patient making an otherwise satisfactory recovery following an acute myocardial infarction, who suddenly develops severe central chest pain similar to that experienced when the infarction occurred. The majority of cases occur within the first 10 days following infarction. Clinically, electro-mechanical dissociation is highly suggestive of rupture, and may be supported by other signs of acute tamponade. The most definitive diagnostic investigation is echocardiography, which should show the presence of fluid around the heart. Treatment should be immediate pericardiocentesis, introducing a large-bore cannula from a subxyphoid approach and at the same time making preparations for transfer to the operating theatre for immediate thoracotomy and relief of the tamponade.

Despite its high frequency there are only a few reported instances of successful surgical management.[14-16] This is not surprising in view of the nature of the defect, since unless surgery can be immediately instituted the patient is unlikely to survive.

Where facilities for cardiopulmonary bypass exist, these should be employed. However, time must not be lost since the principal objective is firstly to relieve the tamponade. A left anterolateral thoracotomy through the fifth intercostal space will provide excellent access to the whole of the left ventricle, allowing easy release of the pericardial tamponade and initially digital control of the bleeding point. If a facility for cardiopulmonary bypass exists on site, then it is probably best to continue with digital control until a median sternotomy can be performed and bypass set up between the right atrium and ascending aorta. Otherwise an attempt will have to be made to suture the defect, which is extremely difficult given that the tissues are necrotic and the beating heart makes accurate placement of a suture difficult. In the absence of cardiopulmonary bypass a monofilament suture mounted on a large (20 mm or greater) round-bodied needle should be selected. Strips of Teflon felt should be used to buttress the suture, incorporating a large bite of myocardium. If at all possible, the suture should be located in healthy myocardium, but if the infarction is large this may be technically impossible to achieve.

On full cardiopulmonary bypass, the technique of repair depends on the location and site of the defect. Small defects through relatively small infarction can be sutured directly by the technique described already. This is especially true if the defect is located anteriorly. For larger defects or those located on the inferior or lateral wall, the heart will have to be elevated, requiring crossclamping of the aorta. The patient should be whole-body cooled to 28–31°C and preferably the heart protected by infusion of cold cardioplegia after crossclamping the aorta. The infarcted tissue can then be resected wholly and the defect repaired using a patch of prosthetic material secured with buttressed sutures placed through the whole thickness of the myocardium (Figure 5.1). If there is known coincidental significant stenoses of other coronary arteries, then they

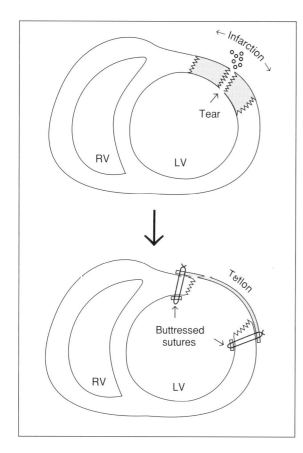

**Figure 5.1**
*The choice of material for patching is not important, but if Teflon is used it would be advisable to pre-clot. The same applies to Dacron, unless it is of low porosity. The most important feature is that all sutures placed in the myocardium should, where possible, be located in healthy tissues and be securely buttressed on pledgets of Teflon or similar material.*

cardiopulmonary bypass, a left atrial pressure line should be inserted to monitor left ventricular filling pressures postoperatively, and the chest closed after meticulous haemostasis with at least two drainage tubes in position. Postoperatively the patient's management should be as for any other major cardiac operation.

## False aneurysm

Occasionally, rupture may be contained either by layers of myocardium or because the pericardial space is obliterated. As such it is likely to go undiagnosed and present later as a false aneurysm. Unlike with a true aneurysm of the ventricle, the risk of subsequent rupture is high, so surgical repair should be performed.[17] The difficulty relates to the timing of surgery if the false aneurysm is detected within a few days or weeks of the infarction. From a technical point of view, repair is much easier after the infarction has healed and a fibrotic scar developed which facilitates suturing. Using two-dimensional echo, a false aneurysm can be observed and its progress carefully monitored. If it remains stable through the acute and healing phase of the infarction, then it is reasonable to wait until scar formation has occurred in 6–8 weeks. During that time the patient should be treated for any hypertension and restricted to light exercise. Repair should be carried out through a median sternotomy on cardiopulmonary bypass with resection of the infarcted tissue and replacement with prosthetic material secured on buttressed sutures. Any coincidental coronary artery stenoses should be bypassed at the same time.

Any echocardiographic evidence of expansion of a false aneurysm during the acute or healing stage should constitute an indication for immediate surgical repair. Also, recurrent chest pain should arouse suspicion of extension

should be bypassed, but if coronary angiography has not been performed previously, then it is wise not to extend the duration of the operation or to blindly perform coronary bypass surgery. Having weaned the patient from of the false aneurysm and not be attributed solely to myocardial ischaemia.

## Ventricular septal rupture

Rupture of the interventricular septum is the second most common form of rupture complicating acute myocardial infarction. It accounts for approximately 2 per cent of deaths following myocardial infarction[2,18] and is more common in older women than one might expect, given the incidence of myocardial infarction in females as a whole.[5,8,9] There does not appear to be any relationship with the extent of coincidental coronary artery disease,[5] but it is more likely to occur where there has been no previous myocardial infarction[1] and most especially where little or no coronary collateral circulation exists to the infarction territory.[19] Often it is the mode of presentation of the infarction which has otherwise been silent.[5] As with free wall rupture, our experience is that these patients were all in good haemodynamic condition prior to the occurrence of the rupture and not suffering any significant ventricular failure. In the literature the site of the septal rupture is variously described as anterior, posterior, inferior, apical or various permutations of these. This has led to confusion in analysing these patients from a prognostic point of view. It is better to define the ventricular septal defect (VSD) as either anterior or inferior, based on the precipitating infarction, which is almost always the result of occlusion of the left anterior descending in the case of anterior VSDs, or occlusion of a dominant right coronary artery in the case of inferior VSDs.

Where the posterior descending artery is a terminal branch of the circumflex, occlusion there will result in an inferior infarction and any consequent VSD should be analysed as inferior.

In most published series the rate of anterior to inferior appears to be approximately 2 : 1.[16,19] Whether this is a true reflection of the actual incidence or instead reflects the proportion of patients who present is unclear. What is very clear is that the prognosis for an anterior VSD is much better than that for an inferior VSD,[6,20,21] and therefore the explanation for the lower number of inferior VSD presentations may be that many of them die before diagnosis can be confirmed.

Rupture of the interventricular septum follows a similar timescale to other ruptures, with the peak around the third or fourth day, but can occur anywhere from 1 to 10 days following the acute infarction. Clinically, a sudden severe chest pain may accompany rupture with rapid development of cardiogenic shock, shortness of breath and signs of pulmonary congestion. Central venous pressure is elevated and oliguria or anuria may quickly ensue, depending on the severity of cardiogenic shock. In a small number of patients, the rupture is well tolerated and they remain relatively stable. On examination the most pertinent sign is the presence of a systolic murmur. The differential diagnosis would therefore be between a ventricular septal rupture and papillary muscle rupture, causing mitral incompetence. Nowadays the most simple investigation is echocardiography, which should easily distinguish one from the other.[22] The addition of colourflow mapping with pulsed and continuous wave Doppler enhances diagnostic accuracy to a point where cardiac catheterization is not required. In addition, the technique is especially useful in postoperative management where a recurrent VSD is suspected.[23] If that facility is not available, then passage of a Swan-Ganz catheter with serial oximetry should identify a step-up in oxygen saturations at right ventricular level, confirming the presence of a left-to-right shunt.

From those measurements a calculation of the shunt can be made, but that seems to have little bearing on the prognosis.[21] Instead, the pulmonary artery pressure recorded seems to be a more significant indicator of prognosis—the higher it is the better.[6] The absence of cardiogenic shock, not surprisingly, is a favourable factor.[6] A clear difference in prognosis is seen between anterior and inferior VSDs, with approximately a 75 per cent survival rate in anterior and anywhere from 20 to 30 per cent survival in inferior defects.[6] A plausible explanation for this difference is that occlusion of the right coronary artery may well cause infarction of the right ventricle, which is rarely the case with occlusion of the LAD. Right ventricular function could therefore be significantly impaired and the sudden imposition of a volume and pressure load would precipitate acute right ventricular failure.[6,24] This would secondarily lead to a low pulmonary artery pressure, whereas a right ventricle that was functionally less impaired might be able to handle the volume and pressure overload and generate a higher pulmonary artery pressure.

Treatment should initially be resuscitative with appropriate inotropic therapy to augment cardiac function. The use of the intra-aortic balloon pump is reasonable since afterload reduction theoretically should increase forward flow from the left ventricle and hence reduce the tendency for left-to-right shunting. Balloon pumping, however, has been shown to be only a temporary measure allowing preparations to be made for surgical repair.[18,25] Theoretically, pharmacological agents which reduce afterload would be helpful for the same reasons, but many of these patients have such low blood pressures that they simply will not tolerate such therapy and instead are very dependent on vasoconstrictors to maintain adequate perfusion pressure. Low-dose dopamine should be instituted in order to try and maintain renal function. Mechanical ventilation should be used where blood gas analysis shows deteriorating respiratory function. Gentle positive end expiratory pressure (PEEP) may also help to reduce the development of pulmonary oedema.

Without treatment, or even with maximum medical therapy, the prognosis for acute ventricular septal defect is very poor. Experience prior to surgical intervention showed that 25 per cent died within 24 h, 70 per cent within 1 week and 90 per cent within 2 months.[26] About 5 per cent might be expected to survive a year. Whether this prognosis would be improved with currently available medical therapy has never been tested, but it seems unlikely that a really major improvement could be achieved.

Controversy surrounds the need for coronary angiography and our view is that this should only be performed if the patient is relatively stable and can tolerate the procedure. If cardiogenic shock is established, then coronary angiography is not advisable and instead arrangements should be made for immediate surgical correction of the rupture.

The first successful treatment for a ventricular septal rupture published in 1957[27] was performed on a patient 6 weeks following the incident, by which time the infarction was well healed and surgical repair was relatively easy from a technical point of view. After that, several reports appeared in the literature of successful surgery and an opinion developed that every effort should be made to delay surgery until 6 weeks following the occurrence of the ventricular septal defect, as surgery before that was almost certain to fail, owing to the necrotic tissues and the unstable nature of the patient. While this observation of good surgical results at a late stage was quite correct, it overlooked the fact there was a very high mortality in the waiting period. It had already been shown that in the natural history of acute ventricular septal rupture 75 per cent of patients were dead within 1 week and 90 per cent within 1 month. Therefore, at 6 weeks the patients going to surgery were self-selected survivors who might be expected to do well anyway. We would now recommend a policy of immediate surgery once the diagnosis has been confirmed. It is rare to encounter a patient who tolerates the lesion so well that surgery can be delayed for several weeks.

However, if that situation does exist, then it is not unreasonable to allow the infarction to heal, but the patient should be monitored closely and any signs of developing cardiogenic shock or deteriorating renal function should constitute an indication for surgical repair.

It is not necessary to delay surgery in order to insert an intra-aortic balloon pump. If an operating theatre is available then the patient should be transferred immediately and if necessary the intra-aortic balloon pump introduced at the end of the operation in order to successfully wean the patient from cardiopulmonary bypass. The operation should be performed through a median sternotomy using cardiopulmonary bypass.

Depending on the preference of the surgeon, cardioplegia can be used or instead the operation can be performed on a perfused fibrillating heart. This is especially true of anterior defects, but for inferior defects surgical access may be difficult on the perfused fibrillating heart and instead it may be easier to use cardioplegia with moderate whole-body cooling. The geometry of the two defects is quite different and should be borne in mind when undertaking repair.

### Repair of the anterior defect *(Figure 5.2)*

These are technically the easier to repair. An incision is made into the left ventricle, through the infarction, parallel to the left anterior

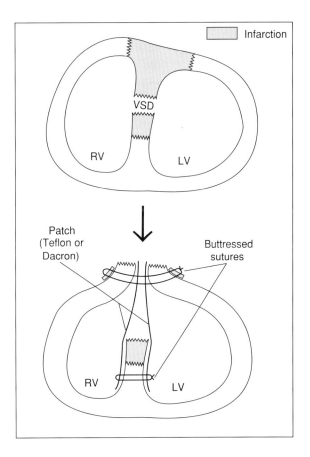

**Figure 5.2**
*The diagram shows the two-patch technique as described in the text. It is also possible to use a single patch but buttressing material must be employed for sutures placed on the ventricular septum, which should themselves be located in healthy myocardium if at all possible.*

descending coronary artery. The VSD should then be easily identified. Any loose necrotic septal tissue should be removed and margins of the defect clearly defined. Often there is not a perfect punched-out hole but rather a series of slit-like tears. In such a situation exact definition of the extent of the defect may be difficult. It is therefore useful to open the right ventricle in parallel to the left anterior descending artery. The defect can then be closed using two patches, one on each side of the ventricular septum, and secured using interrupted mattress sutures. Patches are brought out through the ventriculotomies, which are then closed using further buttressing material on the external surface of the ventricular wall.

### Repair of the inferior defect *(Figure 5.3)*

The important difference between anterior and inferior defects, apart from the involvement of the right ventricle, is the geometry of the ventricular septum in relation to the inferior or diaphragmatic wall of the heart. The ventricular septum is more perpendicular to the inferior wall than it is to the anterior wall of the left ventricle. This should be borne in mind when repairing the defect. The heart will be elevated and again an incision made into the left ventricle, through the infarction, parallel to the posterior descending coronary artery. A similar incision can be made on the right ventricular aspect and the defect then closed in a similar manner to that described for the anterior VSD, using one or two patches secured with interrupted mattress sutures. The patches are brought out through the ventriculotomies, but instead of simply securing the free walls of the ventricle to the patch a second patch should be employed to repair the infarction zone. These patches are placed on the outside of the free wall and secured using mattress sutures buttressed on Teflon from within the ventricle. The patch is then secured to the VSD patches to effect a final closure of the ventriculotomy. The importance of this technique is that it preserves the natural geometry of the ventricular septum in relation to the inferior wall of the

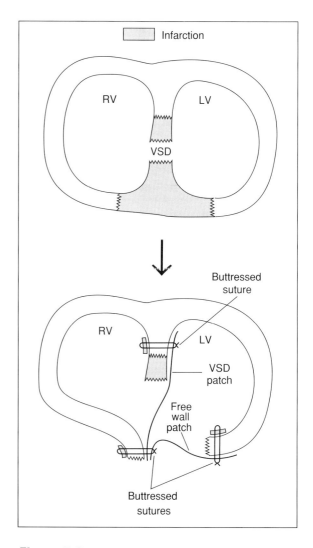

### Figure 5.3
*The technique shown here describes the single patch, but two patches can be used instead of simple buttressing material as shown here. As with other repairs, it is crucial to buttress all sutures placed in the myocardium and to locate them in healthy tissues where possible.*

left ventricle. If the ventricular wall is directly applied to the patch, the distortion will place stresses upon the wall and, owing to the infarcted nature of the tissue, it is highly likely that the free wall will tear under the stress of ventricular systole.

Postoperatively, the intra-aortic balloon pump may be required to wean the patient from cardiopulmonary bypass. Inotropic agents should be used as appropriate and positive pressure ventilation maintained until there is cardiovascular stability and satisfactory respiratory function. In extreme cases a ventricular assist device may be required to wean from bypass. Recovery should be otherwise managed as for any patient undergoing open heart surgery. In the long term the results of repair for anterior defects seem to be very good, with patients recovering a satisfactory quality of life and with a good prognosis.[6,28] However, for inferior defects the experience is not so good. The operative mortality is very high and of those patients who survived a 30-day period many subsequently died within the next several months.[6] There is therefore considerable room for improvement in the management of acute ventricular septal rupture to optimize survival.

The developing field of interventional cardiology offers some intriguing possibilities for alternative management of acute ventricular septal rupture. A report describes the introduction of a balloon into the main pulmonary artery[25,29] which on inflation reduced the left-to-right shunt, improved the systemic blood pressure and restored urine flow. The balloon was maintained inflated for a period of time during which the patient improved and was then successfully operated on. This is analogous to banding of the pulmonary artery used in the management of congenital VSDs. Another report[30] describes the introduction of an occlusion device across the ventricular septum, through the rupture, which again abolished the left-to-right shunt, allowed an improvement in systemic cardiac output and facilitated safe repair of the defect at a later stage. These are interesting and intriguing

reports and warrant further consideration, as the current results, particularly for inferior defects, are so disappointing that an alternative strategy should be sought.

## Mitral incompetence

The mitral valve is very much a three-dimensional structure, both in its anatomy and functional performance. Ventricular systole causes closure of the valve, which depends on the two leaflets opposing and forming a secure seal. This is facilitated by the functional integrity of those two leaflets so that they move freely. In addition, the so-called mitral annulus contracts with ventricular systole as a further contribution to secure apposition of the leaflets. Finally, the subvalvular tension apparatus of the fibrous chords suspended from the papillary muscles ensures that the valve leaflets do not prolapse. This complex function can easily be disrupted, resulting in varying degrees of valve incompetence. Firstly, myocardial infarction may compromise the contractility of the ventricle and allow an increase in the diastolic volume, with stretching of the mitral annulus leading to incompetence. This is known as functional mitral incompetence and can often be treated successfully by afterload reduction or inotropic therapy to improve contractility and reduce the end-diastolic dimensions of the left ventricle.

Infarction of a papillary muscle may result in inability of that muscle to contract and therefore that part of the valve may tend to prolapse again, leading to incompetence. At the extreme end is a situation where the infarcted papillary muscles actually rupture under the stress of ventricular systole, which leads to gross incompetence and is a very serious condition.

Clinically, mitral incompetence, after myocardial infarction, may present variably.

On the one hand the patient may be asymptomatic and only on careful auscultation may a murmur be heard. The murmur may be intermittent, depending on left ventricular function. At the other extreme, usually associated with papillary muscle rupture, there may be instant pulmonary oedema with circulatory collapse. Treatment depends entirely on the clinical status of the patient, from a situation where no specific treatment is required, to one where full-scale resuscitative measures are needed. Mild to moderate degrees of mitral insufficiency are well tolerated and probably best managed with medical therapy. Papillary muscle rupture, however, is usually a serious event, with up to 70 per cent mortality within 24 h.[31] Fortunately, it is the least common form of structural failure of the myocardium.[2]

Either papillary muscle may rupture but most commonly (80 per cent) it is the posteromedial which is involved. The explanation may be that this muscle derives its blood supply solely from the posterior descending coronary artery, while the anterolateral papillary muscle may have a dual supply, either from the obtuse marginal branches of the circumflex coronary or from the diagonal branches of the left anterior descending. Not surprisingly, infarction always involves the subendocardium, but in about half of the cases extends to full thickness.

This is unlike the case in free wall or septal rupture, where infarction is always transmural. In addition, the area of infarction need not be large and indeed can be confined solely to the papillary muscle. In some instances, however, papillary muscle rupture may coexist with a free wall rupture[17] or ventricular septal defect.[32,33]

### Treatment of papillary muscle rupture

Most patients who suffer this complication of myocardial infarction were stable prior to the occurrence of rupture. The exact precipitating factor is unknown but it is logical to implicate hypertension in the same way that it is implicated in other forms of myocardial rupture. Either of the two papillary muscles may rupture, and this may involve the whole papillary muscle or one of the heads. The result is immediate severe mitral incompetence with rapidly developing pulmonary oedema and circulatory collapse. The patient who had previously been stable will have a tachycardia, be dyspnoeic, cold and clammy and show all features of cardiogenic shock. Oliguria or anuria is a frequent finding. Examination of the chest will reveal a systolic murmur at the apex and there will be coarse crackles throughout the lungfields consistent with pulmonary oedema. The chest X-ray will confirm bilateral pulmonary oedema. Secondary right ventricular failure with elevated pulmonary artery pressure will lead to elevated jugular venous pressure. The differential diagnosis is from rupture of the interventricular septum and this difference can easily be defined either by serial oximetry using a Swan–Ganz catheter or less invasively by two-dimensional echocardiography. An important clinical difference is that patients with acute VSDs can tolerate lying flat while those with acute mitral incompetence cannot. Initial treatment would depend on the patient's clinical condition, but positive pressure ventilation may be required. Theoretically it would be beneficial to employ afterload reduction in the form of vasodilator therapy, but since these patients often have critically low blood pressure, such treatment may be impossible and rather they may require vasoconstrictors such as adrenaline. Low-dose dopamine should be used to try and maintain renal function. The intra-aortic balloon pump is a useful tool to improve systemic cardiac output. The only real solution to the problem is to restore competence to the mitral valve and this will require surgical intervention, which should be arranged as a matter of urgency. Depending on the patient's clinical condition, it may be possible to carry out coronary angiography prior to surgery, but in severely compromised patients this should not be undertaken as it may cause further haemodynamic deterioration. However, if possible, coronary angiography should be carried out and significant stenoses bypassed at the time of mitral valve surgery.

Surgery for acute mitral valve incompetence is difficult owing to the small size of the left atrium and the poor haemodynamic condition of the patient prior to operation. The operation should be performed through a median sternotomy with full cardiopulmonary bypass and venous cannulae in each of the two cavae. Cardioplegia should be used with moderate whole-body cooling. If coronary arteries require bypassing this should be performed and it is not unreasonable to use the internal mammary artery, but if the patient is very unstable it may not be safe to delay the operation while the mammary artery is harvested.

The mitral valve can be approached in a variety of ways, but the most common is through a vertical incision in the interatrial groove. If necessary, after placing snares around the caval cannulae the right atrium can be opened, which will give better access to the mitral valve by incising the interatrial septum. Conservative operations on the mitral valve have been reported and theoretically offer an advantage over prosthetic replacement.[34,35] However, it would be inadvisable to prolong the operation unnecessarily in an attempt to achieve repair of the valve, which may in any event suffer early failure. The type of prosthetic replacement is not critical, but if a biological prosthesis is selected then great care must be taken as the struts of the prosthesis projecting into the ventricular cavity could easily perforate the infarcted zone on the ventricular wall. In replacing the valve it is only necessary to excise the anterior leaflet and the infarcted ruptured papillary muscle. The posterior leaflet and its suspensory apparatus can be preserved but if a mechanical prosthesis is used great care must be taken to ensure that none of the subvalvular apparatus will interfere with the action of the valve leaflet.

Having successfully replaced the valve, it may be difficult to wean the patient from cardiopulmonary bypass. In order to facilitate this, the left atrial pressure should be measured by a cannula placed directly in the atrium. A pulmonary artery pressure catheter is also of considerable help. The intra-aortic balloon pump should be used if there is any difficulty and appropriate inotropic therapy. A prolonged period of support bypass may be necessary, even to the point of using a left ventricular assist device. Postoperative management should be the same as for any other patient undergoing mitral valve replacement with or without coronary bypass surgery.

*Results*

Few centres have reported a large experience of surgical treatment for acute mitral insufficiency. Furthermore, analysis of results is complicated by the fact that there is a variety of pathology included, ranging from acute rupture of the whole papillary muscle to situations where there is no rupture but rather severe papillary muscle dysfunction causing the incompetence.[36] Nevertheless, it is apparent that these patients, whether they have complete rupture of the papillary muscle or severe dysfunction, constitute a high-risk group where surgical treatment is carried out because of cardiogenic shock.[36,37] Early operative mortality varies but is reported to be as high as 50 per cent. However, where patients survive the early operative period to leave hospital, the long-term results appear to be satisfactory.[37]

The problem nevertheless remains that, as with other forms of rupture, these patients were often in good haemodynamic condition and in some cases their infarction was silent. There is little that can be done to diagnose the silent infarction, especially as it generally occurs outside a hospital environment. However, where infarction has occurred, and the patient is stable, making an otherwise uncomplicated recovery, greater awareness is needed of the possibility of myocardial rupture in just such a situation. The current results of surgical treatment of acute papillary muscle dysfunction or rupture leave considerable room for improvement. Loisance et al[37] suggest that an alternative strategy may be the use of more aggressive circulatory support, such as left ventricular assist devices, before surgical intervention. Theoretically this is an attractive proposition but is as yet unproven and the complication rate from applying such a device may well counterbalance any clinical benefit that might accrue from improved operating conditions.

## What if I had acute myocardial rupture?

Given the very poor prognosis for any one of the three forms of rupture, my immediate reaction is that I wish it had been prevented. Ultimately, prevention lies in preventing the infarction in the first instance and I do not propose to analyse how that may be achieved. Presuming, however, that an infarction had occurred, early application of fibrinolytic therapy must surely be sensible to try to prevent at least a transmural infarction. That should significantly reduce if not abolish altogether the likelihood of free wall or ventricular septal rupture, providing that thrombolysis can occur before the whole thickness of the myocardium is no longer salvageable.

Rest, both from physical exertion and emotional stress, must still form an important part of recovery following an established infarction. This, I hope, would reduce rises in blood pressure which might cause rupture of the infarcted myocardium until such time as it had stabilized and scar formation had begun. To this end, beta-blockade therapy would be appropriate and also serve to lessen the chance of arrhythmias.

If these simple measures fail and rupture nevertheless occurs, I would have to hope that I was in a centre where a cardiac surgical facility existed together with astute, clinically aware clinicians who would immediately recognize what had happened. With left ventricular free wall rupture there is no alternative but rapid surgical decompression and repair. For acute ventricular septal rupture, unless I were fortunate enough to sustain the event without major haemodynamic deterioration, I would be willing to allow the technique of Grant or Hachida[23,25] to be tried, but only to maintain or recover stability before transfer to surgical correction. For acute mitral insufficiency, the intra-aortic balloon pump seems to be the most efficacious method of achieving haemodynamic stability or even improvement. Again, it should not be used on a prolonged basis and after 12–24 h or sooner if no improvement had occurred, I would go forward for surgery to replace the mitral valve rather than to attempt repair.

The thought of all these surgical options and interventions brings me round again to the old adage that 'prevention is better than cure' and to that end we must surely strive more diligently.

# References

1    Reddy SG, Roberts WC, Frequency of rupture of the left ventricular free wall or ventricular septum among necropsy cases of fatal acute myocardial infarction since introduction of coronary care units, *Am J Cardiol* (1989) **63**:906–11.

2    Davies MJ, Woolf N, Robertson WP, Pathology of acute myocardial infarction with particular reference to occlusive coronary thrombi, *Br Heart J* (1976) **38**:659–64.

3    Edmonson HA, Hoxie HJ, Hypertension and cardiac rupture, *Am Heart J* (1942) **24**:719–33.

4    ISIS-1 (First International Study of Infarct Survival) Collaborative Group, Randomised trial of intravenous Atenolol among 16,027 cases of suspected acute myocardial infarction: ISIS-1, *Lancet* (1986) **2**:57–65.

5    Naeim F, de la Maza LM, Robins SL, Cardiac rupture during myocardial infarction, a review of 44 cases, *Circulation* (1972) **45**:1231–9.

6    Anderson DR et al, Post-infarction ventricular septal defect: the importance of site of infarction and cardiogenic shock on outcome, *Eur J Cardiothorac Surg* (1989) **3**:554–7.

7    Schuster EH, Bulkley BH, Expansion of transmural myocardial infarction: a pathophysiologic factor in cardiac rupture, *Circulation* (1979) **60**:1532–8.

8    Spiekerman RE et al, The spectrum of coronary heart disease in a community of 30,000, a clinico-pathologic study, *Circulation* (1962) **25**:57–65.

9    Dellborg M et al, Rupture of the myocardium—occurrence and risk factor, *Br Heart J* (1985) **54**:11–16.

10   ISIS-2 (Second International Study of Infarct Survival), Collaborative Group, Randomised trial of intravenous streptokinase, oral aspirin, both, or neither among 17,187 cases of suspected acute myocardial infarction: ISIS-2, *Lancet* (1988) **2**:349–60.

11   Harvey W, *Complete works* (Willis R, translated) (London: Sydenham Society 1847) 127.

12   Becker AE, Vanmantgem JP, Cardiac tamponade—a study of 50 hearts, *Eur J Cardiol* (1975) **3**:349–58.

13   Bates RJ et al, Cardiac rupture—challenge in diagnosis and management, *Am J Cardiol* (1977) **40**:429–37.

14   Cobbs BW, Hatcher CR, Robinson PH, Cardiac rupture: three operations with 2 long-term survivals, *JAMA* (1973) **223**:532–5.

15   Nunez L et al, Diagnosis and treatment of subacute free wall ventricular rupture after infarction, *Ann Thorac Surg* (1983) **35**:525–9.

16   Pappas PJ et al, Ventricular free wall rupture after myocardial infarction. Treatment and outcome, *Chest* (1991) **99**:892–5.

17   Voldaver Z, Coe J, Edwards JE, True and false left ventricular aneurysms: propensity for the latter to rupture, *Circulation* (1975) **51**:567.

18   Buckley MJ et al, Surgical management of ventricular defects and mitral regurgitation complicating acute myocardial infarction, *Ann Thorac Surg* (1973) **16**:598–609

19   Skehan JD et al, Patterns of coronary artery disease in post infarction ventricular septal rupture, *Br Heart J* (1989) **62**:268–72.

20   Loisance DY et al, Ventricular septal defect after acute myocardial infarction, *J Thorac Cardiovasc Surg* (1980) **80**:61–7.

21   Moore CA et al, Post infarction ventricular septal rupture: the importance of site of infarct and right ventricular function in determining survival, *Circulation* (1986) **74**:45–55.

22   Panidis IP et al, Acquired ventricular septal defect after myocardial infarction: detection by combined two-dimensional and doppler echocardiography, *Am Heart J* (1986) **111**:427.

23   Smyllie J et al, Diagnosis of ventricular septal rupture after myocardial infarction: value of colourflow mapping, *Br Heart J* (1989) **62**:260–7.

24   Fananpazir L et al, Right ventricular dysfunction and surgical outcome in post-infarction ventricular septal defect, *Eur Heart J* (1983) **4**:155–67.

25  Gold HK et al, Intra-aortic balloon pumping for ventricular septal defect or mitral regurgitation complicating acute myocardial infarction, *Circulation* (1973) **47**:1191.

26  Sanders RJ, Kern WH, Blout SG, Perforation of the intraventricular septum complicating myocardial infarction: a report of 8 cases, one with cardiac catheterisation, *Am Heart J* (1956) **51**:736.

27  Cooley DA et al, Surgical repair of ruptured interventricular septum following acute myocardial infarction, *Surgery* (1957) **41**:930–7.

28  Jones MT et al, Surgical repair of acquired ventricular septal defect. Determinants of early and late outcome, *J Thorac Cardiovasc Surg* (1987) **93**:680–6.

29  Grant P, Patel P, Singh SP, Balloon catheter used in the treatment of a ventricular septal rupture following a myocardial infarction, *New Engl J Med* (1986) **314**:60–1.

30  Hachida M et al, Percutaneous transaortic closure of post-infarctional ventricular septal rupture, *Ann Thorac Surg* (1991) **51**:655–7.

31  Wei JY, Hutchins GM, Bulkley BH, Papillary muscle rupture and fatal acute myocardial infarction, *Ann Intern Med* (1979) **90**:149–53.

32  Nishimura RA et al, Papillary muscle rupture complicating acute myocardial infarction: analysis of 17 patients, *Am J Cardiol* (1983) **51**:373–7.

33  Radford MJ et al, Survival following mitral valve replacement for mitral regurgitation due to coronary artery disease, *Circulation* (1979) **60**(suppl. 1): I-39–47.

34  Rankin JS et al, A clinical comparison of mitral valve repair versus valve replacement in ischaemic mitral regurgitation, *J Thorac Cardiovasc Surg* (1988) **95**:165–77.

35  Gula G, Yacoub MH, Surgical correction of complete rupture of the anterior papillary muscle, *Ann Thorac Surg* (1981) **32**:88–91.

36  Tepe MA, Edmunds LH, Operation for acute post-infarction mitral insufficiency and cardiogenic shock, *J Thorac Cardiovasc Surg* (1985) **89**:525–30.

37  Loisance DY et al, Are there indications for reconstructive surgery and severe mitral regurgitation after acute myocardial infarction? *Eur J Cardio-Thorac Surg* (1990) **4**:394–7.

# 6

# Asymptomatic left ventricular dysfunction

*Graham Jackson*

## *Introduction*

Chronic heart failure (CHF) due to systolic dysfunction is a common problem, increasing progressively with age and rising in incidence dramatically in those aged over 75 years[1] (Figure 6.1). It is a condition with a particularly poor prognosis and high recurrent hospitalization rate. Mortality data before the angiotensin converting enzyme inhibitors

(ACE) became available revealed only a 25 per cent chance of surviving 3 years after referral to hospital for treatment.

Clinical trials documented improved survival with the addition of enalapril[2] or hydralazine and isosorbide dinitrate[3,4] to digoxin and diuretics in severe and moderate heart failure. Impressive presentation of the data in terms of risk reduction tends, however, to hide the fact that, even on ACE therapy, mortality at 2 years

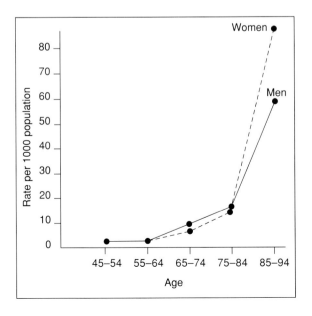

**Figure 6.1**
*Incidence of heart failure. (From Kannel WB, Belanger AJ, Am Heart J (1991) **721:925.**)*
*By the year 2001 there will be 22 per cent of people aged over 75 years, and a massive 69 per cent increase in those aged over 85 years. The potential benefits of successful therapy for this condition can be easily seen.*

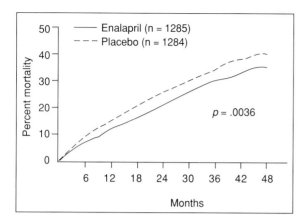

**Figure 6.2**
*SOLVD Treatment Study. Enalapril significantly reduced mortality compared to placebo but there still remains a 35 per cent death rate at 2 years. (From SOLVD Investigators,* N Engl J Med *(1991)* **535:**209–302.)

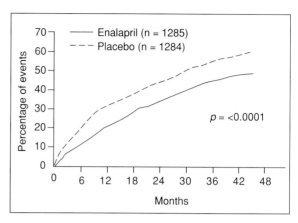

**Figure 6.3**
*SOLVD Treatment Study. Death or hospitalization for heart failure identifying a significant benefit from enalapril at 2 years (p < 0.0001) but there remains a high morbidity and mortality. (From SOLVD Investigators,* N Engl J Med *(1991)* **325:**293–302.)

was 35.2 per cent in the SOLVD treatment trial (moderate failure) (Figure 6.2). Combining death or hospitalizations for heart failure at 2 years, the risk reduction from enalapril versus placebo was 26 per cent (*p* < 0.0001) but the actual figures of 57.3 per cent for placebo and 47.7 per cent for enalapril should not invite complacency and most emphatically reinforce the poor prognosis and increased morbidity from CHF even when patients are receiving ACE therapy (Figure 6.3).

It would be wrong to underestimate the benefits of ACE inhibitors in the treatment of heart failure. It has been calculated from the SOLVD trial that ACE inhibitor therapy given to 1000 CHF patients for 12 months would save 17 premature deaths and 67 hospitalizations for CHF. The ACE strategy is undoubtedly a major advance in the therapy of symptomatic heart failure. To progress *further*, however, a switch in emphasis is necessary, with the focus of attention being the *prevention* of heart failure, with studies of therapy in patients with asymptomatic left ventricular dysfunction. Before discussing these trials we need to step back and look at the rationale.

# *Pathophysiology of left ventricular dysfunction post-myocardial infarction*

Prevention trials have focused on post-infarction patients, as they represent the leading cause of heart failure, certainly up to age 75 years. They also represent a ready and large pool of patients who can be screened for left ventricular dysfunction, e.g. by echocardiography, either to enter studies or subsequently to benefit from them.

Dzau and Braunwald[5] summarized the pathophysiological chain of events, as illustrated in Figure 6.4. This emphasized the importance of reducing the extent of infarction rather than purely attending to the prevention and treatment of malignant arrhythmias, which had been the focus of attention in the 1970s and early 1980s. Hammermeister et al[6] showed in 1979 that in patients with coronary artery disease there was a highly significant correlation between end systolic volume and cardiac death after 2 years and White et al[7] identified a similar correlation post-infarction, leading to the speculation that therapy aimed at reducing infarction size and preventing left ventricular dilatation (remodelling) might be of significant patient benefit.

The concept of remodelling[8] of the left ventricle revolves around left ventricular dilatation and hypertrophy post-infarction as a means of maintaining stroke volume becoming counterproductive. As compensatory mechanisms fail, performance declines, dilatation progresses and performance deteriorates further. McKay and colleagues[8] proposed a model to explain the development of remodelling which in turn identifies potential sources of intervention (Figure 6.5).

Following myocardial damage there is initially sympathetic stimulation and after 2–3

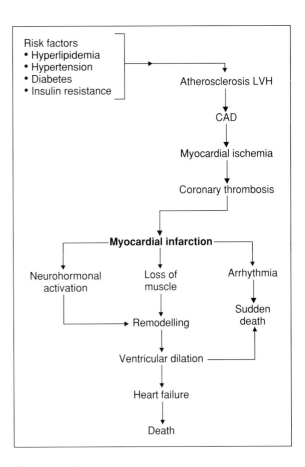

**Figure 6.4**
*Chain of events leading to cardiovascular mortality. (Adapted from Dzau V, Braunwald E, Am Heart J (1991)* **121:**1244–636.)

days activation of the renin–angiotensin system. As can be seen from Figure 6.6, the neurohormonal response to reduced left ventricular function may establish the so-called 'vicious circle' of heart failure with further reduction in left ventricular function and increasing left ventricular size. It can be seen

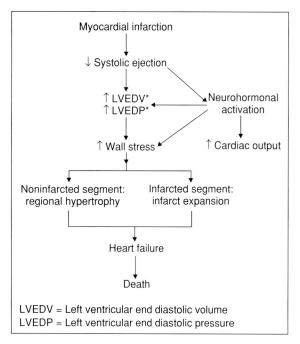

**Figure 6.5**
*Mechanism of left ventricular remodelling.
Intervention at (a) and/or (b) may prevent heart
failure developing. (Adapted from McKay RG et
al, Circulation (1986) **74**:693–702.)*

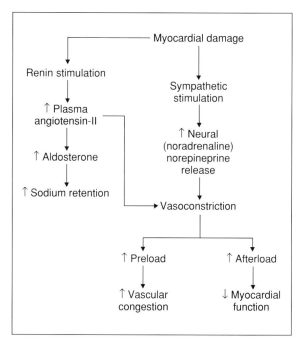

**Figure 6.6**
*Neurohormonal activation following myocardial
damage identifies sites for intervention. Adapted
from Cohn JN, ed. Drug Treatment of Heart
Failure (Advanced Therapeutics Communications
Int. (1988) 50.)*

that if excesses of sympathetic stimulation
and/or renin–angiotensin activation can be
ameliorated, it may be possible to reduce the
neurohormonal effects on LVEDV and wall
stress (Figure 6.5) and therefore prevent the
progression of left ventricular function to heart
failure and premature death.

We need therefore to look at evidence for
benefit from beta-blockade and ACE inhibition
if the concept of remodelling and interruption
of neurohormonal activation is valid with
regard to mortality reduction and cessation of
left ventricular failure progression.

# Beta-blockade

Beta-blockers are to some extent 'old hat' and
their benefits are often overlooked as the newer
and 'sexier' drugs are developed and evaluated.
In my last three lectures on managing myocardial
infarction (MI), with a pooled audience of
300 junior and senior doctors, not one gave
intravenous beta-blockade as a routine post-
infarction treatment. This may be a good
example of the perversity of clinical trials—to
enter them the patient may have to forego
benefits already achieved. This is a slight

digression but a practical one, for it relates to the discrepancies between establishing benefit from theory and then translating the benefit into both short-term and long-term usage.

There is no doubt that beta-blockers improve survival post-infarction whether given intravenously[9,10] or orally.[11-13] Intravenously (Figure 6.7), the benefit reflects a reduction in cardiac rupture and ventricular fibrillation. In addition to thrombolysis,[14] metoprolol IV also decreased myocardial ischaemia and re-infarction if given within 2 h of initiation of thrombolytic therapy.

Orally, in the β-Blocker Heart Attack Trial,[13] after just over 2 years the mortality in the propranolol group was 7.2 per cent compared to 9.8 per cent with placebo, a reduction of 26 per cent ($p < 0.005$). In the metoprolol trial[12]

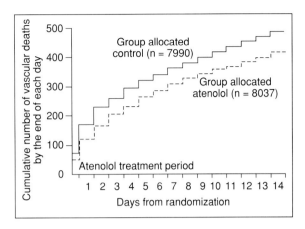

**Figure 6.7**
*Intravenous beta-blocker therapy post-infarction—intravenous and oral atenolol reduced cardiovascular mortality by 15 per cent. (From ISIS-1 (First International Study of Infarct Survival) Collaborative Group, Lancet (1986) 2:57–65.)*

| | Intravenous | Oral |
|---|---|---|
| Metoprolol | 5 mg over 2 min, three doses[a] | 50 mg every 6 h for 2 days; then 100 mg twice daily[b] |
| Propranolol | 0.033 mg/kg over 2 min, three doses* | 20–80 mg every 6 h[b] |
| Atenolol | 5 mg over 5 min, two doses[a] | 50 mg every 12 h for 2 days; then 50 or 100 mg as a single daily dose[b] |
| Esmolol | 500 µg/kg over 1 min; then 50–250 µg/kg/min infusion (effects are rapidly titratable; each upward titration should be preceded by repeat bolus of 500 µg/kg over 1 min) | – |

[a]5 min of observation between boluses
[b]Oral dosing should begin 15 min after final intravenous bolus

**Table 6.1**
*Beta-blocker regimes for acute myocardial infarction.*

the 2-year placebo mortality was 17.2 per cent compared with 13.2 per cent on metoprolol, a reduction of 23 per cent ($p < 0.043$). The beta-blockers reduce infarction size, residual ischaemia, arrhythmias and re-infarction.

Providing there are no contraindications to intravenous beta-blockade, Table 6.1 summarizes the regimes to be considered. If unsure of suitability, the short-acting agent esmolol can be used as a test dose, as the drug effects are completed in 15–30 min and any adverse effects will be short-lived.

## ACE inhibitors

There are three major studies of ACE inhibitors in asymptomatic left ventricular dysfunction. Smaller-pilot studies had shown that captopril attenuated left ventricular dilatation in patients with anterior infarctions when compared to placebo,[15] and similarly, when compared to frusemide and placebo, attenuated left ventricular dilatation in patients with q-wave MI who had symptomatic left ventricular dysfunction.[16]

### SAVE[17]

The survival and ventricular enlargement trial (SAVE) rationale encompassed the assumption that attenuation of ventricular remodelling, i.e. prevention of significant dilatation, following an infarction would improve survival and clinical outcome. Patients were enrolled 3–16 (median 11) days post-MI and followed up for 2–5 (average 3.5) years. Ejection fraction was ≤40 per cent and 1116 were randomized to placebo and 1115 to captopril. The target captopril dose was 50 mg tds, which was achieved in 79 per cent. Captopril significantly reduced cardiovascular mortality (21 per cent, $p = 0.014$) (Figure 6.8), hospitalization for heart failure (22 per cent, $p = 0.019$) (Figure 6.9) and

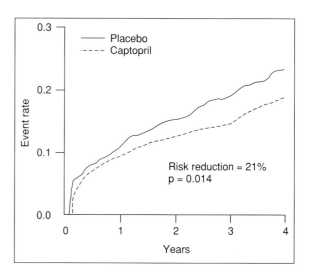

**Figure 6.8**
*Cardiovascular mortality—SAVE. (Adapted from Pfeffer MA et al,* N Engl J Med *(1992).)*

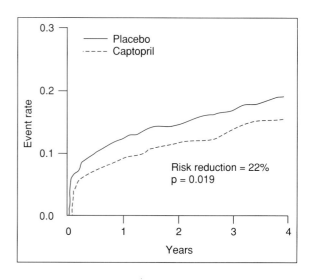

**Figure 6.9**
*Hospitalization for heart failure—SAVE. (Adapted from Pfeffer MA et al,* N Engl J Med *(1992).)*

recurrent MI (25 per cent, $p = 0.015$). Adverse effects were low, with discontinuation of therapy for cough (2.4 per cent captopril, 0.8 per cent placebo, $p = 0.003$) being the only significant variable.

SAVE focused almost certainly on the optimum time post-infarction for the initiation of ACE inhibitors and the implications for post-MI care are extremely important. Translated into clinical practice, an echocardiogram or nuclear LV assessment should be performed on all asymptomatic patients post-MI. If the ejection fraction (EF) is ≤40 per cent and there is no residual ischaemia justifying specific intervention, captopril should be initiated. Importantly, the benefits occurred during long-term follow-up, throwing some doubt on the validity or relevance of short-term trials. The benefits were independent of and in addition to beta-blockade and thrombolysis.

## SOLVD—prevention[18]

In the Studies of Left Ventricular Dysfunction (SOLVD) prevention trial, enalapril or placebo was given to patients with chronic left ventricular dysfunction who were asymptomatic. Eighty per cent had sustained a previous infarction but not within the previous 30 days (median delay 1 year). The study is therefore quite different from SAVE, looking at a much later stage of left ventricular dysfunction when benefits might expect to be less, i.e. remodelling has already occurred. Therefore it may or may not be the case that enalapril can be used with equal certainty of benefit as captopril in the early stage of MI convalescence, as it has not been fully evaluated in this environment. Patient follow-up was 3.3 years and survival benefit was a non-significant 8 per cent from enalapril. However, the drug significantly prevented the development of heart failure (37 per cent), but we do not know

whether this was a symptomatic benefit or a benefit due to the slowing of disease progression. We therefore do not have the mandate we would like to use enalapril or other ACE inhibitors at this later stage of left ventricular dysfunction in the absence of symptoms, as it may simply be effective when symptoms develop and we know that already.

This is a great pity because it clouds a logical story and counsels us against widespread screening for asymptomatic left ventricular dysfunction other than 3–16 days post-MI. We may, however, draw comfort from the consistent benefit symptomatically and the trend prognostically.

## CONSENSUS II[19]

The Co-operative New Scandinavian Enalapril Survival Study II[19] concerned enalapril given within 24 h of an acute MI. Therapy began intravenously and then switched to oral enalapril for a relatively short 6 months of follow-up. Enalapril was administered immediately, i.e. at the time of sympathetic stimulation and not renin–angiotensin activation. No survival benefit occurred and the trial was halted prematurely. A possible explanation for a failure to benefit may stem from early hypotension (<90 mm Hg systolic 12 per cent enalapril, 3 per cent placebo $p < 0.001$), increasing infarction size at a time of sympathetic stimulation, with a critically adverse effect on the supply–demand equation.

It appears that the time window for ACE post-MI is going to be extremely important and an early intravenous approach is not to be recommended (compare with beta-blockers). The premature cessation of this trial because of concerns over an adverse trend towards enalapril prevents us from making comparisons with the longer term studies SAVE and SOLVD. All we have learnt is that an early intravenous plus oral strategy is not advantageous at 6 months. We will never know if the benefit lost initially would have been regained at, say, 2–3 years of oral therapy, which is a great pity.

## Summary

Of the three large ACE trials, only SAVE adds to our therapy post-MI, although SOLVD prevention supports the symptomatic benefits already established for ACE inhibitors. SAVE's important benefits were additive to beta-blockade, allowing us to develop from our knowledge of beta-blockade, both intravenous and oral. Similarly, SAVE's benefits were in addition to thrombolysis. Where, therefore, have these studies taken us?

The theory we started with looks to be relevant to clinical practice in that responding to the post-infarction neurohormonal changes *at the right time* improves prognosis and reduces heart failure hospitalizations. We should use ACE inhibition (captopril) in patients with left ventricular systolic dysfunction who are recovering from a myocardial infarction, and beta-blockade should be continued. We should take note of the target doses used (captopril 50 mg tds in SAVE and enalapril 20 mg daily in SOLVD) and establish these as *our* targets. The tendency to dabble with lower doses may be emotionally comfortable but it is not scientifically sound.

We cannot extend these observations to other classes of vasodilators without further study.

We do not have a mandate to initiate widespread screening for asymptomatic left ventricular dysfunction other than 3–16 days post-infarction. However, as the incidence of heart failure rises sharply at age 75 years, a screening and intervention trial in the 70–75 year olds might be of major clinical importance.

## If I had ...

If I had a myocardial infarction I would want to receive thrombolysis and intravenous beta-blockade. The latter would need to be cautious as I have a slight tendency to bronchospasm—I would like a trial of esmolol. I would assume that as I am under 50 years of age a routine interval coronary angiogram would be performed and I would take aspirin and atenolol orally until then.

I would be disappointed if my echocardiogram on the third or fourth day showed a reduced EF as I would know my prognosis was not as good as anticipated and thrombolysis was unlikely to have been successful. I would commence captopril, hoping to avoid the coughing side-effect, which can be very limiting. I would still push for an angiogram to rule out operable residual coronary artery disease which might affect my prognosis.

Based on my coronary anatomy and quality of left ventricular function I would make important lifestyle changes relating to workload and leisure time in the sure knowledge that I should have done this much earlier.

I believe that dilatation of my left ventricle (remodelling) could be contained, my heart failure delayed and my life expectancy improved by captopril combined with beta-blockade. What I do not know is if my lifestyle could be remodelled to help prevent it happening again.

# References

1   Kannel WB, Belanger BAJ, Epidemiology of heart failure, *Am Heart J* (1991) **121**:951–7.

2   The SOLVD Investigators, Effects of enalapril on survival in patients with reduced left ventricular ejection fractions and congestive heart failure, *N Engl J Med* (1991) **325**:293–302.

3   Cohn JN et al, Effect of vasodilator therapy on mortality in chronic congestive heart failure: results of a Veterans Administration Co-operative Study, *N Engl J Med* (1986) **314**:1547–52.

4   Cohn JN et al, A comparison of enalapril with hydralazine—isosorbide dinitrate in the treatment of chronic congestive heart failure, *N Engl J Med* (1991) **325**:303–10.

5   Dzau V, Braunwald E, Resolved and unresolved issues in the presentation and treatment of coronary artery disease: a workshop consensus statement, *Am Heart J* (1991) **121**:1244–63.

6   Hammermeister KE, DeRouen TA, Dodge HT, Variables predictive of survival in patients with coronary disease: selection by univariate and multivariate analyses from the clinical, electrocardiographic, exercise, arteriographic and quantitative angiographic evaluations, *Circulation* (1979) **59**:421–30.

7   White HD et al, Left ventricular end-systolic volume as the major determinant of survival after recovery from myocardial infarction, *Circulation* (1987) **76**:44–51.

8   McKay RG et al, Left ventricular remodelling after myocardial infarction: a corollary to infarct expansion, *Circulation* (1986) **74**:693–702.

9   ISIS-1 (First International Study of Infarct Survival) Collaborative Group, Randomised trial of intravenous atenolol among 16,027 cases of suspected acute myocardial infarction: ISIS-1, *Lancet* (1986) **2**:57–65.

10  The MIAMI Trial Research Group, Metoprolol in acute myocardial infarction (MIAMI). A randomised placebo-controlled international trial, *Eur Heart J* (1985) **6**:199–226.

11  The Norwegian Multicenter Study Group, Timolol-induced reduction in mortality and reinfarction in patients surviving acute myocardial infarction, *N Engl J Med* (1981) **304**:801–7.

12  Herlitz J et al, Goteborg metoprolol trial: mortality and causes of death, *Am J Cardiol* (1984) **53**:9D–14D.

13  Beta Blocker Heart Attack Trial Research Group, A randomised trial of propanolol in patients with acute myocardial infarction: mortality results, *JAMA* (1982) **247**:1707–14.

14  Roberts R et al for the TIMI Investigators, Immediate versus deferred beta blockade following thrombolytic therapy in patients with acute myocardial infarction: results of the Thrombolysis in Myocardial Infarction (TIMI) 11-B Study, *Circulation* (1991) **83**:422–37.

15  Pfeffer MA et al, Effect on captopril on progressive ventricular dilatation after anterior myocardial infarction, *N Engl J Med* (1988) **319**:80–6.

16  Sharpe E et al, Treatment of patients with symptomless left ventricular dysfunction after myocardial infarction, *Lancet* (1988) **1**:255–9.

17  Pfeffer MA et al, The effect of captopril on mortality and morbidity in patients with left ventricular dysfunction following myocardial infarction: results of the Survival and Ventricular Enlargement Trial, *N Engl J Med* (1992) **327**:669–77.

18  The SOLVD Investigators, Effect of enalapril on mortality and the development of heart failure in asymptomatic patients with reduced left ventricular ejection fractions, *N Engl J Med* (1992) **327**:685–91.

19  Swedberg K and the Consensus II Study of Group Effects of Early Administration of Enalapril on Mortality in Patients with Acute Myocardial Infarction, Results of the Co-operative New Scandinavian Enalapril Survival Study II (Consensus II), *N Engl J Med* (1992) **327**:678–84.

# 7

# Dyslipidaemia—regression, progression and drug therapy

*D John Betteridge*

## Introduction

There is no doubt that these are exciting times for the physician interested in the detection and treatment of dyslipidaemia. On the one hand the epidemiological link between increasing plasma cholesterol concentrations and coronary heart disease (CHD) is considered by many to point to a causal relationship; the primary prevention trials of lipid lowering taken together have unequivocally shown reduction of coronary morbidity and mortality; the nature of the interaction of atherogenic lipoprotein particles with cells important in atherogenesis is increasingly understood; the angiographic trials have pointed not only to reduced progression of coronary atherosclerosis but also regression; dramatic advances in the understanding of lipoprotein metabolism at the molecular level have facilitated the development of novel therapeutic agents and the first attempts at gene therapy for homozygous familial hypercholesterolaemia.

On the other hand, controversy still exists. An article published in the *British Medical Journal* in 1992[1] entitled 'Should there be a moratorium on the use of cholesterol lowering drugs?' led to headlines in the lay press such as 'Murder linked to lipid drugs'; the failure of the primary prevention trials of lipid lowering to demonstrate a reduction in overall mortality

has been highlighted by some despite the fact that the trials did not have the statistical power to assess this; the undoubted epidemiological association between low plasma cholesterol levels and increased morbidity and mortality from a variety of non-cardiac causes has been linked by some to the 'adverse' effects on non-cardiac mortality seen in the primary prevention trials; probably related to the above, the rate of detection and appropriate therapy of lipid risk factors in individuals with established CHD where benefit is beyond question is disappointingly low.

In this chapter I will discuss in detail the epidemiological and clinical trial evidence supporting an important role for the modification of plasma lipid levels in the secondary prevention of CHD. In addition the recent exciting results of the angiographic trials will be described. Finally I will give some pointers to optimum therapy for lipid and lipoprotein disorders in CHD patients.

## Lipids, lipoproteins and CHD

### Low-density lipoprotein

The evidence linking plasma cholesterol and particularly low-density lipoprotein (LDL) cholesterol, the major carrier of plasma cholesterol, to CHD has been strengthened considerably over the last decade. Advances have occurred in many different areas, including epidemiology, and animal and clinical studies. Of particular interest is the follow-up of the MRFIT screenees.[2] This massive amount of data involving over 360 000 men has confirmed the relationship between increasing plasma cholesterol concentrations and increasing CHD mortality. Furthermore, data from Chinese populations, where mean cholesterol concentrations are much lower than those in Western industrialized societies, point to a continuous gradient of CHD risk with increasing plasma cholesterol.[3] The epidemiology studies taken together emphasize the strength of the relationship between plasma cholesterol and CHD; the 'dose–response' nature of the link, independence from other risk factors, impressive consistency between and within various population groups, and the predictive nature of the relationship. The epidemiological data are supported by spectacular progress in the understanding of lipoprotein metabolism and lipoprotein–cell interactions, particularly the description of the LDL receptor and the acetyl-LDL receptor (scavenger receptor) by Goldstein and Brown and their colleagues.[4,5] Identification of the LDL receptor, the activation of which largely determines plasma LDL concentrations, was facilitated by the study of cultured fibroblasts derived from patients with familial hypercholesterolaemia. In this condition, the most severe of the hyperlipidaemias, the genetic defect is at the LDL receptor gene, producing absent or defective LDL receptor activity and, as a consequence, high plasma LDL concentrations. This experiment not only enabled Brown and Goldstein to make their Nobel prize-winning observations but also emphasizes the link between LDL and atherosclerosis, as young people with this

condition have a 100-fold increased CHD risk without the presence of other risk factors.[6] This work, taken together with recent studies of experimental atherosclerosis in non-human primates, has enabled the identification of highly plausible mechanisms of arterial foam cell formation, the early lesion of atherosclerosis. Briefly, when monkeys are fed a high-fat, high-cholesterol diet, the first identifiable lesion is the adhesion of circulating blood monocytes to arterial endothelium. At a later stage monocytes penetrate into and accumulate in the subendothelial space. Later these cells acquire the characteristics of macrophages, take up lipid and become lipid-laden foam cells typical of the fatty streak. At this stage the overlying endothelium is disrupted, possibly because of the toxic effects of the foam cells. This allows platelet adhesion and aggregation to take place with release of growth factors, smooth muscle cell proliferation and progression to a fibrous plaque.[7]

The apparent central role for the monocyte/macrophage in the formation of the foam cell has concentrated attention on the interaction of lipoproteins with these cells. Native LDL does not produce foam cells when incubated with monocyte/macrophages in culture. However, when LDL is modified chemically (e.g. by acetylation) the lipoprotein is avidly internalized through a receptor-mediated process leading to massive cellular cholesterol accumulation.[5] The macrophage receptor responsible for interaction with modified LDL has been termed the scavenger receptor. Unlike the classical LDL receptor, the scavenger receptor is present in cells isolated from patients homozygous for familial hypercholesterolaemia and its expression is not regulated by cellular cholesterol content. The scavenger receptor has recently been cloned.[8]

Steinberg's group[9] has provided considerable evidence that the 'physiological' modification which occurs in LDL such that it becomes a ligand for the scavenger receptor is peroxidation. In addition to uptake by the scavenger receptor, oxidatively modified LDL may contribute to atherogenesis in other ways; it is cytotoxic and stimulates monocyte adhesion and monocyte chemotaxis, amongst its other properties. In keeping with the hypothesis that the essential modification of LDL is peroxidation, it has been shown that antioxidants such as α-tocapherol and butylated hydroxytoluene inhibit LDL modification by cultured cells. It is of interest that the hypocholesterolaemic agent probucol has antioxidant properties and also blocks the oxidative modification of LDL in vitro.[9] Furthermore, in experimental animals probucol treatment is associated with reduced LDL uptake in macrophage-rich fatty streaks and reduced atherogenesis.[10]

## High-density lipoprotein

Approximately 20–30 per cent of cholesterol in plasma is transported in high-density lipoproteins (HDL), the smallest of the lipoprotein species. The HDL fraction is perhaps the most heterogeneous of all lipoprotein classes; this heterogeneity reflecting direct synthesis of nascent HDL particles by the liver and intestine, the transfer of surface components from triglyceride-rich lipoprotein particles to HDL during hydrolysis by the enzyme lipoprotein lipase and the exchange of cholesteryl ester formed on HDL for triglyceride between HDL and lipoproteins of lower density through lipid transfer proteins.[11,12] Lecithin:cholesterol acyltransferase (LCAT), a key enzyme in cholesterol metabolism, catalyses the formation of cholesteryl ester from free cholesterol using a fatty acyl residue derived from lecithin. HDL is the major site of activity of this enzyme, and

apoprotein A-I, the principal apoprotein of HDL, is an important activator of LCAT. The free cholesterol for the LCAT reaction may come from other lipoproteins or cell membranes. It is the ability of HDL to act as an acceptor of free cholesterol with subsequent esterification and transfer either to other lipoproteins or directly back to the liver that facilitates the potential role of HDL in reverse cholesterol transport, removal of cholesterol from the periphery and its return to the liver, the major site of cholesterol excretion. The LCAT reaction is responsible for the maturation of nascent HDL particles which are secreted as bilayer discs containing apoprotein and phospholipid. As these particles accept free cholesterol it is esterified by LCAT and the bilayer discs become spherical as the cholesteryl ester forms a hydrophobic droplet in the core of the particle. The ability of the HDL fraction to accept free cholesterol appears to be a property of a small subpopulation of the lipoprotein class and involves particles which are rich in apoprotein A-I with only a small amount of lipid. The nature of the interaction between HDL and peripheral cells remains to be fully determined but it is likely that specific receptors are involved.[13,14]

The lipoproteins LDL and VLDL contain a lot of cholesteryl esters but cholesterol on these particles is not a substrate for the enzyme LCAT. This observation suggested that cholesteryl ester can transfer between lipoproteins. Cholesteryl ester exchange protein[15] enables a mole-for-mole exchange of triglyceride for cholesteryl ester between lipoproteins. Thus the major part of the cholesteryl ester formed within the HDL fraction by the LCAT reaction eventually returns to the liver in VLDL and LDL and is taken up by the LDL receptor. However, HDL may deliver cholesterol back to the liver directly but this pathway in quantitative terms is less important. The triglyceride-rich HDL resulting from the exchange process with lipoproteins of lower density is a substrate for hepatic triglyceride lipase. Triglyceride is hydrolysed, resulting in smaller HDL particles (HDL$_3$) which can recycle and accumulate more cholesteryl ester (HDL$_2$).

Lipoprotein particles within the HDL fraction are intimately related to the metabolism of triglyceride-rich lipoproteins. They serve as a reservoir for apoproteins E and C, which are important in triglyceride metabolism. Furthermore, surface components, principally phospholipid and apoproteins A-I and A-II, of triglyceride-rich lipoproteins transfer to HDL during their hydrolysis by lipoprotein lipase. It has been calculated that up to 50 per cent of circulating HDL mass can be obtained through transfer of these surface components. As a result, larger, less dense HDL particles (HDL$_2$) are formed.[16]

Although the association between HDL cholesterol and coronary disease was first documented in the early 1950s, it was not until the landmark paper of Miller and Miller in 1975[17] that interest arose in this relationship. Unlike with LDL cholesterol, the relationship between HDL and CHD risk is inverse; low levels are associated with increased risk of CHD whilst high levels appear to be protective. This association was confirmed in many different major epidemiological studies, including the Framingham, Honolulu and Tromso heart studies.[18] The relationship was strong and independent of other risk factors. Gordon and colleagues analysed the relationship between HDL cholesterol and cardiovascular disease in data from four prospective American studies and showed that for an increase in HDL of 1 mg/dl (0.026 mmol/l) there was a decrease in CHD risk of 2.5 per cent.[19] This relationship was seen at all age groups and even more strongly in women. There appeared to be some inconsistency with data from Britain collected as

part of the British original Regional Heart Study, where the association between increasing levels of HDL cholesterol and decreased CHD risk did not persist after adjustment for other factors, including age, smoking, blood pressure, body mass index and levels of non-HDL cholesterol.[20] This was not seen in other prospective population studies and it appears that this difference was due to a statistical artefact because when the British data were analysed using total cholesterol as opposed to non-HDL cholesterol levels the results were consistent with those of the majority of the other studies.[19]

In studies between countries, particularly when non-industrialized countries are included which tend to have low rates of CHD and low total and HDL cholesterol, the inverse relationship between HDL cholesterol and CHD disappears.[21] However, when industrialized countries alone are studied then the inverse correlation holds.[22] It would appear therefore that low levels of HDL are more strikingly a risk factor in Western populations where dietary saturated fat intake is high and plasma total cholesterol is high.

There is no doubt about the strong epidemiological association between HDL cholesterol and CHD but the mechanism(s) by which HDL influences risk remain to be fully determined.[23] The role of HDL cholesterol in reverse cholesterol transport is an attractive hypothesis but this remains to be proven and other potential protective mechanisms for HDL do not involve the lipoprotein class in a direct role. As has been discussed, HDL is intimately related to the catabolism of triglyceride-rich lipoproteins. It is a possibility that this is the primary association although this is not strongly supported by epidemiological data linking plasma triglycerides to CHD. However, it has been suggested that a low plasma HDL may reflect the accumulation of triglyceride-rich remnant particles which are known to be highly athero-genic. HDL may also be implicated in other aspects of atherosclerosis. Inhibitory effects on platelet aggregation, for instance, have been demonstrated. Furthermore, HDL may inhibit the modifications of LDL and the interaction of modified LDL with cells.

## Triglycerides and CHD

The role of plasma triglycerides in CHD risk remains a confused area. Many studies, both prospective population studies and cross-sectional studies performed in the 1970s, showed a strong relationship between the level of plasma triglyceride and CHD. However, when the statistical technique of multivariate analysis was applied to these studies and other risk factors were entered into the mathematical model, the relationship between triglyceride and CHD disappeared.[24] Failure to demon-strate an 'independent' role for plasma triglyc-erides led to a reduced interest in triglycerides as a CHD risk factor and many laboratories stopped routinely measuring plasma triglyc-erides. However, this was probably inappropri-ate. There is inherent variability in plasma triglyceride measurement and because of this it does not come out strongly in mathematical models. Furthermore, the metabolism of plasma triglycerides is closely related to HDL metabolism and it would seem inappropriate to enter these factors separately into a mathemat-ical model when they are so intimately bound together metabolically.

There are other confounding factors when trying to determine the role of plasma triglyc-erides in CHD risk. The triglyceride molecule is unlikely to be involved in atherogenesis. However, plasma total triglycerides reflect several important lipoprotein particles in blood which contain triglyceride. These particles also contain cholesteryl esters and it is likely that

some of these triglyceride-rich particles are atherogenic while others are not. It is known that chylomicron remnants and VLDL remnant particles accumulate in type III hyperlipopro-teinaemia, or dysbetalipoproteinaemia. This condition is strongly associated with premature vascular disease.[25] It is of interest that remnant particles can directly interact with monocyte/macrophages to form foam cells in tissue culture. The accumulation of these triglyceride-rich remnant particles has been demonstrated in several hypertriglyceridaemic states. However, there is no simple measure of these particles and currently they are only measured in research studies. A useful develop-ment for future assessment of patients would be a simple, easy measure of these remnant parti-cles. Triglycerides are traditionally measured in the fasting state and it is possible that impor-tant alterations in triglyceride metabolism which may be associated with atherosclerosis may be missed by only measuring fasting triglycerides. It is likely that the individuals will respond differently in the postprandial metabolism of triglyceride-rich lipoproteins and in the future it is likely that more detailed assessment of patients may involve postprandial studies of triglyceride metabolism.

Perhaps it is artificial to try and look at HDL independent of triglyceride and independent of cholesterol and this is emphasized by data from two recent prospective studies; the Procam Study in Germany[26] and the follow-up of the placebo-treated group of the Helsinki Heart Study.[27] Both these studies have pointed to the very high risk of CHD in those individuals with hypertriglyceridaemia associated with a low HDL, and an LDL/HDL cholesterol ratio >5. In the Helsinki Heart Study this subgroup of individuals had a relative risk of 3.8 per cent for developing a coronary event.[27] In the Procam Study the association of hypertriglyc-eridaemia with an LDL/HDL cholesterol ratio of >5 was seen in 4.3 per cent of the study population of 4559 males aged 40–64 years. However, this particular lipoprotein profile accounted for one-quarter of all CHD events observed.[26]

Another factor confounding the relationship between plasma triglyceride and CHD risk is the association of increased plasma triglycerides and alterations in other lipoprotein particles. I have already discussed the association with low HDL cholesterol levels. However, increased plasma triglycerides are also associated with changes in the LDL fraction. It has been known for some years that the LDL fraction is heterogeneous and there is considerable evidence pointing to the increased risk of CHD associated with the smaller dense LDL particles.[28] Why the smaller denser LDL particles may be more atherogenic is not fully understood, but one potential reason is that they seem more susceptible to alteration by lipid oxidation.[29] In one study over two-thirds of the variance in the LDL subfractions could be explained by plasma triglyceride and HDL cholesterol changes.[30]

An important further potential role that plasma triglycerides may have in atherosclerosis and CHD is their relationship to coagulation factors and there is substantial evidence that hypertriglyceridaemia represents a procoagulant state. The coagulation factor VII has been found to be associated with plasma triglycerides and in fact levels of factor VII follow quite closely alterations in plasma triglycerides following a fatty meal.[31,32] It is likely that the surfaces of the triglyceride-rich particles activate the intrinsic coagulation pathway. Hypertriglyceridaemia has also been linked to impaired fibrinolysis through increased levels of plasminogen activator inhibitor 1 (PAI-1), which is the fast-acting inhibitor of tissue type plasminogen activator.[33]

It can be seen that the relationships between triglyceride and CHD are complex and are confounded by different triglyceride-rich particles which may have different effects, associated abnormalities in HDL metabolism and LDL subfractions, and also interactions with thrombotic factors. Plasma triglyceride should not be ignored when assessing the CHD risk in an individual but it would appear to be particularly important in the presence of a low HDL cholesterol concentration and an LDL/HDL cholesterol ratio of >5.[26,27] These parameters are regularly available in the clinical situation. More detailed individualization of the risk attributable to triglycerides will come with improved techniques to identify remnant particles and thus the ability to demonstrate the presence of small dense LDL particles and possibly to assess thrombotic factors. These aspects of the link between triglycerides and CHD have been reviewed by a recent consensus panel and guidelines have been published for a clinical approach to hypertriglyceridaemia.[34]

## Lipoprotein (a)

Lipoprotein (a) is LDL to which an extra apoprotein, namely apoprotein (a), is joined to apoprotein B100 of LDL by disulphide bridges.[35] The increasing interest in lipoprotein (a) over the past few years stems from the fact that there is striking homology between apoprotein (a) and the zymogen of the coagulation and fibrinolytic system, plasminogen.[36] Apoprotein (a) consists of the protease region of plasminogen together with kringle 5 and then a variable number of internal repeats of kringle 4 (Figure 7.1). There is striking size heterogeneity within lipoprotein (a), depending on the number of internal repeats of the kringle 4 domain, ranging from 15 to 40. Much still needs to be understood about the metabolism

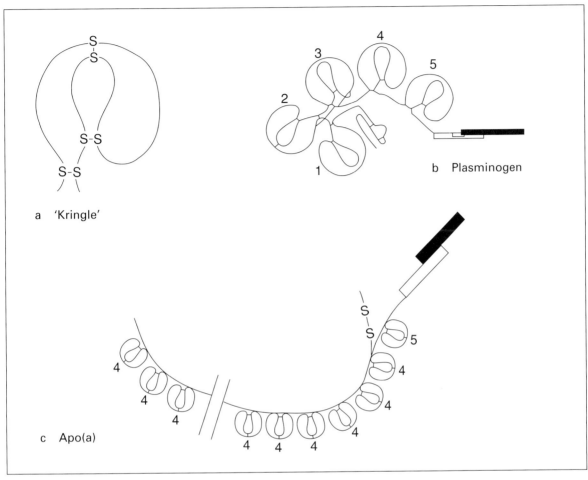

**Figure 7.1**
*Schematic representation of (a) single kringle domain characterized by three disulphides and four loops; (b) plasminogen with five kringles numbered from 1 to 5 followed by the protease region, and (c) apo(a) characterized by multiple internal repeats of kringle 4, one kringle 5 and the protease region. (From Scanu,[35] with permission.)*

of lipoprotein (a). Plasma levels appear to be largely determined by the rate of synthesis, predominantly in the liver. Although in vitro studies suggest that lipoprotein (a) can bind to the LDL receptor it would appear that the catabolism of lipoprotein (a) via LDL receptors plays only a minor role in lipoprotein (a) catabolism.

Plasma concentrations of lipoprotein (a) show immense variation within and between populations but tend to remain fairly stable throughout life. In Caucasian populations the great majority of individuals will have low levels of lipoprotein (a). (Blacks have elevated levels compared to whites.) However, high levels of lipoprotein (a) have been shown to be a strong independent risk factor for the development of CHD.[37] It would seem that lipoprotein (a) is important only when plasma cholesterol levels are in the range seen in Western populations. In patients with familial hypercholesterolaemia, high lipoprotein (a) levels are associated with an increased prevalence of CHD in this high-risk group.[38] In addition to CHD, lipoprotein (a) has been shown to be independently related to stroke.[39] Of considerable interest are studies that have looked at the offspring of individuals suffering from a myocardial infarction. Children of these patients showed significantly increased lipoprotein (a) levels.[40] In fact, lipoprotein (a) is amongst the most prevalent of the inherited risk factors for CHD and a substantial proportion of the genetic component of risk of CHD in the absence of traditional risk factors probably relates to lipoprotein (a) levels.

The mechanism whereby lipoprotein (a) increases the risk of CHD and stroke remains to be fully determined.[41] Certainly lipoprotein (a) is deposited in the arterial wall and lipoprotein (a) has been detected in atheromatous lesions. The homology with plasminogen suggests a possible role for lipoprotein (a) in thrombosis. Lipoprotein (a) can inhibit plasminogen activation. Furthermore, lipoprotein (a) has been shown to bind tissue plasminogen activator, interfering with its ability to activate plasminogen. However, it has been more difficult to demonstrate correlations in vivo between lipoprotein (a) concentrations and measures of fibrinolytic activity. Lipoprotein (a) levels do not appear to influence plasminogen activator therapy in acute myocardial infarction. However, lipoprotein (a) levels are a risk factor for restenosis after coronary artery bypass surgery. Lipoprotein (a) can behave like an acute phase protein and increased levels have been observed in subjects with unstable angina compared to stable angina.

Lipoprotein (a) levels seem to be little affected by diet although there is some evidence that long-term treatment with omega-3 polyunsaturated fatty acids may reduce lipoprotein (a).[42] Conventional lipid-lowering drugs seem to have little effect apart from nicotinic acid.[43] There is some preliminary evidence that fibrate therapy may be associated with reduction in lipoprotein (a) levels in the longer term but these initial reports need to be confirmed. High alcohol intake is associated with very low lipoprotein (a) levels. Recent work suggests that both type I and type II diabetics are more likely to have elevated levels of lipoprotein (a) compared to normal individuals. Those diabetics with microalbuminuria have increased lipoprotein (a) levels and in fact other types of kidney disease are also associated with increased lipoprotein (a) levels. In the diabetics, lipoprotein (a) levels fall as glycaemic control is improved. The mechanism of these changes in lipoprotein (a) levels remains to be determined.[41]

## Lipoproteins and coronary risk in subjects with established clinical coronary disease

Surveys to determine the number of individuals with established CHD receiving therapy designed to modify lipid risk factors have shown very low treatment rates.[44] It is difficult for a lipidologist to understand the reluctance of many cardiologists to instigate aggressive lipid-modifying therapy in these individuals, as the evidence of benefit would appear to be considerable. Perhaps some of the reluctance to embark on such therapy stems from the idea that lowering plasma cholesterol in someone with established disease is akin to closing the stable door once the horse has bolted! There is no doubt that data from early studies, particularly the Coronary Drug Project, pointed to myocardial damage as being a better predictor of subsequent re-infarction or death than plasma lipid levels.[45] This is particularly true in the early stages after myocardial infarction. However, what perhaps has not been appreciated amongst cardiologists is the long-term association between serum cholesterol, particularly LDL cholesterol, and re-infarction. This has been found to be the case in many longitudinal studies.[46] As would be expected also, high HDL cholesterol is inversely related to subsequent re-infarction.

Perhaps another reason for lack of enthusiasm in treating plasma cholesterol is that some studies have shown that the relative risk of individuals with high cholesterol compared to a low cholesterol for re-infarction was not large. This was certainly true in the Coronary Drug Project, where the relative risk for those in the highest quintile compared to the lowest was 1.5.[47] However, when assessing the potential for reducing coronary events in those with established disease it is important to consider not only relative risk but the absolute risk in these individuals, which is high. It is likely that there will be considerable benefit of treating raised cholesterol levels even if the relative risk across the cholesterol concentrations is relatively low, when this is superimposed on individuals at high absolute risk.

The high absolute risk in those with established CHD is well established from many different population studies. For instance, in the British Regional Heart Study the re-infarction rate was 14 per cent over a follow-up period of just over 4 years in those with ECG evidence of previous definite infarction compared to 2 per cent in individuals with no

such evidence.[48] Furthermore, in the control groups of the various secondary prevention trials that have been performed, re-infarction rates were about 6 per cent per annum.[46] This compares to a figure of 1–2 per cent seen in primary prevention trials. Despite the advances in management of the post-infarction patient and the more widespread use of aspirin and beta-blockers, it is likely that the re-infarction rate will remain high. To return to the relative risk associated with increase in cholesterol and those with established disease, more recent studies have pointed to a similar relative risk in those with established disease as in those without disease, and in the Lipid Research Clinics follow-up study the relative risk in those with established disease was considerably higher than in those without established disease, 10.4 versus 4.2.[49]

The potential for reducing the rate of re-infarction with lipid-lowering therapy has been well argued by Roussouw et al.[46] They calculate, for instance, that in the Lipid Research Clinics follow-up study the excess risk of death from CHD over a 10-year period in men with established disease with cholesterol levels above 6.2 mmol compared to those with cholesterol levels below 5.2 mmol/l was 154 : 1000. Even if the data from the Coronary Drug Project are used, where the relative risk attributable to cholesterol was much lower, using similar calculations the potential for reducing CHD death by cholesterol lowering was 67 : 1000. Of course these impressive figures may not materialize if cholesterol lowering is instigated. It is possible that the potential benefit from calculations of the epidemiological data may not be fully attained by intervention. However, from reviews of the secondary prevention trials it does appear that the risk of subsequent re-infarction and coronary death can be reduced. Although the numbers of events tend to be higher for obvious reasons in the secondary prevention trials, still some of the studies did not have adequate power to determine differences in the intervention group compared to the control group. To overcome this problem Roussouw et al performed a meta-analysis of eight secondary prevention trials which included at least 100 individuals in the control and in the intervention groups, lasted for at least 3 years, followed a randomized design and were free of confounding interventions to address other risk factors.[46] Trials using early known toxic drugs such as D-thyroxine and oestrogens were not included for obvious reasons. The overall analysis shows a significant reduction in both non-fatal and fatal re-infarction. From these trials it was apparent that a 10 per cent reduction in serum cholesterol level was associated with a 15 per cent reduction in total myocardial infarction, with a 19 per cent reduction in non-fatal myocardial infarctions and a 12 per cent reduction in fatal myocardial infarctions.

The early trials used available therapy which led to only small reductions in plasma cholesterol. The current secondary prevention trials with newer agents which can lower cholesterol by 30 per cent are anticipated with great interest. Of course, subjects for secondary prevention trials are survivors in the sense that they were not recruited until at least 3 months following infarction and, of course, those individuals with severe myocardial damage may well have died within this 3-month period. However, the numbers of individuals surviving 3 months after myocardial infarction is still large. Another point to make about the secondary prevention trials is that individuals were not recruited on the basis of having a high plasma cholesterol and in fact the average cholesterol levels at baseline in these studies were modest, ranging between 6.3 and 7.6 mmol/l. No doubt related to the importance of coronary death in individuals with established disease, the secondary prevention trials were associated not only with a reduction in coronary mortality but also with a trend for a reduction in overall deaths. There was no significant increase in cancer deaths and no significant increase in non-cardiovascular, non-cancer deaths.[46,50] On the basis of these studies it is likely with modern therapy that cholesterol lowering will have as good as if not a better effect in reducing subsequent re-infarction and coronary death than aspirin therapy or beta-blocker therapy.

## Angiographic trials

In addition to the evidence from the secondary prevention trials there is no doubt that the recent angiographic trials have provided additional exciting information with regard to the potential benefits of modifying plasma lipid levels in the patient with established CHD. Two of these trials involved diet and lifestyle measures only. The Leiden Intervention Trial, published in 1985,[51] involved 39 CHD patients with >50 per cent stenosis in at least one coronary artery. This was an uncontrolled study and all patients received dietary intervention over a 2-year period. The diet was principally vegetarian with a high polyunsaturated/saturated fat ratio (>2) and a dietary cholesterol intake of <100 mg/day. The mean plasma total cholesterol concentration at baseline was 6.9 mmol/l and the dietary measures were associated with a reduction in plasma cholesterol of approximately 10 per cent. HDL cholesterol was little changed. Angiography was performed at baseline and after approximately 2 years using non-quantitative techniques. Forty-six per cent of patients showed no new lesion growth after 2 years. In lesions that did progress, plaque enlargement correlated well with the total cholesterol/HDL cholesterol ratio.

In the recent lifestyle heart trial[52] more substantial changes were obtained in plasma lipid levels but at the price of a very strict diet programme involving a reduction of total calories from fat to only 10 per cent and a substantial reduction in cholesterol intake. Other lifestyle measures included stress management, advice against smoking and an exercise programme. Twenty-two individuals with angiographically documented CHD were included in the intervention group and 19 individuals in the control group. In fact the recruitment to this study was somewhat disappointing and a criticism of the study is that originally 53 subjects were randomly assigned to the intervention group and 43 to the control group but many did not agree to participate in the study following the randomization. LDL cholesterol fell by 37 per cent in the intervention group from a baseline level of approximately 3.9 mmol/l compared to a 6 per cent reduction in the control group. Along with the reduction in LDL cholesterol there was a 24 per cent reduction in apoprotein B. Probably related to the high carbohydrate content of the intervention diet, plasma triglyceride levels rose by 22 per cent in the intervention group. HDL cholesterol fell slightly in both groups by 3 per cent. Unfortunately, HDL cholesterol levels were not well matched between the control and treatment groups at baseline, being significantly higher in the control group. Repeat quantitative coronary angiography was performed after 1 year. In the intervention group there was a 2.2 per cent reduction in stenosis compared to a 3.4 per cent increase in the control group ($p < 0.001$). When the effects on lesions showing >50 per cent stenosis were examined separately, a 5.3 per cent reduction was seen in the intervention group compared to a 2.7 per cent progression in the control group ($p = 0.03$). Although this study has been criticized because of randomization problems

and the rigour of the dietary and lifestyle measures applied, it is encouraging to see that in as short a time as a year changes can be observed using quantitative angiography.[52]

Several early trials of the effects of hypolipidaemic drug treatment on atherosclerosis progression/regression involved relatively small numbers of patients. However, more recently, larger trials have been performed, some using the new technology of quantitative angiography. In 1984 the encouraging results of the National Heart, Lung and Blood Institute Type II Hyperlipidaemia Trial were published.[53] In this trial 116 hypercholesterolaemic patients all received diet therapy and either placebo or the anion-exchange resin cholestyramine for a 5-year period. During the course of the study cholestyramine therapy was associated with a 26 per cent reduction in LDL cholesterol and an 8 per cent increase in HDL cholesterol. In the placebo group there was a 5 per cent fall in LDL cholesterol. Non-quantitative coronary angiography was performed at baseline and after 5 years. When lesions showing >50 per cent stenosis at baseline were analysed it was apparent that there was a significant difference in the progression of these lesions between the treated group and the placebo group. Thirty-three per cent of patients taking placebo showed progression of these lesions compared to 12 per cent of the intervention group. Significant associations were seen between the degree of plaque progression and LDL reduction and HDL increase. This trial was encouraging to the extent that lipid-lowering therapy could possibly halt progression, but no evidence of regression was seen.[53]

The Cholesterol-Lowering Atherosclerosis Study (CLAS), first published in 1987,[54] was a landmark angiographic trial in that it was the first study to suggest the possibility of plaque regression. Patients included in this trial were non-smoking men aged 40–59 years who had undergone previous coronary artery bypass surgery. The investigators were able to identify 188 individuals who could tolerate colestipol, an anion-exchange resin, and nicotinic acid at high dose. All individuals were given a lipid-lowering diet, half being randomly allocated to combination drug therapy and half to placebo preparations. In the intervention group there were dramatic alterations in cholesterol-rich lipoproteins, with a 43 per cent reduction in LDL cholesterol and a 37 per cent increase in HDL cholesterol. Plasma triglycerides were reduced by 22 per cent. Non-quantitative coronary arteriography was performed at baseline and at 2 years and the results are based on 162 individuals. In the intervention group there was a significant reduction in the average number of lesions per subject which progressed. In addition, new plaque formation was also significantly reduced both in native vessels and in the grafts. Furthermore, by using a global score analysis actual regression in native vessels in 16 per cent of the intervention group was observed.[54]

Evidence for atherosclerosis regression in response to aggressive lipid-lowering therapy supporting the findings of the CLAS study has come from three recently published trials. The Familial Atherosclerosis Treatment Study (FATS) involved 146 men under the age of 62 years who had a family history of premature cardiovascular disease and angiographically demonstrated CHD with at least one coronary stenosis ≥50 per cent or three lesions ≥30 per cent stenosis.[55] Baseline apolipoprotein B levels were greater than 125 mg/dl. Subjects were randomly assigned to one of three treatment groups. All three groups were given dietary counselling by professional dieticians. In the conventional treatment group patients received placebo. However, if plasma LDL cholesterol levels were greater than the 90th percentile for the US population, the anion-exchange resin

colestipol was prescribed. The other two groups received alternative intensive lipid-lowering therapy: colestipol in high dose (30 g/day) together with nicotinic acid (4 g/day) or high-dose colestipol with the HMG-CoA reductase inhibitor lovastatin (40 mg/day). Quantitative computer coronary angiography was performed at baseline and after 30 months. In the conventional treatment group LDL cholesterol fell by 9 per cent and HDL cholesterol increased by 3 per cent. In the colestipol/nicotinic acid group, there was a 34 per cent reduction in LDL cholesterol and a 41 per cent increase in HDL cholesterol. The dramatic increase in HDL in this group is attributable to nicotinic acid, which is highly effective in increasing HDL cholesterol levels. In the colestipol/lovastatin group there was a 48 per cent reduction in LDL cholesterol and a 14 per cent increase in HDL cholesterol. The LDL cholesterol/HDL cholesterol ratio was comparable in the two intensive intervention groups. Along with changes in lipoprotein cholesterol concentrations there were highly significant reductions in apoprotein B in these groups.

Assessment of progression/regression was based on visual and computerized, quantitative assessment of nine standard proximal segments and the two principal measures were the minimum lumen diameter and the percentage stenosis. The primary end-point was the average change in percentage stenosis for the most severe lesion in each of nine proximal segments. In the conventionally treated group, definite lesion progression was observed in at least one proximal segment in 46 per cent of patients. By contrast, lesion regression was observed in 11 per cent. In the aggressive intervention groups, 21 per cent of patients had definite lesion progression in the colestipol/lovastatin group and 25 per cent in the colestipol/nicotinic acid group. Lesion regression was observed in 32 per cent of patients in the colestipol/lovastatin group and in 39 per cent in the colestipol/nicotinic acid group. These differences were highly statistically significant.

When lipid risk factor alterations were analysed in relation to regression of coronary lesions, significant associations were seen for apoprotein B, LDL cholesterol and HDL cholesterol. Along with the important changes in angiographically demonstrable disease, differences in clinical events were noted during the study. In the conventionally treated group, 10 of the 52 patients suffered clinical events, including coronary death, myocardial infarction or the need for further surgery, compared to 3 out of 46 individuals in the colestipol/lovastatin group and 2 out of 48 individuals in the colestipol/nicotinic acid group.[55]

Further evidence for atheroma regression comes from the University of California San Francisco intervention trial.[56] This was an open study in 72 patients with heterozygous familial hypercholesterolaemia. A control group was treated with diet alone or diet and low-dose resin therapy and the treatment group received high-dose anion-exchange resin therapy plus nicotinic acid or lovastatin. Some individuals were treated with triple drug therapy. In the intervention group, LDL cholesterol levels fell from an average of 7.32 mmol/l to 4.45 mmol/l. The primary outcome variable was change in cross-sectional percentage area stenosis after an average 26-month follow-up period. In the control group this was +0.80, indicating progression, whilst in the treatment group this was −1.53, indicating regression. It is of interest that this study also involved women, and significant changes were seen when women were analysed separately.[56]

The most recent of the regression trials is the St Thomas' Atherosclerosis Regression Study (STARS).[57] Ninety men with CHD were studied and the average plasma cholesterol at baseline was 7.2 mmol/l. Patients were randomly allocated to one of three groups: a control group, a diet group given low-cholesterol, low-saturated-fat eating advice, and a third group received similar dietary advice together with the anion-exchange resin cholestyramine. Follow-up was for an average of 39 months and quantitative coronary angiography was performed at baseline and at the end of the study. Coronary lesions in these patients were less severe than in most of the other studies and only 8 per cent showed >50 per cent stenosis.

Compared to the control group, dietary therapy led to a 13 per cent reduction in LDL cholesterol, whereas HDL cholesterol remained unchanged. The addition of cholestyramine led to a 33 per cent reduction in LDL cholesterol. Significant reductions in the percentage of patients showing progression of atherosclerosis were seen in both the diet group and the diet plus cholestyramine group. Similarly, the percentage of patients showing regression was increased in these two groups compared to the control. Despite the fact that a more substantial reduction in LDL cholesterol was seen in the group taking cholestyramine, there was no difference between these two groups with regard to the percentage of patients who showed progression or regression. However, the mean luminal diameter overall showed significantly more improvement in those taking diet and cholestyramine. These changes correlated significantly with LDL cholesterol and the LDL/HDL cholesterol ratio. The dietary measures involved in this study were certainly less strict than the diet used either in the Leiden diet trial[51] or the lifestyle trial[52] and involved a reduction in total calories from fat to 27 per cent with a P/S ratio of approximately 1 and a daily cholesterol intake of 100 mg daily. In addition to the beneficial effects of the diet and diet plus cholestyramine on the angiographic data, significant reductions were also noted in clinical events in these two groups compared to the control group.[57]

The largest regression trial so far reported is the Programme on the Surgical Control of the Hyperlipidaemias (POSCH) Study.[58] The study has provided very useful information on the effect of lipid lowering on atherosclerosis but the plasma cholesterol reduction was achieved by partial ileal bypass. This procedure, which involves bypass of the distal third of the small intestine or the distal 200 cm (whichever is greater) with restoration of bowel continuity by end-to-end ileocaecostomy, was used in the past for the treatment of severe hypercholesterolaemia in those individuals who responded to resin therapy but were unable to take resins at effective dosage long term. The surgical procedure acts in a similar way to the resins by interrupting the enterohepatic circulation of the bowel; however, it is now not part of clinical practice since the advent of newer, more potent therpeutic agents. Eight hundred and thirty-eight men and women (91 per cent men) who had suffered a myocardial infarction were recruited for this study. Of these, 421 were randomly assigned to undergo surgery; of these 5 per cent refused but were still included in the surgical group for data analysis. Repeat coronary angiography was performed after 5–10 years follow-up in approximately 85 per cent of the surgery group. In the group that did not receive surgery, 32 per cent were taking one or more cholesterol-lowering drugs. LDL cholesterol fell by 38 per cent in the surgical group and there was a 4 per cent increase in HDL cholesterol. Both the surgical group and the control group received dietary advice along the lines of the American Heart Association phase II diet guidelines. The surgery was not without problems and reversal of the bypass was required in 23 patients, mainly due to intractable diarrhoea. This study was large enough to be able to look at outcome in terms of CHD events and there was a 28 per cent reduction in CHD mortality in the surgery group. This was not significant but when non-fatal myocardial infarctions and CHD deaths were combined the overall reduction in CAD was highly significantly reduced in the group that underwent surgery. Repeat angiograms were analysed non-quantitatively and there was significantly less progression of atherosclerosis in the surgical group compared to the control group.[58]

There is no doubt that the encouraging data from the regression trials points to a role for intensive lipid-lowering therapy in the individual with established coronary disease. There are several large regression trials currently in progress using powerful lipid-lowering regimens based on the statin drugs, which are better tolerated than those involving resins or nicotinic acid. The results of these trials are awaited with interest, with regard to the impact of therapy not only on lesions but also on clinical outcome. However, our current information from the existing trials is highly encouraging.

## Target lipid levels in secondary prevention

Various guidelines and consensus documents have been produced giving goals of therapy in terms of plasma lipids in various situations. For instance, the current National Cholesterol Education Programme guidelines for patients with established coronary disease suggest diet therapy if LDL cholesterol is ≥130 mg/dl, drug therapy for an LDL cholesterol level ≥160 mg/dl.[59] In view of the emerging evidence from the regression trials and from the analysis of the secondary prevention trials, are these LDL levels appropriate for therapy of this important group of patients in the 1990s? Certainly there is a view amongst many lipidologists treating these individuals that more aggressive targets should be set. La Rosa et al argue for such an approach in a recent special report of the National Cholesterol Education Programme.[60] They suggest that in the patient with established disease the primary target of therapy should, of course, be LDL cholesterol but that the optimal level for LDL cholesterol should be <100 mg/dl and if necessary drug therapy should be instigated to achieve this goal. Furthermore, based on the emerging evidence with regard to HDL cholesterol and triglycerides they suggest that drug therapy might be considered in patients with established coronary disease who have HDL cholesterol levels <35 mg/dl or triglycerides >250 mg/dl.[60]

## Assessment and treatment of hyperlipidaemia in the patient with clinical coronary artery disease

From the previous discussion it is clear that a full lipid profile should be determined in all patients with clinically apparent coronary artery disease. After an overnight fast, blood should be taken for measurement of plasma cholesterol, triglyceride and HDL cholesterol. From these data LDL cholesterol can be calculated using the Friedewald[61] calculation (Figure 1.2) so long as the fasting total triglyceride does not exceed 4.5 mmol/l. Although LDL cholesterol remains the main therapeutic target, it is clear that, in those with disease, attempts should be made to increase plasma HDL cholesterol levels and to decrease plasma triglycerides. Some specialist lipid clinics are introducing measurements of lipoprotein (a) into clinical practice as a further indication of risk. Furthermore, apoprotein B is another useful measure and may be elevated in some patients when the total cholesterol is not dramatically increased. Care should be taken in the interpretation of lipid and lipoprotein results if the blood is sampled when the patient is in the postoperative period or acutely ill with myocardial infarction, as illness tends to lower total cholesterol. In fact the author has seen patients with familial hypercholesterolaemia whose cholesterol usually runs at 10 or 11 mmol/l untreated but who, when sampled in the postoperative period, showed cholesterol levels below 6 mmol/l. It is conventional to assess the plasma lipid profile 3 months after myocardial infarction or surgery.

$$\text{LDL cholesterol} = \text{total cholesterol} - \text{HDL cholesterol} - \frac{\text{total triglyceride}}{2.19}$$

(i)  All concentrations in mmol/l
(ii) This formula gives a good estimate of LDL cholesterol so long as the total triglyceride does not exceed 4.5 mmol/l

**Figure 7.2**
*Friedewald[61] calculation of LDL cholesterol.*

| Principle | Amount | Food sources |
|---|---|---|
| Decreased total fat<br>Decreased saturated fat | <30% energy<br>7–10% of energy | Avoid butter, hard margarine, whole milk, cream, ice cream, high-fat cheese, fatty meats and poultry, sausages, pastries, coffee whitener, products containing hydrogenated oils, palm oil and coconut oil |
| Increased use of high-protein food (low in saturated fat) | | Fish, chicken and turkey; veal, game, spring lamb |
| Increased complex carbohydrate; increased fruit and vegetable fibre; increased legumes | About 35 g/day of fibre, one-half derived from fruit and vegetables | All fruit, including dried fruit, all fresh and frozen vegetables; lentils, dried beans, chick peas; unrefined cereal food, including oats |
| Decreased dietary cholesterol | <300 mg/day | Allowance up to two egg yolks per week and liver up to twice monthly; other offal avoided |
| Moderately increased use of mono- and polyunsaturated oils and products | Mono: 10–15% of energy<br>Poly: 7–10% of energy | Olive oil, sunflower oil, corn oil and products based on these |

Recommendations of the European Atherosclerosis Society prepared by the International Task Force for Prevention of Coronary Heart Disease.[62]

**Table 7.1**
*The lipid-lowering diet.*

It cannot be overemphasized that the treatment of plasma lipid levels is part of an overall strategy to reduce risk factors for vascular disease in the CHD patient. Dietary and lifestyle measures are the cornerstone of treatment in this group as with any other patient group. However, the threshold for using hyperlipidaemic agents in this group is much lower than when contemplating primary prevention. Dietary measures include attempts to try and achieve ideal body weight and the reduction of calories from fat in the diet, particularly saturated fat. The dietary guidelines of the European Atherosclerosis Society[62] are shown in Table 7.1. There is wide variation in response to dietary measures.

Obviously this will depend on the previous diet taken by the patient but genetic factors determine response to diet also. However, overall in clinical practice we see reductions in total cholesterol of between 10 and 15 per cent. In the author's opinion dietary measures are much more likely to be successful if the patients are seen and counselled by a dietitian on a one-to-one basis. The formal dietary advice should be backed up by literature and practical help in assessing and cooking appropriate foods. The patient's partner should attend the dietary sessions. The diet should be a family affair and it goes without saying that those with premature vascular disease should have their children assessed for dyslipidaemia at an age when blood sampling will not be a major imposition on the child. In the author's practice children with dyslipidaemia can follow a low-fat, low-cholesterol diet from the age of 4–5 years. Ramsey et al[63] have drawn attention to the minimal effect of dietary measures (step 1 dietary advice of the US National Cholesterol Education Program) in an overview of 16 published controlled trials. In the author's view this probably reflects poor adherence to the diet. In secondary prevention trials, where motivation may be greater, various dietary regimes have proved more effective, as in the recent St Thomas' Atherosclerosis Regression Study, for instance.[57]

The role of monounsaturated fatty acids, such as found in olive oil, has received considerable attention recently and has been the subject of many dietary clinical trials. There is no doubt that monounsaturated fat appears to be as good a substitute for saturated fat as polyunsaturated fat.[64] Furthermore, HDL cholesterol levels, which tend to fall with conventional low-fat, low-cholesterol diets, tend not to do so when monounsaturated fat is increased. The use of monounsaturated fat has the theoretical advantage that it is less sensitive to lipid peroxidation because of fewer double bonds. Emerging evidence from animal and human studies suggests that this is the case.[65]

There is no doubt from epidemiological studies that dietary intake of fish and fish oils is associated with reduced coronary events and there are prospective studies in coronary patients which appear to indicate the benefit of regular fish eating.[66] It is my policy to encourage the eating of fish as part of the prudent diet.

Appropriate exercise regimes are an important part of lifestyle measures to prevent CHD.[67] Exercise regimes, as well as acting as an aid to weight reduction, can affect the lipid profile principally by increasing plasma levels of HDL cholesterol and decreasing plasma triglycerides. However, the amount of exercise required for the effects on plasma lipoprotein levels is high.

## Lipid-modifying drug therapy

If target levels for plasma lipid and lipoprotein concentrations are not reached by dietary and lifestyle measures alone, then hypolipidaemic drugs should be prescribed in the patient with clinically overt coronary artery disease. Market research analyses performed in the UK show that the general appreciation of appropriate lipid-lowering drug therapy for the differing dyslipidaemias is poor and many clinicians need to learn more about the appropriate indications for the different lipid-lowering drugs. It is convenient to think of these agents as drugs which lower cholesterol principally, drugs which lower triglyceride principally, and drugs which will lower both cholesterol and triglycerides.

# Drugs which lower plasma cholesterol

## Bile acid sequestrant resins

The bile acid sequestrants have been available for clinical use for many years. Cholestyramine was introduced in the 1960s and colestipol in the 1970s. They are basic anion-exchange resins which are hydrophilic but insoluble in water. They are administered as flavoured powders mixed with water or fruit juice. After oral administration they remain unabsorbed in the gastrointestinal tract and bind bile acids, resulting in increased faecal elimination of bile acids. This interruption of the enterohepatic circulation of bile acids results in the synthesis of more bile acid in the liver from cholesterol. Furthermore, the absorption of dietary cholesterol is reduced because of the binding of the bile acids and additional cholesterol is lost in the faeces. Cholesterol is needed for the increased hepatic production of bile acids and this comes from two sources: firstly, hepatic LDL binding and uptake is increased, leading to a decrease in plasma LDL levels;[68] secondly, hepatic cholesterol synthesis de novo is increased.

In patients who can take resins at high doses, LDL cholesterol may fall by up to 30 per cent.[69] HDL cholesterol tends to increase slightly. Triglyceride levels may increase slightly with resin therapy, particularly in those who have raised triglycerides. In those with previously normal levels the increases are transient; however, they may be more sustained in patients with pre-existing elevations of VLDL. The effect of treatment on plasma LDL levels is usually evident after a week and is maximum after 2 weeks of therapy.

The fact that the resins have been used in clinical practice for many years and the fact that they are not absorbed are obvious benefits; however, compliance with these agents may be poor, principally due to gastrointestinal side-effects, including nausea, abdominal discomfort, indigestion and constipation. To a certain extent the effects on the gut may be overcome by starting resin therapy in low dose and gradually increasing the dose. It is of interest that in placebo-controlled trials transient elevations of liver enzymes have been observed with resins; the mechanism of this action is unknown but presumably it is related to the interruption of the enterohepatic circulation of bile. There is a theoretical risk of steatorrhoea and malabsorption of folate and fat-soluble vitamins with resins at high dose but this does not seem to be a problem in clinical practice.

The resins may bind to and decrease the absorption of concomitantly administered drugs and in clinical practice it is best to take other agents at least 1 h before or at least 4 h after resin therapy. The resins have been shown to interfere with the absorption of the oral anticoagulants, corticosteroids, digitalis preparations, iron, thyroid hormones and thiazide diuretics amongst others.

In my opinion the current place of resins is in low dosage, administered once a day, preferably before the evening meal for mild to moderate hypercholesterolaemia. They are also very useful in combined therapy for more severe hypercholesterolaemia in combination particularly with the HMG-CoA reductase inhibitors and also fibrates and nicotinic acid. They have been used in both primary and secondary prevention trials of CHD and also in regression studies and have been shown to decrease morbidity from CHD and to prevent progression of atheromatous plaques and in some instances induce regression.[53,54,57,70]

## Probucol

Probucol is a lipophilic bis-phenol compound which is structurally unique amongst the hypolipidaemic agents. It leads to moderate reduction of total and LDL cholesterol (10–20 per cent). It also reduces HDL cholesterol (10–30 per cent) and for this reason has not been a first-line agent. Plasma triglycerides are unaffected. The mechanism of action of probucol is not well defined. However, it would appear that the compound is transported in plasma in LDL[71] and probably as a result of this leads to changes in the lipoprotein surface proteins and increased LDL catabolism, probably through LDL receptor-independent mechanisms.[72] Probucol lowers HDL by inhibiting the synthesis of apoproteins A-I and A-II, the major lipoproteinsof HDL, and both the HDL subfractions $HDL_2$ and $HDL_3$ are reduced. However, despite the effects on HDL, probucol in clinical studies has been shown to mobilize tissue deposits of cholesterol, particularly in tendon xanthomata,[73] and it is likely that probucol exerts an effect on reverse cholesterol transport independent of its effects on plasma HDL levels.

There has been considerable interest in the role of LDL oxidation in atherogenesis recently and probucol has powerful antioxidant activity. Probucol has been shown in vitro to delay the oxidation of LDL and its subsequent incorporation into monocyte macrophages to form foam cells.[72] It has also been shown to reduce atherogenesis in animal models of atherosclerosis. However, as yet there is no evidence of an anti-atherosclerotic effect of probucol in man.

Probucol is generally well tolerated and there are very few adverse effects. However, some patients do complain of diarrhoea and other minor gastrointestinal disturbances. Probucol treatment is not associated with any abnormalities of liver function. ECG changes have been described, including prolonged QT intervals. In addition, fatal arrhythmia has occurred in laboratory animals fed high-dose probucol over the long term. In a small but detailed study in probucol-treated patients the QT and the QTC intervals were significantly prolonged during probucol therapy; however, the QT/QS2 ratio was unchanged.[74] Based on the supposition that the QT/QS2 ratio is a more accurate predictor of arrhythmia risk, this study suggests that the clinical significance of the effects of probucol on the ECG is small.

Probucol is highly lipophilic and accumulates in the body, particularly in adipose tissue. For this reason it should be stopped in women at least 6 months prior to attempted conception.

## Drugs which lower plasma cholesterol and plasma triglyceride

### Fibric acid derivatives

These drugs have been available for over 20 years for clinical use. Clofibrate, the first drug of this class, was introduced in 1962 and was found to be more effective in lowering plasma triglycerides (~20 per cent) than in lowering plasma cholesterol. Clofibrate was chosen for the WHO primary prevention trial, and although it reduced coronary morbidity, there was no effect on coronary mortality, and all-cause mortality was increased, with a higher incidence of death due to liver, gallbladder, intestinal and pancreatic disease.[75] For this reason clofibrate has largely become obsolete. However, the recent re-analysis of the WHO trial findings on an intention-to-treat basis does not show significant increases in violent or accidental deaths or cancer.[76] Nevertheless, there is no doubt that clofibrate increases the lithogenicity of bile and therefore precipitates gallstone formation. Newer agents of this class are more effective on plasma lipids and have less effect on biliary cholesterol concentration.

The precise mechanisms of action of the fibrates remain to be fully determined and certainly from their differing effects on lipid and lipoprotein concentrations it is likely that the various fibrates differ quantitatively if not qualitatively in their impact on important aspects of lipoprotein metabolism. The most well documented effect is on the stimulation of the lipoprotein lipase enzyme which is responsible for the catabolism of triglyceride-rich particles.[77] In addition, they may reduce VLDL production in the liver and this may be partly explained by their effect in decreasing the flow of free fatty acids, the major substrate for hepatic triglyceride production. Effects have also been demonstrated on the clearance of plasma LDL cholesterol, possibly through non-specific effects in decreasing cholesterol synthesis and therefore increasing receptor activity or through the modification of LDL such that it is more likely to be taken up by the LDL receptor.[78] Some of the fibrate class have been demonstrated to have effects on other factors important in vascular risk such as fibrinogen, and some fibrates have a small effect in decreasing blood glucose concentrations.

The major effects of the fibrates are on plasma triglycerides, with reductions of 50–60 per cent. They also increase HDL cholesterol levels by 15–20 per cent. The effect of fibrates on LDL cholesterol depends on the type of hyperlipidaemia. In isolated hypercholesterolaemia or mixed hyperlipidaemia, reductions in LDL cholesterol of 10–25 per cent have been demonstrated. However, in isolated hypertriglyceridaemia (WHO type IV), where LDL concentrations tend to be low, LDL can actually increase on fibrate therapy. There is no doubt that the newer fibrates are more potent than the original member of this class, clofibrate, and the fibrates certainly differ in their effect on LDL cholesterol.

The fibrates are generally well tolerated and, fortunately, serious side-effects are very rare.

Abnormalities of liver function are sometimes noted and myopathy has been reported occasionally, particularly in patients with impaired renal function. Care needs to be taken when fibrates are used in patients taking anticoagulants, as the fibrates may potentiate the anticoagulant activity.

It is encouraging that the Helsinki Heart Study, which used gemfibrozil,[79] showed considerable reduction in coronary events in the gemfibrozil-treated group and the concerns raised in terms of safety in the WHO clofibrate trial[75] did not appear to be a feature in this study.

### Nicotinic acid

The lipid-lowering activity of nicotinic acid was first described in the 1950s.[80] Its lipid-lowering activity is only seen at high dose and is completely separate from its role as a vitamin. It needs to be distinguished from nicotinamide, which lacks lipid-lowering ativity. At high dose, nicotinic acid inhibits hepatic VLDL production. However, the detailed mechanisms leading to this effect are not fully understood. At doses of 3 g/day significant reductions are observed in both plasma cholesterol and triglyceride, with often a marked increase in HDL cholesterol. In fact, in terms of effects on the lipid profile, nicotinic acid can be considered a broad-spectrum agent. However, its use is limited by its acceptability to patients. Many patients have uncomfortable flushing reactions with the drug and this leads to discontinuation of therapy in many individuals. With perseverance there is tachyphylaxis to flushing but this will return immediately if dosage is omitted. Gastrointestinal upsets are also common, with nausea, vomiting, diarrhoea and abdominal cramps. The cutaneous flushing seems to be prostaglandin mediated in that it can be blocked partly by aspirin. Nicotinic acid treatment may also adversely affect glucose tolerance, it may increase uric acid levels, and, rarely, serious hepatotoxicity has been described.

Nicotinic acid was part of the combination therapy used in some regression trials[54–56] and was one of the modalities of treatment tested in the Coronary Drug Project, where it was associated with a reduced incidence of non-fatal myocardial infarction.[81] Furthermore, the long-term follow-up of the nicotinic acid group of the Coronary Drug Project showed a reduced overall mortality.[82] Nicotinic acid analogues have been developed in an attempt to overcome some of the side-effects with nicotinic acid. Acipimox, 5′-methylpyrazine carboxylic acid 4-oxide, is chemically related to nicotinic acid and probably has a similar mechanism of action. It appears to be better tolerated than nicotinic acid; however, it is probably not as potent.

## HMG-CoA reductase inhibitors

The introduction of this new class of agents into clinical practice represents a landmark in the treatment of hyperlipidaemia.[83] They were discovered in the 1970s in the culture broths of various fungus species. They are specific competitive inhibitors of the enzyme HMG-CoA reductase, which catalyses the first committed step in cholesterol synthesis. This is important in the sense that previous inhibitors of cholesterol synthesis which acted at a much later stage in the synthetic pathway led to the accumulation of large sterol intermediates and were found to be toxic. These intermediates do not occur with the HMG-CoA reductase inhibitors. The main action of the drugs is on the liver, which is the major organ for LDL catabolism, and as a result of decreased hepatic cholesterol synthesis the LDL receptor activity is upregulated and this leads to increased removal of plasma LDL

through the physiological LDL receptor pathway. As a result, plasma LDL concentrations are reduced by over a third. There is some evidence that these compounds may also decrease hepatic lipoprotein production. In addition to the dramatic effects on LDL cholesterol, modest effects are seen in reducing plasma triglycerides (10–20 per cent) and small increases in HDL have been observed (5–10 per cent).

The reductase inhibitors can be given once daily in the evening and are generally well tolerated. Occasionally elevated hepatic enzymes are observed which appear to be readily reversible without any clinical consequence. Very rarely, myositis has been observed with muscle pain and marked elevation of plasma creatine kinase. These isolated reports have tended to be in patients on multiple drug regimes, particularly involving cyclosporin, nicotinic acid and gemfibrozil. Myositis is also more likely to occur if the drugs are used in patients with hepatic disease, which is a relative contraindication. Concern was raised about the possibility of these inhibitors of cholesterol synthesis giving rise to cataract based on previous experience with inhibitors of cholesterol synthesis at a much later stage in the synthetic pathway. However, there is no clinical evidence of there being a problem of cataract formation with the HMG-CoA reductase inhibitors. In addition there is no evidence of clinically significant effects of the drugs on other major products of the cholesterol synthetic pathway, particularly steroid hormones, ubiquinones and dolichols.[84] There are ongoing studies looking at the effects of these new agents in both the primary and secondary prevention trials. The FATS regression trial[55] and also the regression trial in familial hypercholesterolaemia[56] incorporated an HMG-CoA reductase inhibitor into the combination drug therapy used.

## Drugs which lower plasma triglyceride alone

### Omega-3 fatty acids

Fish oil capsules containing principally eicosa-pentanoic acid and docosahexanoic acid are available for clinical use in several countries, including the UK. In high dose, fish oils reduce hepatic VLDL production. At the recommended dosage (10 capsules/day) these agents are effective in lowering triglyceride, particularly when triglyceride levels are very high, such as in type V hyperlipidaemia. At this dose no effect on plasma cholesterol levels is observed.

## An approach to drug therapy

The epidemiological and clinical findings from both the secondary prevention trials and the regression trials point to an important role for lipid-lowering therapy in the patient with established coronary disease. Nevertheless, lipid-lowering therapy should be seen as part of an overall risk-reduction strategy and should only be introduced after appropriate dietary therapy. However, the threshold for use of hypolipidaemic agents should be lower in these high-risk patients. The choice of hypolipidaemic agent will depend on the individual lipoprotein profile.[85] I have summarized the actions of the various hypolipidaemic agents in Table 7.2 and have given a guide to the use of these agents in the different lipoprotein abnormalities (Table 7.3). In severe hyperlipidaemia, combination drug therapy using agents that have complementary actions on lipoprotein metabolism can often achieve satisfactory lipid levels.[86]

## If I had ...

This would be a somewhat embarrassing proposition in the sense that my academic and clinical life has been spent in advocating measures designed to prevent the development of early coronary heart disease. However, I suppose it would be possible in a loose sense to attribute this to the stresses and the strains of medical life, both clinical and academic, in London post-Tomlinson Report. Assuming after my coronary that my myocardium could remember to a certain extent what its function was, I would be keen to correct all the possible risk factors that I could correct. I am entirely convinced about the relationship of lipids and lipoproteins to risk of subsequent events and to this end I would endeavour to achieve not just the targets of the recent consensus statements as indicated in this chapter but would rather go along with the suggestions of La Rosa and colleagues.[60] I am taken with the view that in someone who has established coronary disease an alteration towards a less atherogenic lipoprotein profile should be advocated whatever the initial levels and that reducing what in the healthy individual would be only a modest elevation in LDL cholesterol, for instance, is likely to be beneficial. I would wish therefore to have my own LDL cholesterol reduced to around 2 mmol/l if my primary abnormality was hypercholesterolaemia. By achieving such a low LDL cholesterol level I would expect not only to delay progression of my atherosclerosis but to actually induce regression. How would I achieve this? Well, I would try very hard with lifestyle measures, particularly weight reduction and reducing dietary saturated fat. As I like fish and poultry and game I think I could still eat very well despite the diet guidelines. If I had to take lipid-lowering agents and I only needed to achieve a small additional LDL

| Drug class | Mechanism of action | Metabolic effects | Plasma lipoproteins | | |
|---|---|---|---|---|---|
| | | | LDL | HDL | VLDL |
| Bile-acid sequestrants | Interruption of enterohepatic circulation of bile salts leading to increased hepatic bile acid synthesis and enhanced LDL receptor activity | Increased LDL clearance through the LDL receptor | ↓↓↓ | ↑ | →↑ |
| Nicotinic acid | Inhibition of adipose tissue lipolysis and reduction of free fatty acid flux to liver | Decreased VDL and LDL synthesis; decreased clearance of HDL | ↓↓ | ↑↑↑↑ | ↓↓↓ |
| Fibric acid derivatives | Increased lipoprotein lipase; reduced hepatice VLDL and apolipoprotein B production; ? increased LDL receptor activity | Increased VLDL catabolism; increased synthesis of HDL | ↓ | ↑↑ | ↓↓↓ |
| Probucol | LDL modification; antioxidant | Enhanced LDL clearance through non-receptor pathways; ? decreased synthesis of HDL | ↓ | ↓ | ↑ |
| HMG-CoA reductase | Competitive inhibition of early stage in cholesterol synthesis leading to increased LDL receptor activity | Enhanced LDL clearance through the LDL receptor | ↓↓↓ | ↑ | → |

*Source*: Betteridge.[86]

**Table 7.2**

| Dyslipoproteinaemia | Drug therapy | | |
| --- | --- | --- | --- |
| | First-line agents | Second-line agents | Combination therapy |
| Familial lipoprotein lipase deficiency | None | None | None |
| Heterozygous familial hyperlipidaemia | Reductase inhibitors, resins, nicotinic acid | Fibrates, probucol | Resins + reductase inhibitors, resin + nicotinic acid, resins + fibrates |
| Familial combined hyperlipidaemia | Fibrates, nicotinic acid | Reductase inhibitors | Resins + fibrates, resins + nicotinic acid, (statins + fibrates) |
| Remnant particle disease (type III, dysbetalipoproteinaemia) | Fibrates, nicotinic acid | Reductase inhibitors | |
| Familial hypertriglyceridaemia | Fibrates, nicotinic acid | | Fibrates + nicotinic acid |
| Polygenic hypercholesterolaemia | Resins, reductase inhibitors | Fibrin probucol | |

Source: Betteridge.[86]

**Table 7.3**
*Therapeutic options for treatment of primary dyslipidaemias.*

reduction then I would take a low-dose resin, no more than two packets before my evening meal. Anything beyond this and I would take a low-dose statin. If I had severe hypercholesterolaemia I would take the combination of the resin and the statin.

I would be on less sure ground if my lipid abnormality consisted of hypertriglyceridaemia with a low HDL cholesterol. Having said that I think the balance of evidence points to an important role for this dyslipidaemia in atherosclerosis, I would take comfort from some of the secondary prevention trials, particularly the Stockholm study, which suggested an important relationship between reducing triglyceride levels and reducing subsequent risk.[87] Therefore, if dietary measures failed to reduce my triglycerides below 2.3 and to increase my HDL cholesterol above 0.9, I would take a hypolipidaemic agent and I would choose to take one of the fibrate compounds. I would tell myself that in addition to correcting the lipid abnormality this compound would be likely to lower my fibrinogen and, if preliminary reports are to be believed, also lower my lipoprotein (a) slightly.

Perhaps the most difficult lipid abnormality to treat is severe mixed hyperlipidaemia and this is the abnormality I would least like to have to deal with personally. There is no doubt that theoretically the combination of a statin and a fibrate is attractive in this situation but the risk of side-effects is increased. However, despite this I would happily take a statin and a fibrate if I had premature coronary disease and severe mixed dyslipidaemia. I would be on the look out for muscle symptoms particularly, and would have a 3-monthly check of my liver enzymes and my creatine phosphokinase (CPK). Second best would be a resin and a fibrate.

Like all my patients with severe dyslipidaemias I would hope that my cardiology colleagues would submit me to an annual exercise electrocardiogram and I would trust their skill with the angioplasty balloon as necessary and if appropriate would submit myself to the surgeon. As a mere physician I never cease to marvel at seeing patients who appear so well just a few days after coronary artery bypass surgery.

# References

1 Smith GD, Pekkanen J, Should there be a moratorium on the use of cholesterol lowering drugs? *Br Med J* (1992) **304**:431–4.

2 Martin MJ et al, Serum cholesterol, blood pressure and mortality: implications from a cohort of 361,662 men, *Lancet* (1986) ii:933–6.

3 Chen Z et al, Serum cholesterol concentration and coronary heart disease in a population with low cholesterol concentrations, *Br Med J* (1991) **303**:276–82.

4 Brown MS, Goldstein JL, Receptor-mediated control of cholesterol metabolism, *Science* (1986) **191**:150–4.

5 Goldstein JL et al, Binding site on macrophages that mediates uptake and degradation of acetylated low density lipoprotein producing massive cholesterol deposition, *Proc Natl Acad Sci USA* (1979) **76**:333–7.

6 Scientific Steering Committee on behalf of the Simon Broome Register Group, Risk of fatal coronary heart disease in familial hypercholesterolaemia, *Br Med J* (1991) **303**:893–6.

7 Ross R, The pathogenesis of atherosclerosis—an update, *New Engl J Med* (1986) **314**:488–500.

8 Kodama T et al, Type I macrophage scavenger receptor contains α helical and collagen-like coils, *Nature* (1990) **343**:531–5.

9 Steinberg D et al, Beyond cholesterol. Modifications of low density lipoprotein that increase the atherogenicity, *New Engl J Med* (1989) **320**:915–24.

10 Kita T et al, Probucol prevents the progression of atherosclerosis in Watanabe heritable hyperlipidaemic rabbit, an animal model for familial hypercholesterolaemia, *Proc Natl Acad Sci USA* (1987) **84**:5928–31.

11 Tall AR, Plasma high density lipoproteins. Metabolism and relationship to atherosclerosis, *J Clin Invest* (1990) **86**:379–84.

12 Miller NE, High density lipoprotein: a major risk factor for coronary atherosclerosis. *Clin Endocrinol Metab* (1987) **1**:603–22.

13 Oram JF, Brinton EA, Bierman EL, Regulation of HDL receptor activity in cultured human skin fibroblasts and human arterial smooth muscle cells, *J Clin Invest* (1983) **72**:1611–21.

14 Oram JF, Johnson CJ, Brown T-N, Interaction of high density lipoprotein with its receptor on cultured fibroblasts and macrophages, *J Biol Chem* (1987) **262**:2405–10.

15 Swenson TL, The role of the cholesteryl ester transfer protein in lipoprotein metabolism. *Diabetes Metab Rev* (1991) **7**:139–53.

16 Chen Y-DI, Reaven GM, Intestinally-derived lipoproteins: metabolism and clinical significance. *Diabetes Metab Rev* (1991) **7**:191–208.

17 Miller GJ, Miller NE, Plasma high density lipoprotein concentration and development of ischaemic heart disease, *Lancet* (1975) i:16–19.

18 Gordon DJ, Rifkind BM, High density lipoprotein—the clinical implications of recent studies. *New Engl J Med* (1989) **321**:1311–16.

19 Gordon DJ et al, High density lipoprotein cholesterol and cardiovascular disease: four prospective American studies, *Circulation* (1989) **79**:8–15.

20 Pocock SJ et al, High density lipoprotein cholesterol is not a major risk factor for ischaemic heart disease in British men, *Br Med J* (1986) **292**:515–19.

21 Knuiman JT et al, Total cholesterol and high density lipoprotein cholesterol levels in populations differing in fat and carbohydrate intake, *Arteriosclerosis* (1987) **7**:612–19.

22 Simons LA, Interrelations of lipids and lipoproteins with coronary artery disease mortality in 19 countries, *Am J Cardiol* (1986) **57**:5G–10G.

23 Betteridge DJ, High density lipoprotein and coronary heart disease, *Br Med J* (1989) **298**:974–5.

24 Hulley SB et al, Epidemiology as a guide to clinical decisions: the association between triglyceride and coronary heart disease, *New Engl J Med* (1980) **302**:1383–418.

25 Mahley RW, Rall SC, Type III hyperlipoproteinaemia (dysbetalipoproteinaemia). The role

of apolipoprotein E in normal and abnormal lipoprotein metabolism. In: Sriver CR, Beaudet AL, Sly WS, Valle D, eds. *The metabolic basis of inherited disease*, 6th edn (McGraw Hill: New York 1989) 1195–213.

26  Assmann G, Schulte H, Relation of high density lipoprotein cholesterol and triglycerides to incidence of atherosclerotic coronary artery disease (the PROCAM experience), *Am J Cardiol* (1992) **70**:733–7.

27  Manninen V et al, Joint effects of serum triglyceride and LDL cholesterol and HDL cholesterol concentrations on coronary heart disease risk in the Helsinki Heart Study. Implications for treatment, *Circulation* (1992) **85**:37–45.

28  Austin MA et al, Atherogenic lipoprotein phenotype: a proposed genetic marker for coronary heart disease risk, *Circulation* (1990) **82**:495–506.

29  Tribble DL et al, Variations in oxidative susceptibility among six low density lipoprotein subfractions of differing density and particle size, *Atherosclerosis* (1992) **93**:189–99.

30  McNamara JR et al, Effect of gender, age and lipid status on low density lipoprotein subfraction distribution. Results of the Framingham Offspring Study, *Arteriosclerosis* (1987) **7**:483–90.

31  Meade TW et al, Haemostatic function and cardiovascular death: principal results of the Northwick Park Heart Study, *Lancet* (1986) **ii**:533–7.

32  Carvalho de Sousa J et al, Coagulation factor VII and plasma triglycerides. Decreased catabolism as a possible mechanism of factor VII hyperactivity, *Haemostasis* (1989) **19**:125–30.

33  Hamsten A et al, Increased plasma levels of a rapid inhibitor of tissue plasminogen activator in young survivors of myocardial infarction, *New Engl J Med* (1985) **313**:1557–63.

34  International Committee for the Evaluation of Hypertriglyceridaemia as a Vascular Risk Factor. The Hypertriglyceridaemias: risk and management, *Am J Cardiol* (1991) **68**:1A–42A.

35  Scanu AM, Lipoprotein (a). *Baillière's Endocrinol Metab* (1990) **4**:939–46.

36  McLean JW et al, cDNA sequence of human apolipoprotein (a) is homologous to plasminogen, *Nature* (1987) **300**:132–7.

37  Utermann G, Lipoprotein (a): a genetic risk factor for premature coronary heart disease, *Curr Opinion Lipidol* (1990) **1**:404–10.

38  Seed M et al, Relation of serum lipoprotein (a) concentration and apolipoprotein (a) phenotype to coronary heart disease in patients with familial hypercholesterolaemia, *New Engl J Med* (1990) **322**:1494–9.

39  Zenker G et al, Lipoprotein (a) as a strong indicator for cerebrovascular disease, *Stroke* (1986) **17**:942–5.

40  Sirinivasan SR et al, Racial (black-white) differences in serum Lp(a) distribution and its relation to parenteral myocardial infarction in children. Bogalusa Heart Study, *Circulation* (1991) **84**:160–7.

41  Kostner GM, Krempler F, Lipoprotein (a), *Curr Opinion Lipidol* (1992) **3**:279–84.

42  Berg-Schmith E et al, The effect of n-3 polyunsaturated fatty acids on Lp(a), *Clin Chim Acta* (1991) **198**:271–8.

43  Brewer HB, Effectiveness of diet and drugs in the treatment of patients with elevated Lp(a) levels. In: Scanu AM, ed. *Lipoprotein (a)* (Academic Press: San Diego 1990) 211–20.

44  Cohen MV et al, Low rate of treatment of hypercholesterolaemia by cardiologists in patients with suspected and proven coronary artery disease, *Circulation* (1991) **83**:1294–304.

45  Schlant RC et al, The natural history of coronary heart disease: prognostic factors after recovery from myocardial infarction in 2789 men: the 5 year findings of the Coronary Drug Project, *Circulation* (1982) **66**:401–14.

46  Roussouw JE, Lewis B, Rifkind BM, The value of lowering cholesterol after myocardial infarction, *New Engl J Med* (1990) **323**:1112–19.

47  Coronary Drug Project Research Group, Natural history of myocardial infarction in the Coronary Drug Project: long term prognostic importance of serum lipid levels, *Am J Cardiol* (1978) **42**:489–98.

48  Shaper AG et al, Risk factors for ischaemic heart disease: the prospective phase of the British Regional Heart Study, *J Epidemiol Commun Health* (1985) **39**:197–209.

49  Pekkanen J et al, Ten year mortality from cardiovascular disease in relation to cholesterol level among men with and without pre-existing cardiovascular disease, *New Engl J Med* (1990) **322**:1700–7.

50  Rossouw JE, Canner PL, Hulley SB, Deaths from injury, violence and suicide in secondary prevention trials of cholesterol lowering, *New Engl J Med* (1991) **325**:1813.

51  Arntzemus AC et al, Diet, lipoproteins and the progression of coronary atherosclerosis. The Leyden Intervention Trial, *New Engl J Med* (1985) **312**:805–11.

52  Ornish D et al, Can lifestyle changes reverse coronary heart disease? *Lancet* (1990) **336**:129–33.

53  Brensike JF et al, Effects of therapy with cholestyramine on progression of coronary arteriosclerosis: results of the NHLB type II coronary intervention study, *Circulation* (1984) **69**:313–24.

54  Blankenhorn DH et al, Beneficial effects of combined colestipol-niacin therapy on coronary atherosclerosis and coronary venous bypass grafts, *JAMA* (1987) **257**:3233–40.

55  Brown G et al, Regression of coronary artery disease as a result of intensive lipid-lowering therapy in men with high levels of apolipoprotein B, *New Engl J Med* (1990) **323**:1289–98.

56  Kane JP et al, Regression of coronary atherosclerosis during treatment of familial hypercholesterolaemia with combined drug regimens, *JAMA* (1990) **264**:3007–12.

57  Watts GF et al, Effects on coronary artery disease of lipid-lowering diet or diet plus cholestyramine in the St Thomas' Atherosclerosis Regression Study (STARS), *Lancet* (1992) **339**:563–9.

58  Buchwald H et al, Effect of partial ileal bypass surgery on mortality and morbidity from coronary heart disease in patients with hypercholesterolaemia, *New Engl J Med* (1990) **323**:946–55.

59  Report of the National Cholesterol Education Program Expert Panel on Detection, Evaluation and Treatment of High Blood Cholesterol in Adults, *Arch Intern Med* (1988) **148**:36–69.

60  LaRosa JC, Cleeman JI, Cholesterol lowering as a treatment for established coronary heart disease, *Circulation* (1992) **85**:1229–35.

61  Friedewald WT, Levy RI, Frederickson DS, Estimation of the concentration of low density lipoprotein cholesterol in plasma without use of the preparative ultracentrifuge, *Clin Chem* (1972) **18**:499–502.

62  Prevention of coronary heart disease: scientific background and new clinical guidelines. Recommendations of the European Atherosclerosis Society prepared by the International Task Force for Prevention of Coronary Heart Disease, *Nutr Metab Cardiovasc Dis* (1992) **2**:113–56.

63  Ramsey L, Yeo W, Jackson P, Dietary reduction of serum cholesterol concentration: time to think again, *Br Med J* (1991) **303**:953–7.

64  Mattson FH, Grundy SM, Comparison of effects of dietary saturated, monounsaturated and polyunsaturated fatty acids on plasma lipids and lipoproteins in man, *J Lipid Res* (1985) **26**:194–202.

65  Riccardi G, Rivellese AA, An update on monounsaturated fatty acids, *Curr Opinion Lipidol* (1993) **4**:13–16.

66  Burr M et al, Effects of changes in fat, fish and fibre intakes on death and myocardial infarction, *Lancet* (1989) **2**:757–61.

67  Berlin JA, Coditz GA, A meta analysis of physical activity in the prevention of coronary heart disease, *Am J Epidemiol* (1990) **132**:612–28.

68  Shepherd J et al, Cholestyramine promotes receptor mediated low density lipoprotein catabolism, *New Engl J Med* (1980) **302**:1219–22.

69  Betteridge DG et al, Treatment of familial hypercholesterolaemia. United Kingdom lipid clinics study of pravastatin and cholestyramine, *Br Med J* (1992) **304**:1335–8.

70  Lipid Research Clinics Program. The lipid research clinics coronary primary prevention trial results. 1. Reduction in the incidence of coronary heart disease, *JAMA,* (1984) **251**:351–64.

71  Dachet C, Jacotot B, Buxtorf JC, The hypolipidaemic action of probucol. Drug transport and lipoprotein composition in type IIa hyperlipoproteinaemia, *Atherosclerosis* (1985) **58**: 261–8.

72  Steinberg D, Studies on the mechanism of action of probucol, *Am J Cardiol* (1986) **57**:16H–21H.

73 Yamamoto A et al, Effects of probucol on xanthomata regression in familial hypercholesterolaemia, *Am J Cardiol* (1986) **57**:29H–35H.

74 Romics L et al, The effects of probucol on QT/QS2 relation and systolic time intervals, *Int J Cardiol* (1988) **19**:303–8.

75 Committee of Principal Investigators, A cooperative trial in the primary prevention of ischaemic heart disease using clofibrate, *Br Heart J* (1978) **40**:1069–118.

76 Heady JA, Morris JN, Oliver MF, WHO clofibrate/cholesterol trial: clarifications, *Lancet* (1992) **340**:1405–6.

77 Heller F, Harvengt C, Effects of clofibrate, bezafibrate, fenofibrate and probucol on plasma lipolytic enzymes in normolipaemic subjects, *Eur J Clin Pharmacol* (1983) **25**:57–63.

78 Larsen ML, Illingworth DR, Triglyceride-lowering agents: fibrates and nicotinic acid, *Curr Opinion Lipidol* (1993) **4**:34–40.

79 Frick MH et al, Helsinki Heart Study: primary prevention trial with gemfibrozil in middle aged men with dyslipidaemia, *New Engl J Med* (1987) **317**:1237–45.

80 Altschul R, Hoffer A, Stephen JD, Influence of nicotinic acid on serum cholesterol in man, *Arch Biochem Biophys* (1955) **54**:558–9.

81 Coronary Drug Project Research Group, Clofibrate and niacin in coronary heart disease, *JAMA* (1975) **231**:360–81.

82 Canner PL et al, Fifteen year mortality in Coronary Drug Project patients: long term benefit with niacin, *J Am Coll Cardiol* (1986) **8**:1245–55.

83 Grundy SM, HMG-CoA reductase inhibitors for treatment of hypercholesterolemia, *New Engl J Med* (1988) **319**:24–33.

84 Mol MJTM, Stalenhoef AFH, HMG CoA reductase inhibitors, *Curr Opinion Lipidol* (1993) **4**:41–8.

85 Betteridge DJ et al, Detection and management of hyperlipidaemia. Guidelines of the British Hyperlipidaemia Association, *Postgrad Med J* (1993) **69**:359–69.

86 Betteridge DJ, Combination drug therapy for dyslipidaemia, *Curr Opinion Lipidol* (1993) **4**:49–55.

87 Carlson LA, Rosenhamer G, Reduction of mortality in the Stockholm Ischaemic Heart Disease Secondary Prevention Study by combined treatment with lofibrate and nicotinic acid, *Acta Med Scand* (1988) **223**:405–18.

# 8

## Wolff–Parkinson–White syndrome
*Ronald WF Campbell*

## Introduction

Why should Wolff–Parkinson–White (WPW) syndrome be included in a textbook devoted to 'difficult cardiology'? Surely more is known and understood about this condition and its management than almost any other cardiovascular problem? In fact, the difficulties arise because of that knowledge. Sudden death is a very rare but well-recognized first presentation of the condition[1,2] but truly curative therapy is theoretically available to all in whom the condition is diagnosed.[3,4] Population screening, accuracy of risk prediction and the safety of curative treatment are some of the 'difficult' aspects of WPW management.[5] To appreciate why these pose a clinical challenge, the facts of WPW syndrome need to be reviewed.

## The arrhythmias

The accessory pathway which is the basis of WPW syndrome supports two arrhythmias—reciprocating tachycardia and atrial fibrillation. Reciprocating tachycardia[6] is the commoner arrhythmia. It is macro re-entrant, and in its usual manifestation as orthodromic reciprocating tachycardia, the wavefront travels from the atria through the AV node to the ventricles, returning to the atria via the accessory pathway. The pathway participates as the link

for ventriculo-atrial conduction, being used in a retrograde direction. As originally defined, WPW syndrome comprises the surface ECG features of a delta wave and a 'short PR' interval (strictly, the PQ (onset of QRS) is short while the PR (R-wave peak in the QRS) is often normal) in association with arrhythmias.[7] Some individuals have accessory pathways capable of conduction in only a retrograde direction: they can have orthodromic reciprocating tachycardia but their surface ECG is normal. It requires anterograde conduction to create the 'short PR' interval and the delta wave. Strictly, then, these individuals do not have WPW syndrome but are usually, although perhaps inaccurately, considered to have the condition. Importantly, because they lack anterograde conduction over the accessory pathway, they are not at risk of rapid ventricular response rates in the event that they develop atrial fibrillation. Patients with concealed accessory pathways, then, are at low or no risk of sudden death related to their pathway.

The mechanism by which atrial fibrillation arises in WPW syndrome is disputed.[8,9] In the event that it occurs, the normal rate-limiting function of the AV node is bypassed, with resultant rapid ventricular response rates.[10] Ventricular activation may be by conduction over either the AV node or the accessory pathway. In the former case, narrow normal QRS complexes are seen, while when the latter is the route of conduction, pre-excited QRS complexes occur. Often there is fusion, which occurs when conduction is in parallel over both routes. The maximum ventricular rate in atrial fibrillation will usually occur when conduction is exclusively over the accessory pathway, in which circumstance fully or maximally pre-excited QRS complexes are produced. The shortest coupling interval between consecutive pre-excited complexes and atrial fibrillation correlates with the refractory period of the accessory pathway and also correlates with the risk of ventricular fibrillation and sudden death.[8,11]

Accessory pathway physiology is sometimes likened to that of conduction over a copper wire, but this gross oversimplification has dangers. Accessory pathway conduction is dynamic. Accessory pathway behaviour is importantly modified by the phenomenon of concealed retrograde penetration or 'linking', whereby impulses which have been conducted over the AV node to the ventricle or which arise spontaneously in the ventricle (e.g. ventricular ectopic beats) invade the ventricular end of the accessory pathway and modify (usually slow) or block anterograde conduction.[12] Thus even 'fast' accessory pathways may appear 'slow' in atrial fibrillation when this phenomenon is modulating anterograde conduction. Release of accessory pathway conduction will occur if retrograde penetration is removed, as for instance if an AV nodal blocking drug is given.[13,14] Ventricular response rates to atrial fibrillation may rise dramatically.

Accessory pathway conduction is also affected by catecholamines, and assessment of accessory pathway conduction capability performed at basal conditions may erroneously identify an accessory pathway as of little intrinsic risk, yet when isoprenaline is given or exercise undertaken a markedly increased conduction capability is exposed.[15] The association of sudden death and ventricular fibrillation with exercise in WPW syndrome patients underscores the importance of sympathetic tone in modulation of the arrhythmias.[11]

The macro re-entrant nature of orthodromic reciprocating tachycardia and its counter-circulating sister—antedromic reciprocating tachycardia—is well established and has been proven by catheter studies[2] and by peroperative mapping.[16] The majority of WPW syndrome arrhythmias are supported by accessory atrioventricular connections which behave electrophysiologically as undifferentiated atrial tissue. Their insertion into atrial and ventricular muscle provides some modest opportunity for decremental conduction to occur but this is not usually evident.[17]

## The surface ECG

The mechanisms for the delta wave and for the 'short PR' interval are well established. The delta wave represents the myocardium which is invaded by the activation wavefront carried by the accessory pathway. This has been shown by peroperative mapping studies. The delta wave characteristics have been used to predict the anatomical site of the accessory pathway.[2] One dimension of the accessory pathway is fixed—it must be in the plane of the atrioventricular ring. The other two dimensions are crudely reflected by the delta wave characteristics. Initially, separation of location of accessory pathways was suggested, as by type A (RBBB type QRS in V1) or type B (LBBB or more 'normal' QRS in V1).[18] Subsequently, there have been many refinements and a surprising degree of accuracy is now possible.[19,20] Nonetheless, there are caveats. Maximal pre-excitation should be present: the more conduction there is over the

AV node, the more the QRS will reflect ventricular activation by the His-Purkinje network rather than by the accessory pathway. The atrial insertion of left lateral accessory pathways is the last part or at least a late part of the atria to be activated by sinus node activation of the atria and thus with these pathways it is notoriously difficult to produce maximal pre-excitation short of pacing the left atrium or coronary sinus.[21] Indeed, the presence of left lateral accessory pathways may be completely masked by AV nodal conduction and exposed only when there is AV nodal block. Left lateral accessory pathways with short refractory periods are as easily concealed by this mechanism as long refractory period accessory pathways. Their concealment is not due to their intrinsic characteristics but to the nature and timing of their electrical input.

The anatomical position of the heart affects the surface ECG but surprisingly this is not incorporated as a correction factor in any of the schemes for predicting accessory pathway location from delta wave characteristics. The presence of multiple accessory pathways (not as uncommon as generally thought,[11] particularly in those at risk of serious arrhythmias) is rarely revealed by delta wave analysis except when one pathway is blocked and the other(s) are exposed. Nonetheless, QRS delta wave analysis is useful for planning diagnostic and therapeutic electrophysiological procedures. In WPW syndrome with delta waves, activation of the heart is abnormal and so too is repolarization. Abnormal T-waves are expected when pre-excitation exists. Isopotential body surface mapping of T-waves may also be used to reveal accessory pathway location and has been suggested as being more accurate and more sensitive than delta wave vector analysis.[22] For the present, and probably for the foreseeable future, isopotential body surface mapping is a field for experts: its analysis is not simple; the analysis equipment is expensive and multipoint data acquisition is not as clinically friendly as with the standard 12-lead ECG.

## Prognosis

The risk of sudden death in WPW syndrome exists, is widely recognized but probably is greatly exaggerated. This phenomenon has been documented by published case reports— usually of those successfully resuscitated from out-of-hospital sudden death events[11,12,23]—or by the observation of electrophysiologically induced reciprocating tachycardia degenerating through atrial fibrillation to ventricular fibrillation. But how great is the risk and can it be predicted? In the past, there have been suggestions that sudden unexpected death in apparently normal individuals in whom post mortems reveal no abnormality might have been caused by WPW syndrome. It is nearly impossible to investigate this hypothesis. Whilst accessory pathways can be found by modern histopathological techniques,[24] these procedures are immensely time-consuming, involving, as they do, serial sections of the complete AV ring and the tedious tracing of myofibrillar strands. Whilst it would be tempting to ascribe at least some of the sudden unexpected deaths in normal individuals to WPW syndrome, there is really little evidence for this. Were it to be true, then significant mortalities might be expected in patient cohorts who are prospectively followed. Such has not proved the case[25] and it seems that the sudden death risk of WPW syndrome has been exaggerated. Nonetheless, patients can and do die because of accessory pathways. These usually are young individuals who, apart from the rogue fibre bridging the AV groove, are

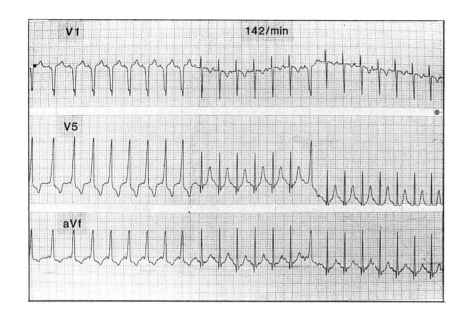

**Figure 8.1**
*Exercise test in patient with WPW syndrome. Note the abrupt disappearance of pre-excitation at a heart rate of 142 beats/min. Later, an electrophysiology study disclosed the antegrade refractory of the accessory pathway to be 380 ms.*

normal and would have had a normal prognosis and an expectation of a high quality of life. With the advent of safe curative therapies for WPW syndrome the problem is *theoretically* soluble.

## Prediction of risk

Obviously, patients who have already suffered a cardiac arrest due to WPW syndrome have a high-risk accessory pathway. The risk of a repetition of the event is near certain as, although accessory pathways may undergo an aging process,[26] this tends to be very slow if it occurs at all. There are no *resting ECG* features which predict sudden death risk other

than that an accessory pathway exists and that it has anterograde conduction capability (delta waves are present). The 'shortening' of the PR interval is not a risk indication—it as much reflects the anatomy of the atrial input as it does any aspect of intrinsic accessory pathway function.

The *exercise ECG* is more useful. If on exercise there is a *sudden* loss of the delta wave, the heart rate at which this occurs roughly correlates with the accessory pathway refractory period and usually a 'safe' pathway can be inferred (Figure 8.1). Gradual loss of the delta wave, which is more commonly seen, reflects changing AV nodal physiology under catecholamine stress and gives *no* information on accessory pathway risk.

Some have advocated that *acute anti-arrhythmic drug administration* can reveal safe (long refractory period) accessory pathways.[27,28] This is based on observations that long refractory period accessory pathways seem more susceptible to anti-arrhythmic agents.[29] Whilst there is a general truth in this, it is not reliable. Even high-risk short refractory period accessory pathways may sometimes be blocked by acute intravenous anti-arrhythmic therapy and so misleadingly suggest that they have a long refractory period. Part of the problem may lie with the lack of catecholamine stress in these tests.

Artificial *induction of atrial fibrillation* by either direct intra-atrial pacing or by transoesophageal atrial pacing is simple and relatively reliable. The shortest RR interval in atrial fibrillation is a good indication of the accessory pathway refractory period[8,11] and, further, the observed clinical response (heart rate, blood pressure, symptoms) reveals much about what might happen in the event of a spontaneous occurrence. A criticism remains that sympathetic activation is not routinely a part of the test.

A *multi-catheter electrophysiological study* will give the most accurate picture of accessory pathway characteristics.[30,31] The antegrade and retrograde refractory period of the pathway and its conduction capabilities can be assessed, as can responsiveness to drugs. Notwithstanding, these assessments are usually made in a resting state and although sedatives are often withheld for electrophysiological studies, it has been less common than is perhaps desirable to administer isoprenaline in the complete assessment of accessory pathway risks. Exercise or even standing may add information about the sympathetic responsiveness of the pathway,[32] but neither are easy to incorporate into invasive electrophysiological studies.

# Treatment

WPW syndrome arrhythmias are eminently treatable. Palliative treatment is provided by drugs given on a regular basis to modify accessory pathway physiology or given intermittently to abort established tachycardias. Curative treatment is also available using either surgery, direct current (DC) ablation or radiofrequency (RF) ablation. Antitachycardia pacing no longer has a place in management.

## Medical therapy

The aim of medical treatment is to block conduction in the accessory pathway or to markedly alter the refractory period of the accessory pathway. Most drugs also alter the echo window or the tachycardia initiation zone but, although of electrophysiological interest, this is of less practical relevance. Medical therapy for WPW syndrome can be very successful. Class Ic drugs such as flecainide and propafenone can provide very satisfactory arrhythmia control.[33,34] For this indication ('SVT' management), there is no evidence of the problem of increased mortality that was observed when flecainide was used in suppressing asymptomatic ventricular ectopic beats in survivors of acute myocardial infarction.[35] In the USA, procainamide, quinidine and disopyramide are used widely for the control of WPW syndrome arrhythmias and, whilst again successful,[29] these agents have the drawback of a moderate incidence of unwanted effects. Beta-blockers have some role to play. They are relatively well tolerated but do little to alter the basal electrophysiology of accessory pathways. Rather they prevent the catecholamine-dependent refractory period changes which may be pivotal in some patients for tachycardia initiation. Calcium entry blocking drugs are also prescribed. They alter the AV nodal component of the circuit, but as they leave the accessory pathway itself unaffected, they will not reduce risk in the event of atrial fibrillation occurring when anterograde accessory pathway function is present. By blocking the AV node and perhaps removing retrograde concealed penetration of the accessory pathway, they may even encourage higher transmission capability across the accessory pathway.[13] Amiodarone is one of the most effective anti-arrhythmic drugs for managing WPW syndrome.[36,37] It is well tolerated and has the advantage that it may stabilize atrial electrophysiology and so provide some protection against the development of atrial fibrillation. Its long half-life is a great advantage as the often young patients afflicted by the syndrome are those most likely to be non-compliant with therapy. Amiodarone does have problems, however. WPW syndrome is a chronic condition necessitating long-term therapy. With time a significant proportion of treated patients will develop unwanted effects of amiodarone therapy and although most, with the possible exception of advanced pulmonary fibrosis and peripheral neuropathy, are reversible on stopping therapy, they nonetheless are potentially dangerous.

## Surgery

Surgery was a remarkable development in the late 1960s.[38] That a conduction pathway invisible to the naked eye could be mapped so precisely as to allow curative surgery, even today represents a great achievement. Surgery is very successful and has until very recently been the treatment of choice for those with life-threatening accessory pathways. Had the surgery been less major it would have been applied much more widely. Large surgical series have been reported.[3,39] Most achieved a better than 95 per

cent success rate for permanent abolition of accessory pathway function (= cure) but most also reported an occasional surgical death. It is naive to expect that such a procedure, necessitating as it usually does normothermic cardiopulmonary bypass, can be performed without risk. The small but measurable surgical risk needs to be placed in perspective with the calculated risk of the condition itself—a comparison that is by no means easy to make.

## DC ablation

With the success of DC AV nodal ablation, attention turned to the possibility of catheter ablation of accessory pathways. Reasonable success rates can be achieved,[40] but there have also been anecdotal reports of disasters, particularly with the blast effect of DC energy delivered in the confines of the coronary sinus. Whilst technically feasible, the procedure has given way to the similar but probably safer radiofrequency technique (RF ablation).

## RF ablation

Radiofrequency ablation of accessory pathway is safe and effective (Figure 8.2). The lesion size is much smaller than that created by DC energy and so localization of the accessory pathway must be much more accurate. Remarkable success rates (99 per cent) have been reported in even the earliest series,[4] though some of the successes involved considerable periods of time in the electrophysiological laboratory (>12 h!). Deaths have occurred with RF ablation and there are anecdotes of cerebral vascular accidents and non-fatal cardiac perforation. These are to be expected. The technique involves the remote delivery of destructive energy. Risks are present but seem very low; almost certainly lower than those of DC ablation and of surgery. RF ablation is now

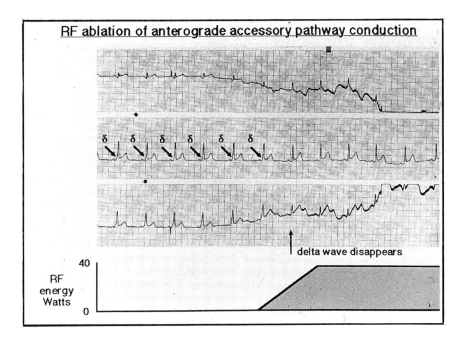

**Figure 8.2**
*Radiofrequency ablation of an accessory pathway. Note that the delta wave disappears within two beats of the start of RF energy delivery. No evidence of the pathway has returned over long-term follow-up and the patient is now asymptomatic.*

being enthusiastically pursued in hundreds of cardiac centres. Its development has revitalized clinical electrophysiology but there is a need for caution if the initially spectacular results obtained by experts are to be repeated by less well-trained cardiologists sometimes working away from surgical rescue facilities.

## WPW syndrome—what are the difficulties?

### Is there any role for medical therapy given the availability of RF ablation?

RF ablation is the treatment of choice for high-risk accessory pathways and for those patients with symptomatic arrhythmias unresponsive to medical therapy. Extending the indications of RF ablation to patients who need to take medical therapy is attractive; it offers a cure rather than palliation and often can be performed as an integral part of an electrophysiological assessment of the patient's condition. Were there *no* risk with RF ablation the decision would be easy, but RF ablation carries a small risk: small, but probably greater than the risk to life posed by the majority of accessory pathways. That risk must be set against the detriments of medical therapy—the need to take therapy regularly; the long-term unwanted effects of therapy; the efficacy of therapy; the medico-legal consequences of taking drugs (some occupations will be excluded)—and also set against the unknown and unpredictable changes which might occur in the accessory pathway. RF ablation gives a true cure which must always be attractive, but the cost of that cure must be recognized.

## Is there any role for surgical therapy?

In many centres where WPW surgery was undertaken, *no* operations are now being performed. Are there any remaining situations where surgery should be considered? This is controversial. Electrophysiologists have shown that with patience (operator and patient) and with sometimes substantial radiation exposure, probably all accessory pathways can be abolished by RF energy. But RF ablation does not repair atrial septal defects, nor manage tricuspid regurgitation in Ebstein's anomaly, nor correct coronary artery disease. When there is coexisting structural cardiac disease, surgical division of accessory pathways may still have a place. Of course, it may be that in the electrophysiological work-up of the patient, it is easier to attempt RF ablation and reduce the complexity of the subsequent surgery to only the grosser anatomical abnormalities. Such a decision will depend upon individual circumstances. Some structural abnormalities are associated with multiple pathways, especially Ebstein's anomaly.[41] RF ablation needs to be individually directed to each accessory pathway, whilst a single surgical approach would tackle all at a stroke. Further, there are accessory pathways which are very difficult to destroy by RF energy. Pride may drive many electrophysiologists to ablate all, regardless of procedure time, but, sooner or later, practical issues may force a management plan that, after a predetermined time, RF ablation is abandoned in favour of a dependable surgical approach. It is certainly alarming to think that the surgical experience in accessory pathway management which has been won over the last 20 years may be lost in a very few years from now.

## Vocational pursuits and medico-legal considerations

Patients whose jobs and livelihood are threatened by diagnosis of WPW syndrome have in the past often been offered surgery to achieve cure. RF ablation is now the technique of choice and its success and relative safety suggests that this approach will now be extended. RF ablation has particular attraction for sportsmen and sportswomen in whom anti-arrhythmic drugs may be relatively ineffective (high catecholamine drive) or precluded by regulations. For them, surgical management has had the great detraction of a median sternotomy. RF risks must never be underestimated and should always be presented in detail to the patient, whose truly informed consent is mandatory.

## Exercise testing in WPW patients

By definition, in WPW patients with delta waves, activation of the ventricle is disturbed and so too is repolarization. T-wave vectors and shapes are abnormal. On exercise, the balance of activation of the ventricle, be it from the AV node and His-Purkinje system or over the accessory pathway, may change. No reliable information on ST-segment displacement or T-wave changes can be obtained. Even if accessory pathway conduction is abruptly lost on exercise (a feature suggesting a relatively long refractory period accessory pathway), the phenomenon of T-wave memory means that ST- and T-wave abnormalities may persist long after normalization of ventricular activation. The exercise ECG has no reliable diagnostic power for the detection of myocardial ischaemia in the setting of pre-excitation.

## Digoxin and WPW syndrome

One of the common presentations of WPW is with arrhythmias in the first year of life. Such 'SVTs' have traditionally been treated with digoxin, and excellent results are achieved. Yet digoxin is considered contraindicated for adult WPW syndrome patients as digoxin can significantly shorten the accessory pathway refractory period[42] (and may further aggravate the problem by its AV nodal effect altering concealed retrograde penetration). There is no consensus on when between the first year of life and adulthood digoxin's benefits turn to risk. I have managed a few adolescent patients who had cardiac arrests and who had had digoxin continued from infancy through childhood. It may be that the pubertal changes in cardiac electrophysiology (principally in the AV node) are a time of special risk posed by WPW. I suggest that the use of digoxin not be abandoned in infants presenting with WPW arrhythmias but that the drug be used for a restricted period of time and the need for represcription substantiated. I believe that digoxin should not be used beyond the age of 8 years for WPW syndrome tachycardia. I have no data to support this strategy but at the very least the suggestion may prompt some research of the problem.

## If I had ...

If I were asymptomatic and WPW syndrome were unexpectedly diagnosed on a routine ECG then:

1 If I were >25 years of age I would ignore it completely.
2 If I were <25 years I would undergo an exercise test. If, on exercise, there was a sudden loss of pre-excitation, I would be reassured and ignore the phenomenon. If pre-excitation persisted, I reluctantly would acknowledge the possibility of a high-risk accessory pathway. Although recognizing that the risk would probably be very small, I would seek an electrophysiological assessment of that risk with RF ablation available if the risks were found to be high.

In most countries there is inadequate provision to offer this approach to all. On that basis, the younger the individual, the more I would favour investigation. Most deaths appear to have been in young teenagers. Moreover, in them the ECG diagnosis could cause significant problems for future employment and insurance.

# References

1   Dreifus LS et al, Ventricular fibrillation: a possible mechanism of sudden death in patients with Wolff–Parkinson–White syndrome, *Circulation* (1971) **43**:520–7.

2   Gallagher JJ et al, The pre-excitation syndromes, *Prog Cardiovasc Dis* (1978) **20**:285–327.

3   Cox JL, Ferguson TB, Surgery for the Wolff–Parkinson–White syndrome: the endocardial approach. In: Cox JL, ed. *Seminars in thoracic and cardiovascular surgery* (W.B. Saunders Company, Harcourt Brace Jovanovich Inc.: Philadelphia 1989) 34–46.

4   Jackman WM et al, Catheter ablation of accessory atrioventricular pathways (Wolff–Parkinson–White syndrome) by radiofrequency current, *N Engl J Med* (1991) **324**:1660–2.

5   Murdock CJ et al, Management of the patient with Wolff–Parkinson–White syndrome, *Cardiology* (1990) **77**:151–65.

6   Wellens HJJ, Durrer D, The role of an accessory atrioventricular pathway in reciprocal tachycardia: observations in patients with and without the Wolff–Parkinson–White syndrome, *Circulation* (1975) **52**:58–72.

7   Wolff L, Parkinson J, White PD, Bundle branch block with short P-R interval in healthy young people prone to paroxysmal tachycardia. *Am Heart J* (1935) **5**:685.

8   Campbell RWF et al, Atrial fibrillation in the pre-excitation syndrome, *Am J Cardiol* (1977) **40**:514–20.

9   Haissaguerre M et al, Frequency of recurrent atrial fibrillation after catheter ablation of overt accessory pathways, *Am J Cardiol* (1992) **69**:493–7.

10  Pietersen AH, Andersen ED, Sandoe E, Atrial fibrillation in the Wolff–Parkinson–White syndrome, *Am J Cardiol* (1992) **70**:38A–43A.

11  Montaya PT et al, Ventricular fibrillation in the Wolff–Parkinson–White syndrome, *Eur Heart J* (1991) **12**:144–50.

12  Gonzalez MD, Greenspan AJ, Kidwell GA, Linking in accessory pathways. Functional loss of antegrade pre-excitation, *Circulation* (1991) **83**:1221–31.

13  Gulamhusein S, Ko P, Klein GJ, Ventricular fibrillation following verapamil in the Wolff–Parkinson–White syndrome, *Am Heart J* (1983) **106**:145–7.

14  Scheinman BD, Evans T, Acceleration of ventricular rate by fibrillation associated with the Wolff–Parkinson–White syndrome, *Br Med J* (1982) **285**:999–1000.

15  Chimienti M et al, Comparison of isoproterenol and exercise tests in asymptomatic subjects with Wolff–Parkinson–White syndrome, *PACE* (1992) **15**:1158 66.

16  Gallagher JJ, Kasell J, Epicardial mapping in the Wolff–Parkinson–White syndrome, *Circulation* (1978) **57**:854.

17  Centurion OA et al, Anterograde and retrograde decremental conduction over left-sided accessory atrioventricular pathways in the Wolff–Parkinson–White syndrome, *Am Heart J* (1993) **125**:1038–47.

18  Rosenbaum FF et al, The potential variations of the thorax and the esophagus in anomalous atrioventricular excitation (Wolff Parkinson White syndrome), *Am Heart J* (1945) **29**:281–326.

19  Reddy GV, Schamroth L, The localisation of bypass tracts in the Wolf–Parkinson–White syndrome from the surface electrocardiogram, *Am Heart J* (1987) **113**:984–93.

20  Bockeria LA, Revishvily AS, Poljakova IP, Body surface mapping and nontraditional ECG leads in patients with Wolff–Parkinson–White syndrome, *PACE* (1990) **13**:1110.

21  Garratt CJ et al, Use of adenosine during sinus rhythm as a diagnostic test for latent preexcitation, *Am J Cardiol* (1990) **65**:868–73.

22  Spach MS, Barr RC, Physiologic correlates and clinical application of isopotential surface maps. In: Hoffman I, Hamby RI, Glassman E, eds. *Vectorcardiography 2* (North Holland Publishing: Amsterdam 1971) 131–41.

23 Prystowsky EN et al, Wolff–Parkinson–White syndrome and sudden cardiac death, *Cardiology* (1987) **74**(suppl 2): 67–71.

24 Gallagher JJ et al, Anatomic substrates of the Wolff–Parkinson–White syndrome. In: Rosenbaum MB, Elizari MV, eds. *Frontiers of cardiac electrophysiology* (Martinus Nijhoff: Boston 1983) 689–701.

25 Krahn AD et al, The natural history of electrocardiographic preexcitation in men. The Manitoba Follow-up Study, *Ann Intern Med* (1992) **116**:456–60.

26 Fan W et al, Age-related changes in the clinical and electrophysiologic characteristics of patients with Wolff–Parkinson–White syndrome: comparative study between young and elderly patients, *Am Heart J* (1991) **122**:741–7.

27 Wellens HJJ et al, Use of procainamide in patients with the Wolff–Parkinson–White syndrome to disclose a short refractory period of the accessory pathway, *Am J Cardiol* (1982) **50**:1087–9.

28 Wellens HJJ et al, Use of ajamaline in patients with the Wolff–Parkinson–White syndrome to disclose a short refractory period of the accessory pathway, *Am J Cardiol* (1980) **45**:130–3.

29 Sellers TD et al, Effects of procainamide and quinidine sulphate in the Wolff–Parkinson–White syndrome, *Circulation* (1977) **55**:15–22.

30 Beckman KJ et al, The predictive value of electrophysiologic studies in untreated patients with Wolf–Parkinson–White syndrome, *J Am Coll Cardiol* (1990) **15**:640–7.

31 Leitch JW et al, Prognostic value of electrophysiology testing in asymptomatic patients with Wolff–Parkinson–White pattern, *Circulation* (1990) **82**:1718–23.

32 Butrous GS, Camm AJ, Effects of postural changes versus exercise on the electrophysiological parameters of the accessory pathway, *Am J Cardiol* (1991) **67**:1237–44.

33 Wiseman MN et al, A study of the use of flecainide acetate in the long-term management of cardiac arrhythmias, *PACE* (1990) **13**:767–75.

34 Breithardt G et al, Effects of propafenone in the Wolff–Parkinson–White syndrome: electrophysiologic finding and long term follow up, *Am J Cardiol* (1984) **54**:29–39D.

35 The Cardiac Arrhythmia Suppression Trial (CAST) Investigators, Preliminary report: effect of encainide and flecainide on mortality in a randomised trial of arrhythmia suppression after myocardial infarction, *New Engl J Med* (1989) **321**:406–12.

36 Feld G et al, Clinical and electrophysiologic effects of amiodarone in patients with atrial fibrillation complicating the Wolf–Parkinson–White syndrome, *Am Heart J* (1988) **115**:102–7.

37 Rosenbaum MB et al, Control of tachyarrhythmias associated with Wolff–Parkinson–White syndrome by amiodarone hydrochloride, *Am J Cardiol* (1974) **34**:215–20.

38 Cobb FR et al, Successful surgical interruption of the Bundle of Kent in a patient with Wolff–Parkinson–White syndrome, *Circulation* (1968) **38**:1018–29.

39 Misaki T, Iwa T, Surgical management of life-threatening arrhythmias, *Jpn Circ J* (1990) **54**:1349–55.

40 Warin JF et al, Catheter ablation of accessory pathways: technique and results in 248 patients, *PACE* (1990) **13**:1609–14.

41 Pressley JC et al, Effect of Ebstein's anomaly on short- and long-term outcome of surgically treated patients with Wolff–Parkinson–White syndrome, *Circulation* (1992) **86**:1147–55.

42 Sellers TD, Bashore TM, Gallagher JJ, Digitalis in the pre-excitation syndrome, *Circulation* (1977) **56**:260–7.

# 9

## Is there a benign form of ventricular tachycardia?

*Jaswinder S Gill and A John Camm*

## Introduction

It has generally become accepted that the presence of ventricular tachycardia (VT) in a patient is of serious prognostic import. Mortality in patients with VT is equivalent to that from some forms of neoplastic disease and may equate to that in patients with cardiac failure. This generalization certainly appears to be true when VT is associated with ischaemic heart disease, hypertrophic cardiomyopathy and dilated cardiomyopathy. However, in some instances, the presence of VT does not always appear to be associated with a poor prognosis, and indeed patients may be at no greater risk of cardiac arrest and sudden death than individuals in the general population. The identification of these forms of VT is examined and discussed in this chapter.

## Malignant forms of VT

### Ventricular tachycardia post-myocardial infarction

There is considerable evidence that patients with sustained VT following a myocardial infarction are at high risk of sudden cardiac death. Sustained VT occurs in approximately 5 per cent of patients hospitalized with acute myocardial infarction and this is the initiating arrhythmia in approximately 20 per cent of

patients with primary ventricular fibrillation in the hospital phase of infarction.[1] In patients with sustained VT not directly associated with acute myocardial infarction, approximately 70 per cent have had a previous myocardial infarction.[2,3] Sustained VT occurs in 5 per cent of patients in the first year after a myocardial infarction.[4] Although episodes of VT are less frequent the further the patient is from the myocardial infarction, VT has been known to present for the first time more than 10 years after the event. There is general agreement that patients with sustained VT following a myocardial infarction are at high risk of sudden cardiac death, and this has been amply documented in the literature.[5,6] In the study from Marchlinski et al,[7] of 40 patients with sustained VT within 3–65 days after myocardial infarction, only 20 were alive after an average follow-up of 20 months and 12 of 20 of these deaths were sudden. Similarly, Di Marco et al[8] report that of 53 patients with sustained VT or ventricular fibrillation 3–60 days after myocardial infarction, 24.5 per cent died in the follow-up period averaging 15–18 months. This is again confirmed by the study of Wilber et al,[9] who examined 166 survivors of out-of-hospital cardiac arrest, the majority of whom had had a previous myocardial infarction, and demonstrated that the incidence of recurrent cardiac arrest was 12 per cent at 1 year and 27 per cent at 5 years (Figure 9.1). Of these patients, sustained monomorphic VT

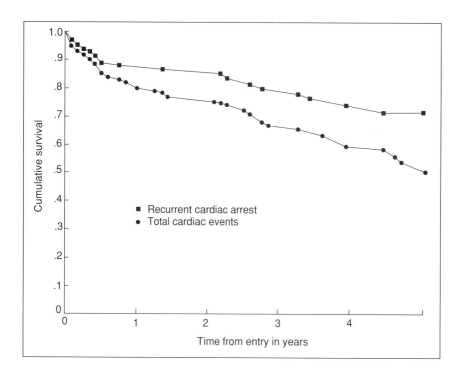

**Figure 9.1**
*Survival in subjects after cardiac arrest. The data represent 166 patients who survived out-of-hospital cardiac arrest, the majority of whom had underlying ischaemic heart disease. The curves demonstrate that approximately 20 per cent have suffered a recurrent cardiac arrest by 5 years, and over 40 per cent had suffered a cardiac event in this time period. (From Wilbor DJ et al, N Engl J Med (1988)* **318:19.***)*

was inducible at electrophysiological testing in 61 patients, ventricular fibrillation in 25 and non-sustained VT in 45, and all of these went on to have serial drug testing. Patients with inducible ventricular arrhythmia who were suppressed by drugs, or were non-inducible, had fewer recurrent cardiac arrests than patients who were inducible but non-suppressed (Figure 9.2). Furthermore, patients with an ejection fraction below 30 per cent had a consistently lower survival in all groups when compared to those with an ejection fraction above this level.

Patients with sustained VT following myocardial infarction, however, form only a small proportion of the patients who develop complex ventricular arrhythmias. A much larger group consists of patients with non-sustained VT identified either on exercise testing or on Holter monitoring. Several recent studies suggest that complex ventricular arrhythmias in the post-infarction patient are independent markers for future risk of sudden cardiac death,[10,11] but their sensitivity and specificity for identification of these cases is low.[12] Nevertheless, the presence of non-sustained ventricular tachycardia (≥3 ventricular ectopic beats (VPCs) at >100 beats/min and lasting <30 s) represents a strong marker for sudden cardiac death.[13–15]

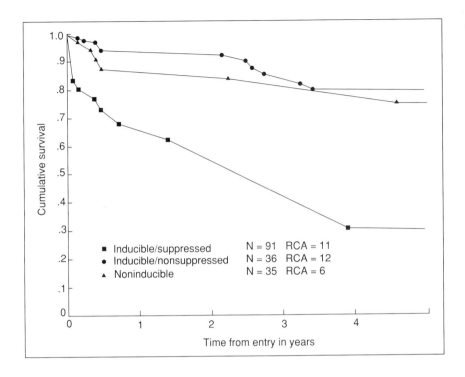

**Figure 9.2**
Survival in patients who were inducible and in those who were non-inducible at programmed stimulation in the same cohort as Figure 9.1. This demonstrates that patients who have ventricular arrhythmia which is inducible by programmed ventricular stimulation and suppressed by drug therapy have a better survival than patients with non-suppressed arrhythmia. RCA = recurrent cardiac arrests. (From Wilber DJ et al, N Engl J Med (1988) **318**:19.)

## Ventricular tachycardia in association with impaired left ventricular function

The majority of studies examining the relationship of ventricular arrhythmia to prognosis in cardiac failure or impaired left ventricular function have included patients with previous myocardial infarction, with some patients having idiopathic dilated cardiomyopathy. These therefore represent mixed aetiologies in the pathogenesis of left ventricular impairment and congestive cardiac failure. Most of the available information concerns non-sustained VT and several recent reviews have summarized the data available in this area. Packer reviewed seven studies in congestive cardiac failure comprising a total of 891 patients[16] in which the occurrence of non-sustained VT varied from 39 to 60 per cent. The overall rate of sudden cardiac death was 14.3 per cent per year. Similarly, eight different studies were reviewed by Surawicz,[17] totalling 398 patients, where the incidence of non-sustained VT varied from 49 to 100 per cent (average 65 per cent). In the majority of these studies, the occurrence of sudden cardiac death was unrelated to the presence of non-sustained VT. A few studies which are more specifically limited to patients with idiopathic

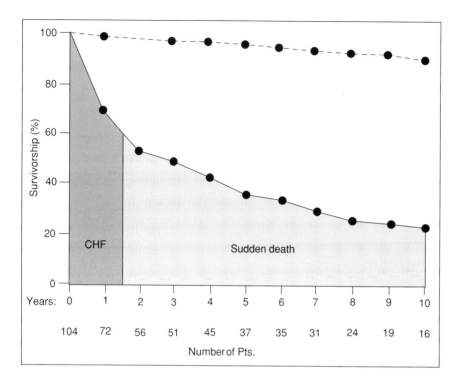

**Figure 9.3**
*Survival in patients with impaired left ventricular function. The group consists of patients with idiopathic dilated cardiomyopathy. This study suggests that early deaths in this group of patients may be due to progressive deterioration of left ventricular function, whereas later deaths are more likely to be related to arrhythmia. (From Fuster V et al, Am J Cardiol (1981) 47:525.)*

dilated cardiomyopathy have reported that non-sustained VT is found in approximately 40 per cent of patients on Holter monitoring, but sustained VT is rare.[18] Most deaths occur in the first 2 years after diagnosis, but these are generally related to progressive heart failure. Thereafter, there is an annual mortality of about 4 per cent, most of the deaths being sudden (Figure 9.3). However, the prognostic implications of ventricular arrhythmias in patients with dilated cardiomyopathy remain controversial. Recent studies suggest that complex ventricular arrhythmias are independent risk factors for sudden cardiac death, although the effect is not large.[19-21] The

study of Huang et al,[22] did not find any relationship between the presence of non-sustained ventricular tachycardia and the occurrence of sudden death. However, the mortality among patients in his study was low, and therefore the validity of judgements on prognostication can be questioned. Presumably, the detrimental effect of poor left ventricular function on survival is so large that it completely overwhelms the effects on survival due to the presence of non-sustained VT. This is in contrast to the implications of non-sustained VT in patients with myocardial infarction, where left ventricular function is not generally severely impaired.

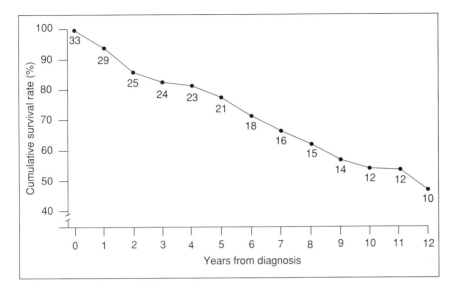

**Figure 9.4**

*Survival in patients with hypertrophic cardiomyopathy. The data are from the 33 young patients with hypertrophic cardiomyopathy. (From McKenna et al, Arch Dis Child (1984* ***59:971.)***

Sustained monomorphic VT is rare in patients with idiopathic dilated cardiomyopathy, except in the small subgroup of patients with predominantly right ventricular disease.[23] For example, in the study of de Maria et al,[24] of 218 patients with idiopathic dilated cardiomyopathy, sustained VT was found in only 3 per cent. However, patients who survive an episode of sustained VT or a cardiac arrest are at particularly high risk for recurrent arrhythmias or sudden death.[25] In the group with isolated right ventricular disease, since left ventricular dysfunction is minimal, aggressive treatment of life-threatening arrhythmia is justified to improve prognosis.

## Ventricular tachycardia in relation to hypertrophic cardiomyopathy

Sudden death in patients with hypertrophic cardiomyopathy is 2–3 per cent per year in adults[26] and 4–6 per cent a year in adolescents and children[27] (Figure 9.4). Non-sustained VT is frequently detected in patients with this condition,[28] although sustained VT is rarely found. VT in these patients is generally slow, non-sustained and asymptomatic. Episodes of VT generally follow periods of relative bradycardia and are not associated with ST segment or QT interval change. One report suggests that when sustained VT occurs, this is associated with aneurysm formation of the ventricle.[29] Aneurysm formation of the ventricle, although rare, can occur in hypertrophic cardiomyopathy in the absence of coronary artery disease.[30,31] At least two groups report that the presence of non-sustained VT on Holter monitoring is associated with the occurrence of sudden death.[32,33] Of the 170 consecutive unoperated patients from the National Institutes of Health, Bethesda, Maryland and the Hammersmith Hospital, London, 13 died suddenly during 3 years. None of the 13 had non-sustained VT on Holter monitoring. The sensitivity of non-sustained VT in this group for prediction of sudden death is 69 per cent, with a specificity of 80 per cent. However, the positive predictive accuracy is low (22 per cent). The low sensitivity in part reflects the inclusion of adolescents who die suddenly, but do not have ventricular arrhythmia. A recent study suggests that spontaneous arrhythmias are rare in children and adolescents and other clinical features may have greater predictive accuracy.[34] Further factors which identify the subgroup of patients with non-sustained VT who are at increased risk of sudden cardiac death are required. There is some evidence that left ventricular ejection rate is significantly reduced in patients who die suddenly, in comparison to patients who survive, suggesting that impairment of left ventricular function may also be important in this group of patients.[35]

## Torsade de pointes

Torsade de pointes is a particular variety of polymorphic VT in which the axis varies, generally over several beats, and there is variation in the QRS morphology. This arrhythmia is frequently, but not invariably, associated with a prolonged QT interval, which may be congenital or acquired. The acquired forms of syndrome can be associated with the use of anti-arrhythmic drugs, bradycardia, hypo-kalaemia or intracranial events such as subarachnoid haemorrhage. Although many attacks of this arrhythmia are non-sustained, there is little doubt that these may degenerate into ventricular fibrillation. In a prospective study of patients with the long QT syndrome, mortality was 1.3 per cent per year,[36] which is high considering that the average age of the population was only 24 years.

# Benign forms of ventricular tachycardia

Ventricular tachycardia appears to be benign when it is not associated with evidence of underlying cardiac disease, when the tachycardia rate is relatively slow and not associated with syncope or haemodynamic compromise and when the tachycardia is relatively easily controlled by drug therapy.

## Ventricular arrhythmias in patients with structurally normal hearts

VT can be identified in the normal healthy population by Holter monitoring approximately 1 per cent of the general population. Subjects with structurally normal hearts do not appear to be at risk of sudden death above that of the general population. Kennedy et al[37] followed 73 asymptomatic individuals, 26 per cent of whom had non-sustained VT, for 3.0–7.5 years, and their mortality was no greater than that of the general population. Similarly, results from the Baltimore Longitudinal Study of Ageing suggest that healthy individuals with frequent and repetitive extrasystoles induced by exercise were at no additional risk of sudden death than healthy age- and sex-matched controls.[38]

Ten per cent of patients with sustained VT

have no obvious underlying structural heart disease.[39] Unfortunately, data in these patients have been marred by the differing numbers and types of investigations which have been utilized by investigators to define the absence of structural heart disease. Currently most groups would define idiopathic VT in patients who present without a prior history of heart disease, but with normal cardiovascular examination, normal resting electrocardiograph and chest X-ray, normal echocardiography and absence of coronary artery disease at cardiac catheterization. However, if members of this group are examined in greater detail, with investigations including right ventricular angiography, detailed right ventricular echocardiography and histological examination of the myocardium by cardiac biopsy, a significant proportion will have an underlying abnormality of myocardial structure or function.[40–42] The predominant abnormality on cardiac histology is the presence of varying degrees of interstitial fibrosis, although fatty infiltration and a mild myocarditis may be found in others. These patients constitute a relatively young group (mean age in most studies being around 30 years) and the male–female distribution is approximately equal (unlike the male predominance of ischaemic heart disease). This group can be subdivided on the basis of numerous criteria, some of which aid classification and others of which do not. The commonest form of classification is based on electrophysiological characteristics, based on dividing the morphology of the VT into two classes—left bundle branch block (LBBB)-like morphology and right bundle branch block (RBBB)-like morphology VT. These two varieties differ in behaviour and characteristics and will be considered separately in this description.

## Left bundle branch block-like morphology VT

These VTs originate from the right ventricle, although the morphology of the arrhythmia is no certain guide as to the site of origin of the arrhythmia. Tachycardias of an inferior axis (normal or rightward) can often be mapped to the right ventricular outflow tract (Figure 9.5), whereas those with a superior axis frequently originate from the other regions of the ventricle, including the inferior wall, septum, right ventricular free wall or apex. In each group, the arrhythmia can be sustained or non-sustained. The arrhythmia is more frequently sustained in the group with superior axes as compared to those with inferior axes. Furthermore, underlying histological abnormality is more likely to be detected in patients with sustained episodes of VT. Recent reports demonstrate that right ventricular outflow VT can be abolished by low-energy discharges or radiofrequency application, suggesting that the anatomical substrate for the arrhythmia is small in these patients.

## Right bundle branch block-like morphology VT

The majority of these patients have arrhythmia originating from the left ventricle. Two distinct forms of arrhythmia appear to occur.

### Fascicular tachycardia

This unusual form of VT is characterized by a RBBB-like VT with generally a leftward axis (Figure 9.6), although forms with a rightward axis have been described. The arrhythmia has distinct characteristics at electrophysiological study, including the following:

1 A relatively narrow QRS complex.
2 The ability to initiate and terminate the arrhythmia by stimulation from both the atrium and ventricle.

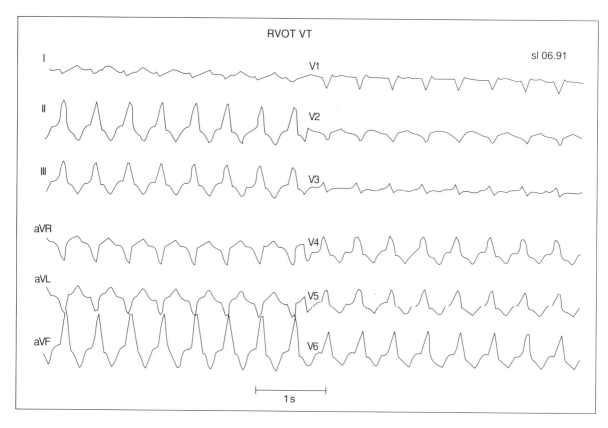

**Figure 9.5**
*A typical example of right ventricular outflow tract tachycardia. The tachycardia is of left bundle branch-like morphology with a rightward axis.*

3 The His bundle deflection can be identified preceding or within each ventricular electrocardiogram on intracardiac recordings (Figure 9.7).
4 The arrhythmia is responsive to calcium entry drugs, suggesting that the mechanism may be triggered activity or calcium-dependent re-entry.

The origin of the VT is from the region of the posterior fascicle of the left bundle or sometimes near the anterior fascicle, and these arrhythmias can be abolished by low-energy DC discharges, or radiofrequency application in these regions, suggesting a localized origin for the VT.

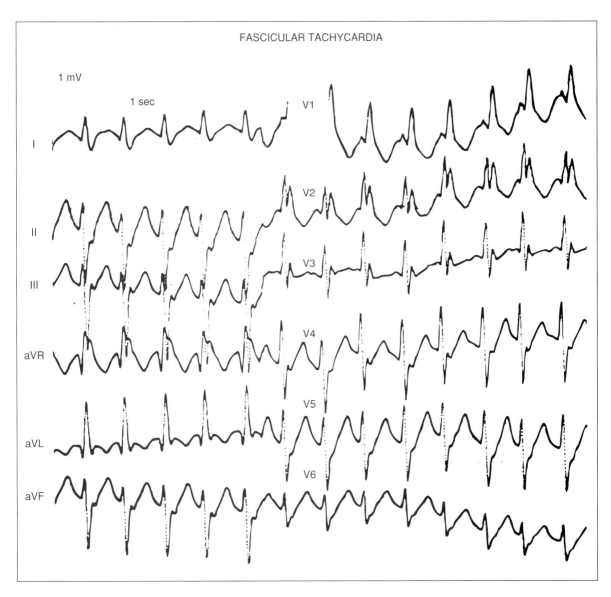

**Figure 9.6**
*Fascicular tachycardia. The VT has a right bundle branch-like morphology with a leftward axis. The QRS complex is relatively narrow and independent P-waves are identifiable.*

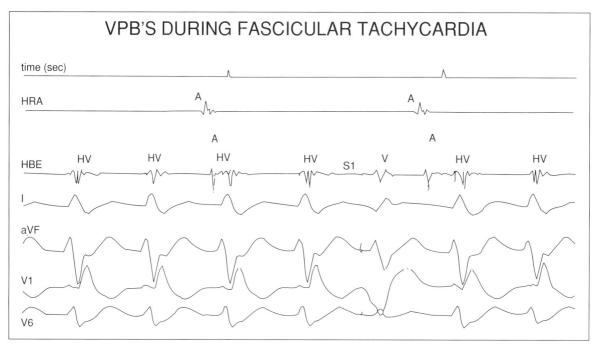

**Figure 9.7**
*The intracardiac recordings from the high right atrium (HRA) and the His bundle region (HBE) in a case of fascicular tachycardia. There is clear dissociation of atrial activity (A) from ventricular activity (V). The His electrode clearly demonstrates a His bundle deflection associated with each V deflection which is brought out of the V by capture from the atrium—the beat following the introduction of a ventricular extrastimulus (S1).*

### Ventricular tachycardia of left ventricular origin, but not of the fascicular variety

A small group of patients have RBBB-like morphology VT, suggesting an origin from the left ventricle, but do not have fascicular tachycardia and usually have no identifiable underlying abnormality. The cause of the VT and its mechanisms are poorly understood.

Studies on prognosis can be subdivided into those which deal with idiopathic VT, where patients with both LBBB-like and RBBB-like morphology VT are included, and the degree of underlying cardiac abnormality is either discussed or not described. The second major group is those patients with right ventricular outflow tract VT, where some patients have some minor degree of abnormality of the cardiac structure. The third group is patients in whom there is no overt abnormality on clinical examination but investigations reveal underlying cardiac abnormality, usually in the form of a right ventricular cardiomyopathy.

## Prognosis in patients with idiopathic VT

Numerous case-series have examined the prognosis in this group of patients. Unfortunately, the documentation of the patients in the case-series has not been uniform, and conclusions must be drawn from the incomplete nature of the data available.

The reports of Rahilly et al[43] and Lemery et al[44] concerned patients with VT associated with a clinically normal heart (both LBBB-like and RBBB-like morphology). No cardiac deaths occurred in the patients in these studies, over a mean follow-up of 2–4 years. There appeared to be no difference in survival of patients with abnormalities detected at investigation in comparison to those with no detectable abnormalities.

Palileo et al[45] and Buxton et al[46] studied specifically right ventricular outflow tract tachycardia. These patients were observed for a mean of 2.5 years (range 0.25–6 years) and no deaths were observed.

Pietras et al[47] examined 38 patients with right ventricular tachycardia, but approximately half the patients had evidence of right ventricular cardiomyopathy, characterized by an abnormal right ventricular volume on cineangiography and abnormal ejection fraction or pressures. On follow-up of these patients (mean 2 years, range 0.25–1.5 years), two patients died, both of whom had obvious right ventricular disease. It is of importance to note that no deaths were observed in the patients with no evidence of right ventricular disease.

These data are in contrast to those studies which present patients with extensive right ventricular disease. Fichett et al[48] described 14 patients with severe right ventricular dilatation of unknown cause, in whom disease was identified by echocardiography or angiography.

Twelve of these patients were observed for a mean of 4.1 years (range 0.5–14 years), of whom 5 died suddenly and 1 with progressive heart failure. Similarly, Deal et al[49] describe 24 patients with VT in the absence of overt heart disease, in whom abnormalities of cardiac size or function were present at cardiac catheterization in 16 of the 23 patients. During a follow-up period of 7.5 years (range 1–20 years), three patients died suddenly. All of the patients who died had evidence of heart disease either at cardiac catheterization or at post mortem, and all had had sustained VT with syncope and inducible sustained VT at programmed stimulation. In patients studied at St George's Hospital, 92 patients with VT and no overt heart disease have been followed for a mean of 2.5 years. Amongst these, two deaths have occurred, both in patients with evidence of abnormality on cardiac histology.

The previous studies have all concentrated on right ventricular tachycardia, although cases of fascicular and left ventricular tachycardia in the absence of myocardial disease have been included in the studies in the first section. There are no clear data on prognosis in patients with fascicular VT or in those patients with left ventricular tachycardia in the absence of identifiable cardiac abnormality. However, most investigators would argue that the risk of sudden death in these patients is low.

All these data would suggest that the risk of sudden death is low in patients with VT who have no evidence of heart disease at invasive and non-invasive investigation. Nevertheless, deaths have been observed in patients who initially appear to be patients with 'clinically normal' hearts, but on closer examination have evidence of heart disease.

The evidence therefore appears to demonstrate that VT is a marker for a poor prognosis in the presence of underlying cardiac disease, and this is applicable to the presence of non-sustained as well as sustained arrhythmia. If this generalization is true, which strategies should be used to identify patients who may have a good prognosis from VT?

# Risk stratification in ventricular tachycardia

Several features of the VT may be useful in classification of the arrhythmia as of serious import or of the prognostically good group.

## History of syncope

Patients with a history of syncope are likely to be at greater risk of sudden death than patients who have never suffered syncope despite many repeated episodes of VT. In the latter group of patients, the arrhythmia tends to be slower, more frequently non-sustained and haemodynamically well tolerated.

## The left ventricular ejection fraction

In patients with an episode of confirmed VT, the ejection fraction of the left ventricle has a considerable bearing on the outcome. Patients with a decreased ejection fraction are at an increased risk of sudden death, when compared to patients with normal or only slightly impaired function.[50] A careful assessment of cardiac function by echocardiography, angiography and radionuclide studies is therefore necessary.

## Signal-averaged electrocardiogram (ECG)

The signal-averaged ECG is recorded by amplification, averaging and filtering of the surface ECG recorded on orthogonal leads.[51] This method allows detection of low-amplitude cardiac electrical signals in the terminal portion of the QRS complex (late potentials), which are thought to represent delayed depolarizations in abnormal/diseased myocardial tissue. There is evidence that the presence of late potentials relates to the presence of histological abnormalities within the myocardium.[42] The same data suggest that late potentials are associated with the presence of sustained VT and evidence of myocardial abnormality by other methods of investigation. This would be consistent with the presence of an anatomical substrate for the occurrence of VT. In patients with sustained VT, the presence of late potentials on signal-averaged ECG relates strongly to the induction of sustained VT at programmed ventricular stimulation.[52,53] Similarly, in patients with non-sustained VT, signal-averaged ECG positive for late potentials was predictive of patients in whom sustained monomorphic VT could be induced at programmed ventricular stimulation (PVS).[54] This therefore allows the selection of patients in whom there is a possibility of the induction of sustained VT by PVS, and therefore the group in whom this test can be used to guide drug therapy.

## Programmed ventricular stimulation

In patients with documented episodes of sustained VT, there is a high rate of induction of VT by PVS (~90 per cent),[55] whereas rates of induction are much lower in patients with non-sustained VT (~10–14 per cent). Induction of VT at PVS carries a poor prognosis, both in patients with sustained,[56,57] and non-sustained VT.[58,59] The major use of PVS is that this method allows guided therapy of the tachyarrhythmia. There is reasonable evidence in the literature that patients who have inducible sustained monomorphic VT at PVS, and are rendered non-inducible by anti-arrhythmic therapy, have an improved prognosis, whereas those who remain inducible are at continued risk of sudden cardiac death.[60] This study also demonstrated that if the VT cycle length could be increased by more than 100 ms and the patient did not suffer symptoms of haemodynamic compromise, then mortality rates were reduced to a similar extent to those rendered non-inducible.

## Drug effects on VT

VT which is easily suppressed by anti-arrhythmic therapy appears to have a better prognosis than VT which remains inducible even when multiple drug trials are attempted. VT which is slowed in rate by therapy by more than 100 ms from untreated values has a better prognosis than in cases where the rate is unaffected (see above).

A potential scheme for the assessment of VT based on these findings is given in Figure 9.8.

# Conclusions

The available data suggest that not all VT is associated with a poor prognosis and certainly the prognosis of some forms of VT is substantially better than that of others. VT associated with underlying cardiac abnormality is more likely to cause sudden death, whereas that associated with major myocardial disease usually carries a grave prognosis. Nonsustained VT appears to be particularly benign in the absence of cardiac disease.

# If I had . . .

If I had VT, I should want to know whether the tachycardia was associated with a substantial risk or not. If I had other heart disease, if I had suffered syncope (or worse) with the arrhythmia or if the arrhythmia was rapid and sustained, I should insist on very detailed assessment and vigorous attempts to prescribe an effective therapy. Nowadays VT can be very well treated with careful drug therapy, implantable devices, and surgical or catheter ablation. Some particular forms of tachycardia are related to transient events, electrolyte disturbances or drug toxicity. I should be relieved to find that this was responsible in my case. Putting right the cause of the arrhythmia would be a simple and very effective therapy. However, I might end up with a diagnosis of 'ventricular tachycardia associated with a normal heart'. I could probably accept this diagnosis if the 12-lead ECG was normal (apart from non-specific T-wave changes and perhaps RBBB), the CXR showed no heart disease and both an echocardiogram and signal-averaged ECG were normal. I should then be concerned more with symptoms than prognosis because arrhythmias such as these are usually 'benign'. A few 24-h Holter ECG recordings would be helpful to define the nature of the arrhythmia, particularly its temporal pattern. Only if the arrhythmia were present for much of the time or if it were associated with distressing symptoms would I consider treatment. I should be loathe to contemplate taking a class 1, or even a class 3, anti-arrhythmic drug to treat a relatively benign rhythm disturbance, but I would consider a beta-blocker or a calcium antagonist such as verapamil. All in all I should be relieved to find that I had a tachycardia which was not going to kill me and I should be determined to ensure that the drugs used to treat the condition would not kill me either.

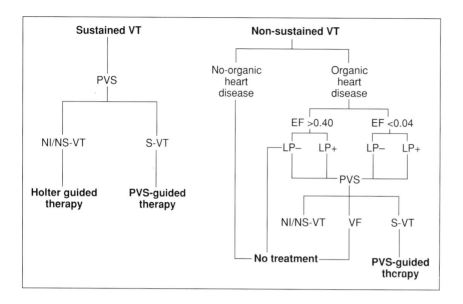

**Figure 9.8**
*A suggested scheme for the assessment of sustained and non-sustained
ventricular tachycardia in order to identify malignant from benign forms.
Patients with sustained VT should undergo programmed ventricular stimulation (PVS) and guided therapy if inducible. Patients with non-sustained
VT with evidence of organic heart disease, with well-preserved ejection
fraction (EF) and negative late potentials (LP) on signal-averaged ECG, can
probably be left untreated, as can those with no underlying organic heart
disease. Those patients with impaired left ventricular function and those
with positive late potentials should undergo programmed ventricular
stimulation (PVS) and, if sustained VT is inducible, should undergo PVS
guided therapy. Those patients who have VF or non-sustained VT or are
non-inducible at PVS may be left untreated.*

# References

1 Lie KI et al, Observations on patients with primary ventricular fibrillation complicating acute myocardial infarction, *Circulation* (1975) 52:755.

2 Spielman SR et al, Predictors of the success or failure of medical therapy in patients with chronic recurrent sustained ventricular tachycardia: a discriminant analysis, *J Am Coll Cardiol* (1983) 401:1.

3 Swerdlow CD et al, Clinical factors predicting successful electrophysiologic–pharmacologic study in patients with ventricular tachycardia, *J Am Coll Cardiol* (1983) 409:1.

4 Kiat H et al, Prediction of late sustained ventricular tachyarrhythmias after myocardial infarction, *J Am Coll Cardiol* (1976) 7:67A.

5 Swerdlow CD, Winkle RA, Mason JW, Determinants of survival in patients with ventricular tachyarrhythmias, *N Eng J Med* (1983) 308:1436.

6 Goldstein S et al, Predictive survival models for resuscitated victims of out-of-hospital cardiac arrest with coronary heart disease, *Circulation* (1985) 5:873.

7 Marchlinski FE et al, Identifying patients at risk of sudden death after myocardial infarction: value of the response to programmed stimulation, degree of ventricular ectopic activity and severity of left ventricular dysfunction, *Am J Cardiol* (1983) 52:1190.

8 Di Marco JP et al, Sustained ventricular tachyarrhythmias within 2 months of acute myocardial infarction: results of medical and surgical therapy in patients resuscitated from the initial episode, *J Am Coll Cardiol* (1985) 6:759.

9 Wilber DJ et al, Out-of-hospital cardiac arrest. Use of electrophysiologic testing in the prediction of long-term outcome, *N Engl J Med* (1988) 318:19.

10 Bigger JT Jr et al, The relationship among ventricular arrhythmias, left ventricular dysfunction and mortality in the 2 years after myocardial infarction, *Circulation* (1984) 69:250.

11 Mukarji J et al, Risk factors for sudden death after acute myocardial infarction: two-year follow-up, *Am J Cardiol* (1984) 54:31.

12 Josephson ME, Treatment of ventricular arrhythmias after myocardial infarction, *Circulation* (1985) 74:963.

13 Anderson KP, DeCamilla J, Moss AJ, Clinical significance of ventricular tachycardia (3 beats or longer) detected during ambulatory monitoring after myocardial infarction, *Circulation* (1978) 57:89.

14 Bigger JT, Weld FM, Rolinzky LM, Prevalence, characteristics and significance of ventricular tachycardia (three or more complexes) detected with ambulatory electrocardiographic recording in the late phase of acute myocardial infarction, *Am J Cardiol* (1981) 48:815.

15 Klieger RE et al, Relationship between clinical features of acute myocardial infarction and ventricular runs 2 weeks to 1 year after infarction, *Circulation* (1981) 63:64.

16 Packer M, Sudden unexpected death in patients with congestive heart failure: a second frontier, *Circulation* (1985) 72:681.

17 Surawicz B, Prognosis of ventricular arrhythmias in relation to sudden cardiac death. Prognostic implications, *J Am Coll Cardiol* (1985) 6:307.

18 Fuster V et al, The natural history of idiopathic dilated cardiomyopathy, *Am J Cardiol* (1981) 47:525.

19 Meinertz T et al, Significance of ventricular arrhythmias in idiopathic ventricular cardiomyopathy, *Am J Cardiol* (1984) 53:902.

20 Holmes et al, Arrhythmias in ischemic and nonischemic cardiomyopathy: prediction of mortality by ambulatory electrocardiomyopathy, *Am J Cardiol* (1985) 55:146.

21 Unverferth DV et al, Factors influencing the one-year mortality of dilated cardiomyopathy, *Am J Cardiol* (1984) 54:147.

22 Huang SK, Messer JV, Denes P, Significance of ventricular tachycardia in idiopathic dilated cardiomyopathy: observation in 35 patients, *Am J Cardiol* (1983) 51:507.

23  Rowland E et al, Ventricular tachycardia of left branch block configuration in patients with isolated right ventricular dilatation. Clinical and electrophysiological features, *Br Heart J* (1984) **51**:15.

24  de Maria R et al, Ventricular arrhythmia in dilated cardiomyopathy as an independent prognostic hallmark, *Am J Cardiol* (1992) **69**:1451.

25  Tamburro P, Wilber D, Sudden death in idiopathic dilated cardiomyopathy, *Am Heart J* (1992) **124**: 1035–45.

26  McKenna WJ et al, Prognosis in hypertrophic cardiomyopathy. Role of age and clinical, electrocardiographic and hemodynamic features, *Am J Cardiol* (1981) **47**:532.

27  Sprito P et al, Clinical course and prognosis of hypertrophic cardiomyopathy in an outpatient population, *N Engl J Med* (1989) **320**:749.

28  Savage DD et al, Prevalence of arrhythmia during 24 hour electrocardiographic monitoring in patients with obstructive and non-obstructive hypertrophic cardiomyopathy, *Circulation* (1979) **59**:866.

29  Alfonso F, Frenneaux MP, McKenna AJ, Clinical sustained uniform ventricular tachycardia in hypertrophic cardiomyopathy: association with left ventricular apical aneurysm, *Br Heart J* (1989) **61**:178.

30  Barbaresi F et al, Idiopathic apical left ventricular aneurysm in hypertrophic cardiomyopathy, *Jpn Heart J* (1985) **26**:481.

31  Maron BJ, Epstein SE, Roberts WC, Hypertrophic cardiomyopathy and transmural infarction without significant atherosclerosis of the extramural coronary arteries, *Am J Cardiol* (1979) **43**:1086.

32  Maron BJ et al, Prognostic significance of 24 hour ambulatory electrocardiographic monitoring in patients with hypertrophic cardiomyopathy. A prospective study, *Am J Cardiol* (1981) **48**:252.

33  McKenna WJ et al, Arrhythmia in hypertrophic cardiomyopathy: 1. Influence on prognosis, *Br Heart J* (1981) **46**:168.

34  McKenna WJ et al, Arrhythmia and prognosis in infants, children and adolescents with hypertrophic cardiomyopathy, *J Am Coll Cardiol* (1988) **11**:147.

35  Newman H et al, Relation of left ventricular function and prognosis in infants, children and adolescents with hypertrophic cardiomyopathy, *J Am Coll Cardiol* (1985) **5**:1064.

36  Moss AJ et al, Hereditable malignant arrhythmias: a prospective study of the long QT syndrome, *Circulation* (1985) **71**:17.

37  Kennedy HL et al, Long-term follow-up of asymptomatic healthy subjects with frequent and complex ventricular ectopy, *N Engl J Med* (1985) **312**:193.

38  Busby JM, Shefrin EA, Fleg JL, Prevalence and long-term significance of exercise-induced frequent or repetitive ventricular ectopic beats in healthy volunteers, *J Am Coll Cardiol* (1989) **14**:1659.

39  Froment R, Gallavardin L, Cahan P, Paroxysmal ventricular tachycardia: a clinical classification, *Br Heart J* (1953) **15**:172.

40  Proclemer A, Ciani R, Feruglio GA, Right ventricular tachycardia with left bundle branch block and inferior axis morphology: clinical and arrhythmological characteristics in 15 patients, *PACE* (1989) **12**:977.

41  Mehta D et al, Echocardiographic and histologic evaluation of the right ventricle in ventricular tachycardias of left bundle branch block morphology without overt cardiac abnormality, *Am J Cardiol* (1989) **63**:939.

42  Mehta D et al, Significance of signal-averaged electrocardiography in relation to endomyocardial biopsy and ventricular stimulation studies in patients with ventricular tachycardia without clinically apparent heart disease, *J Am Coll Cardiol* (1989) **14**:372.

43  Rahilly GT et al, Clinical and electrophysiological findings in patients with repetitive monomorphic ventricular tachycardia and otherwise normal electrocardiogram, *Am J Cardiol* (1982) **50**:459.

44  Lemery R et al, Nonischemic ventricular tachycardia. Clinical course and long-term follow-up in patients without clinically overt heart disease, *Circulation* (1989) **79**:990.

45  Palileo EV et al, Exercise provocable right ventricular outflow tract tachycardia, *Am Heart J* (1982) **104**:185.

46  Buxton AE et al, Right ventricular tachycardia: clinical and electrophysiologic characteristics, *Circulation* (1983) **68**:917.

47  Pietras RJ et al, Chronic recurrent ventricular tachycardia in patients without ischemic heart disease: clinical hemodynamic, and angiographic findings, *Am Heart J* (1983) **105**:357.

48  Fichett DH et al, Right ventricular dilated cardiomyopathy, *Br Heart J* (1984) **51**:25.

49  Deal BJ et al, Ventricular tachycardia in a young population without overt heart disease, *Circulation* (1986) **73**:1111.

50  Mukarji J et al, Risk factors for sudden death after acute myocardial infarction: 2 year follow-up, *Am J Cardiol* (1984) **54**:31.

51  Simpson MB, Use of signals in the terminal QRS complex to identify patients with ventricular tachycardia after myocardial infarction, *Circulation* (1981) **64**:235.

52  Freedman RA et al, Signal-averaged electrocardiographic late potentials in patients with ventricular fibrillation or ventricular tachycardia: correlation with clinical arrhythmia and electrophysiology study, *Am J Cardiol* (1985) **55**:1350.

53  Lindsay BD et al, Improved selection of patients for programmed ventricular stimulation by frequency analysis of signal-averaged electrocardiograms, *Circulation* (1986) **73**:675.

54  Turitto G et al, Value of signal-averaged electrocardiogram as a predictor of the results of programmed stimulation in non-sustained ventricular tachycardia, *Am J Cardiol* (1988) **61**:1272.

55  Josephson ME, *Recurrent ventricular tachycardia in clinical cardiac electrophysiology* (Lea and Febiger: Pennsylvania, 1993).

56  Denniss AR et al, Prognostic significance of ventricular tachycardia and fibrillation induced at programmed stimulation and delayed potentials detected on the signal-averaged electrocardiograms of survivors of acute myocardial infarction, *Circulation* (1986) **74**:731.

57  Richards DA et al, A new protocol of programmed stimulation for assessment of predisposition to spontaneous ventricular arrhythmias, *Eur Heart J* (1983) **4**:376.

58  Buxton AE et al, Prognostic factors in nonsustained ventricular tachycardia, *Am J Cardiol* (1984) **53**:1275.

59  Gomes JAC et al, Programmed electrical stimulation in patients with high grade ventricular ectopy: electrophysiologic findings and prognosis for survival, *Circulation* (1984) **70**:43.

60  Waller T et al, Reduction in sudden death and total mortality by antiarrhythmic therapy evaluated by electrophysiologic drug testing: criteria of efficacy in patients with sustained ventricular tachyarrhythmia, *J Am Coll Cardiol* (1987) **10**:83.

# 10

## The cardiac investigation of transient ischaemic attacks and stroke

*John Chambers*

## Introduction

The aims of cardiac investigation are:

1 To detect a possible, direct source of emboli: thrombus, vegetation, myxoma (Table 10.1).
2 To detect a possible substrate for thrombus formation or platelet aggregation: atrial fibrillation, patent foramen ovale, impaired left ventricular function, aortic atheroma.
3 Occasionally to see whether atypical TIAs are likely to be caused by a cardiac arrhythmia.

The main investigations to be discussed are 12-lead or 24-h ambulatory electrocardiography and echocardiography. Magnetic resonance imaging and computerized tomographic scanning play a limited role in the detection and analysis of intracardiac masses.

## Initial investigation

Cerebral haemorrhage and infarction cannot reliably be differentiated on clinical grounds, and nor can embolic from other causes of ischaemic stroke. For example, abrupt onset of maximal neurological deficit occurs in around three-quarters of patients with an embolic stroke, but also in up to two-thirds of patients with other ischaemic strokes.[1–3] Previous infarctions in other territories suggest emboli, but are seen in at most one-third of all embolic strokes.[3,4] Associated peripheral emboli, although strongly favouring embolic stroke, occur only rarely. There are some clinical types of stroke that make an embolic source likely. Aphasia without hemiparesis and isolated posterior cerebral artery syndromes are usually 'cardio-embolic'. Amaurosis fugax also suggests a cardiac source.[3]

On a CT scan of the brain performed within 7 days of the stroke, cardiac emboli tend to show as cortical, large (>1.5 cm) subcortical or multiple infarctions. Lacunar infarctions are usually caused by thrombosis or occasionally artery-to-artery emboli. Haemorrhagic transformation is more common after embolic stroke and is usually more dense than after cerebral thrombosis.

## How common is a cardiac source for emboli?

In the Framingham study, in which 5184 subjects were followed for 24 years, 2.5 strokes and 0.25 TIA occurred per 1000 population per year.[5] Approximately 80 per cent of strokes are infarctions and in the past it has been estimated that the heart is the source of emboli in about 15–35 per cent of all cases of infarction and in about 15 per cent of TIAs.[3] The diagnosis of a 'cardiac stroke', however, is

- **Common**
  Atrial fibrillation
  Myocardial infarction (anterior > inferior) (Figure 10.4)
  Left ventricular aneurysm
  Globally impaired left ventricular function
  Mitral stenosis (Figure 10.1)
  Left atrial or left atrial appendage thrombus (Figure 10.7)
  Prosthetic heart valve
  Tachybrady syndrome
  ASD
  Aortic atheroma (Figure 10.8)

- **Rare**
  Myxoma or other cardiac tumour (Figure 10.2)
  Infective endocarditis
  Non-infective endocarditis (lupus, marantic endocarditis)
  Restrictive myopathy
  Hypertrophic cardiomyopathy and atrial fibrillation
  Endomyocardial fibrosis
  Left ventricular thrombus with normal left ventricle (lupus,
  malignancy, thrombocythaemia, polycystic kidney disease)
  Left atrial spontaneous contrast (Figure 10.1)
  Pulmonary AV fistulae
  VSD with pulmonary hypertension
  Thoracic aortic dissection

- **Controversial**
  Patent foramen ovale (Figure 10.6)
  Interatrial aneurysm (Figure 10.6)
  Posterior mitral annular calcification
  Mitral prolapse (Figure 10.9)
  Aortic stenosis

*Cardiac abnormalities associated with stroke.*

made only partly on the clinical presentation and on the appearance of CT scanning. It is also suggested by the detection of a potential source for emboli within the heart, the criteria for which vary widely. For example, some authors have included mitral prolapse and others not.

Recent studies using transoesophageal echocardiography have increased the estimate of a cardiac source for emboli in cerebral infarction to at least 50 per cent. This is similar to the figure derived from post-mortem studies.[6] In one study of patients with cerebral infarction and no significant cerebrovascular disease, an incidence of echocardiographic abnormalities as high as 83 per cent was reported.[7] These recent reports need to be placed in their clinical context. We need to know how often a possible source is genuinely likely to have caused cerebral embolism. We also need to know how often these sources coexist and how often they may be associated with extracardiac disease. For example, in one series 19 of 50 (38 per cent) patients with TIA and a potential cardiac source for emboli had severe ipsilateral carotid disease.[8] For the moment, transoesophageal echocardiography is most safely regarded as a research technique in ischaemic stroke (see below).

# The 12-lead electrocardiogram

Good et al[9] found electrocardiographic abnormalities, mostly non-specific, in 58 per cent of patients with stroke and normal cerebral angiography. Evidence of recent anterior infarction, ASD or left ventricular hypertrophy may all give clues to the cardiac source for embolism. For example, stroke occurs in about 6 per cent of all acute anterior infarctions.[3] However, the most common and important abnormality found is atrial fibrillation. This occurs in 20 per cent of patients with a stroke compared with 2–5 per cent of the general population aged over 60 years and up to 10 per cent aged over 75 years.[10–12] In stroke patients, atrial fibrillation is also associated with large infarctions and a high 30-day mortality of around 40 per cent.[13,14]

After the onset of atrial fibrillation in a patient without rheumatic mitral disease, there is no risk of stroke for 2 or 3 days, possibly while thrombogenic factors increase in concentration and platelet function changes.[15] After this, the greatest risk is in the first 2 weeks,

averaging out to 5 per cent per year or a 35–40 per cent lifetime risk.[16,17] This is a relative risk of six times normal[5] (Table 10.1). The effect of atrial fibrillation is dependent on age. There is an attributable risk from atrial fibrillation of 1.5 per cent at age 50–59, which rises to 10 per cent between 70 and 79 years and to 24 per cent between 80 and 89 years.[17] This age dependency may account for discrepancies between studies of lone atrial fibrillation, with some showing a four-fold increase[25] and others an insignificant increase.[18] If lone atrial fibrillation is strictly defined by the absence of all evidence of cardiovascular disease, particularly hypertension, and also by excluding patients aged more than 60 years, there is a low risk of stroke. The risk for both sustained and paroxysmal atrial fibrillation is around 0.5 per cent per year. Stroke occurs in about 2 per cent per year of unselected patients with paroxysmal atrial fibrillation,[19,26] but the risk is higher for tachybrady syndrome, 25 per cent in one 11-year follow-up study.[22] Atrial flutter carries no increased risk of stroke.[27,28]

## Atrial fibrillation as a marker for stroke

Atrial fibrillation is a marker for stroke and not necessarily its underlying cause. Although left or right atrial thrombus can form and lead directly to embolism, atrial fibrillation may also be associated with abnormalities carrying an independent risk of stroke, e.g. cardiomyopathy, ischaemic heart disease or hypertension. Thus, atrial fibrillation is found in 11 per cent of those presenting with haemorrhagic stroke, and in 25–35 per cent of those with cerebral thrombosis defined clinically by a stuttering onset, the presence of a carotid bruit and a lacunar site.[14,16] About 60 per cent of patients with a stroke defined clinically as embolic are in atrial fibrillation.[7]

| | Relative risk[a] | Annual risk (%) | Study (Ref. no.) |
|---|---|---|---|
| Sinus rhythm, no rheumatic disease | 1 | 0.3 | 5 |
| Lone AF (sustained/paroxysmal) | 1 | 0.5 | 18 |
| Paroxysmal AF | | 2.0 | 19 |
| AF sustained | 6 | 4.1 | 5 |
| AF with mitral stenosis | 18 | 4.5 | 5 |
| AF with heart failure | 12 | | 17 |
| AF with hypertension | 12 | | 17 |
| AF with HCM | | 10.0 | 20 |
| AF with normal echo and small LA | | 1.5 | 21 |
| AF with LA > 2.5 cm/m² | | 8.8 | 21 |
| AF with FS < 25% | | 10.7 | 21 |
| AF with regional LV dysfunction | | 9.4 | 21 |
| AF with global LV dysfunction | | 12.6 | 21 |
| AF with LA > 2.5 and moderate LV dysfunction | | 20.0 | 21 |
| Ischaemic heart disease alone | 2 | | 17 |
| Prosthetic mitral valve (on warfarin) | | 3.0 | 3 |
| Prosthetic aortic valve (on warfarin) | | 1.5 | 3 |
| Heart failure alone | 2 | | 17 |
| Hypertension | 3 | | 17 |
| Tachybrady | | 2.3 | 22 |
| Dilated myopathy | | 4.0 | 23 |
| Mitral prolapse | 1 | 0 | 24 |

Abbreviations: AF = atrial fibrillation
FS = fraction shortening
LA = left atrium
HCM = hypertrophic myopathy
LV = left ventricle
[a]Calculated from life tables taking into account the age and risk factors of the population.

**Table 10.1**
*Approximate relative and annual risk of stroke.*

## Does atrial fibrillation affect treatment?

There are now several major trials showing approximately a two-thirds reduction in the incidence of stroke in patients with non-rheumatic atrial fibrillation treated prophylactically with warfarin.[29] The effect of warfarin in secondary prevention is not, however, established.

In patients with rheumatic atrial fibrillation there is a recurrence rate of 30–75 per cent over follow-up periods to 12 years.[34] Some studies have suggested a similar high recurrence rate for non-rheumatic atrial fibrillation,[13] but probably have not adequately excluded valvular disease.

| Study (ref. no.) | n | Patent foramen ovale | | LA thrombus | | Large LA/SC | |
|---|---|---|---|---|---|---|---|
| | | Patient | Control | Patient | Control | Patient | Control |
| 61, 62 | 79 | 13 (16%) | | 6 (8%) | | 13 (16%) | |
| 63 | 50 | 4 (8%) | | 5 (10%) | | 9 (18%) | |
| 64 | 72 | – | | 1 (1%) | | 7 (10%) | |
| 65 | 131 | 27 (21%) | | – | | 25 (19%) | |
| 7 | 40 | 6 (15%) | | 3 (8%) | | 21 (53%) | |
| | 56 | | 13 (23%) | | 1 (2%) | | 3 (5%) |

LA = left atrium
SC = spontaneous contrast

**Table 10.2**
*Transoesophageal echocardiography in ischaemic stroke.*

By contrast, Sandercock et al[14] have shown a recurrence rate of 11 per cent in atrial fibrillation compared to 8.2 per cent in sinus rhythm, results similar to those of Wolf et al.[35] Despite this, there is preliminary evidence that anticoagulation in patients with atrial fibrillation after stroke reduces the risk of recurrence. In a small study, Hart et al[16] showed no recurrence in 18 patients with atrial fibrillation treated with warfarin or in 13 given antiplatelet agents. By contrast, there were 3 (12 per cent) early recurrences in 25 on no therapy. There is also evidence for a beneficial effect in secondary prevention in a study by Koller et al.[36] In the much larger trial by Ezekowitz et al,[33] there were 1002 patients with previous stroke. Recurrences occurred in four on placebo (9.3 per cent per year) compared with two on warfarin (6.1 per cent per year), but the confidence intervals were wide.

The crucial problem of anticoagulation is to balance benefit against the risk of haemorrhage. Significant bleeding occurred in only 1.5–3.0 per cent per patient year in the large trials of prophylactic warfarin, but is more usually around 5–11 per cent per year.[37,38] Some physicians try to stratify patients in terms of risk of recurrence using echocardiography. If the left atrium is large, if there is left ventricular dysfunction or if there is a thrombus, they will be more inclined to anticoagulate the patient in atrial fibrillation after a stroke. Unfortunately there is no firm evidence to support this policy. There is some evidence that a large left atrium increases the risk of a first stroke,[21,30,39] but there are also trials that find no such effect.[4,29] There is also evidence that impaired left ventricular function increases the risk of a first stroke in patients with atrial fibrillation[21] (Table 10.2). The results of the European Atrial Fibrillation Trial are awaited and may help in making balanced judgements about anticoagulation for secondary prevention of stroke. At the present, the decision to anticoagulate must be based on

- **Transthoracic**
  Abnormality on examination, ECG or chest X-ray
  Patient in atrial fibrillation and aged under 60 years
  Suggestion of myxoma (e.g. high ESR, postural syncope)
  Suggestion of endocarditis

- **Transoesophageal**
  Inadequate transthoracic examination
  Mechanical prosthetic mitral valve
  Suggestion of thoracic aortic dissection
  Invasive intervention necessary (cardiac catheter, cardiac surgery)

- **Research**
  Young subject (aged under 60) with no obvious significant risk factors
  Older patients with no evidence of obstructive cerebrovascular disease and in whom anticoagulation is not contraindicated

*Indications for echocardiography in stroke.*

the presence of atrial fibrillation alone and the likely risk of bleeding in the individual patient.

# The role of 24-hour ambulatory monitoring

The yield from 24-hour monitoring is low. In general, atrial fibrillation or sinus node disease are discovered in about 2 per cent of cases.[8,40] Come et al[41] studied 150 patients with stroke for an average of 20 h each. They documented atrial fibrillation in 15 patients, but all had either atrial fibrillation on the 12-lead electrocardiogram on admission or a history of atrial fibrillation. The risk of stroke from paroxysmal atrial fibrillation in the absence of episodes of sinus bradycardia is lower than for sustained atrial fibrillation so there is little need to detect it. There is no increased risk of stroke from AV block unless the atria are fibrillating.[22]

Ambulatory monitoring should be performed if the patient reports syncope or near syncope or when the TIA is atypical, suggesting that it may be caused by cardiac arrhythmia. Atypical features are: disturbances of vision in one or both eyes, a tired or heavy sensation in one or more limb, sensory symptoms alone, brainstem symptoms, and altered consciousness.[42]

# Transthoracic echocardiography

## Normal clinical examination

Although about one-third of patients with ischaemic stroke have an echocardiographic abnormality,[43] in most cases this can be diagnosed clinically. If patients with abnormal electrocardiograms, chest X-rays or clinical signs are excluded, the yield from transthoracic echocardiography is virtually zero.[44–46] Furthermore, those abnormalities detected, e.g. mitral annular calcification or mitral prolapse, tend to be of uncertain significance (see below). Shapiro et al[47] found an abnormality (a pedunculated mitral valve papilloma) in only 1 of a group of 94 patients with transient ischaemic attacks, but who had no clinical evidence of cardiac disease. By comparison, 79 of 106 echocardiograms were abnormal in those patients with clinical heart disease. These findings have been confirmed repeatedly and are not controversial.[9,48,49]

As a note of caution, however, there is one study reporting that as many as 5 of 36 cases of endocarditis presenting with stroke were not accompanied by classical findings, e.g. fever, murmur or vasculitis.[50] There are also occasional reports of mitral stenosis being detected only at echocardiography. Clearly, the accuracy of a normal cardiovascular examination is dependent on the skill of the physician, and it might be tempting to ask for a transthoracic echocardiogram as a 'double check'. There is little excuse for this attitude. However, in groups at special risk, such as immunocompromised patients or intravenous drug abusers, it is reasonable to ask for echocardiography even in the absence of classical signs of endocarditis.

## Abnormal clinical examination

Where the clinical examination, the electrocardiogram or chest X-ray are abnormal, the yield from transthoracic echocardiography is high, with 40–50 per cent of studies revealing abnormalities.[41,49] However, if there are already clinically obvious abnormalities, does echocardiography contribute to the quantification of risk or the decision whether to anticoagulate?

The most common risk factors are adequately diagnosed without echocardiography, notably atrial fibrillation, hypertension and ischaemic disease. Furthermore, some clinical conditions are associated with such a high risk of stroke that failure to detect thrombus or another direct source for emboli would not exclude the clinical likelihood of cardiac stroke. Mitral stenosis is an obvious example, but about one-third of ischaemic strokes in patients with cancer are caused by non-bacterial thrombotic ('marantic') endocarditis.[51,52] The risk of embolism in bacterial endocarditis is 15–20 per cent, usually before or in the first week of antibiotic therapy, and embolism can occur even if no vegetation is imaged at echocardiography.[53]

However, many diagnoses are not adequately made without echocardiography, e.g. endomyocardial fibrosis, myxoma and restrictive myopathy. Confirmation of many clinical diagnoses is also important. If there is a mid-diastolic murmur, an echocardiogram can confirm mitral stenosis (Figure 10.1) and exclude atrial myxoma (Figure 10.2), which is found in about 1 per cent of young patients with strokes.[54]

Echocardiography also refines a clinical diagnosis, possibly improving the risk stratification. For example, in patients with clinical mitral stenosis, a ball thrombus (Figure 10.3) for which surgical removal should be considered cannot usually be detected clinically. As outlined above, there is some evidence that echocardiographic evaluation of left atrial size and of regional and global left ventricular systolic function improves risk stratification in atrial fibrillation at least before the first stroke. In dilated myopathy, the risk of stroke is said to be approximately related to the ejection fraction, and in anterior myocardial infarction the size of the infarction is also related to the risk of stroke.[55] In inferior infarctions, the risk of stroke is low unless the apex is also involved.[55]

Echocardiography can image a direct source for emboli such as a thrombus, but more

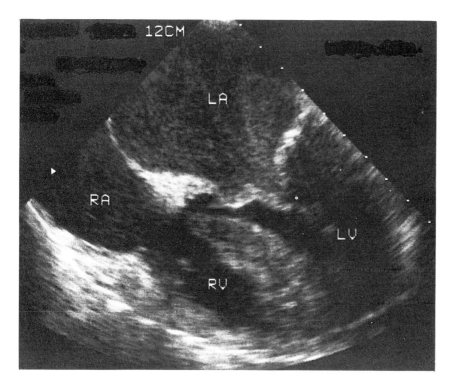

**Figure 10.1**
*Mitral stenosis. A transoesophageal 4-chamber view. There is characteristic thickening of the leaflet tips and elbowing caused by commisural fusion. The interatrial septum bows to the right because of a relatively higher left than right atrial pressure. The left atrium is filled with smoke-like spontaneous contrast formed as fast-flowing blood from the pulmonary veins meets stagnant blood in the left atrium. Differences in density develop at the interfaces between the blood streams possibly by the formation of red cell aggregates.*

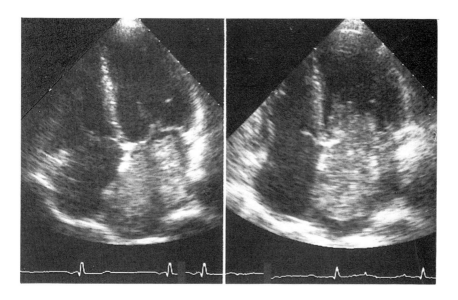

**Figure 10.2**
*Left atrial myxoma. A large mass attached to the interatrial septum virtually fills the left atrium in systole (left-hand panel) and prolapses through the mitral valve in diastole (right-hand panel). It is classical in its heterogeneous echodensity and the fronded appearance of its apex.*

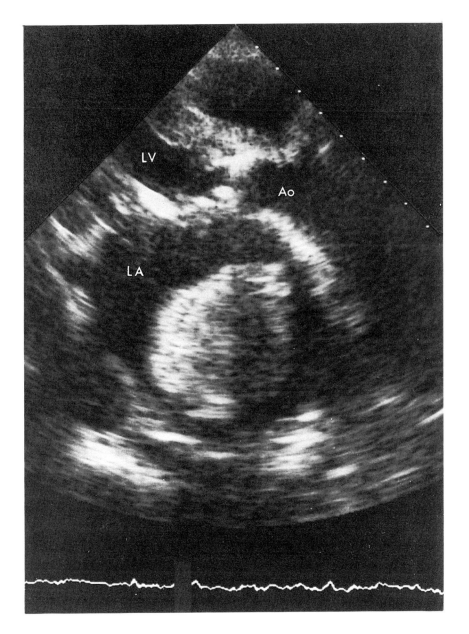

**Figure 10.3**
Ball thrombus. A free-floating ball can be seen in
the left atrium in this parasternal long-axis view.

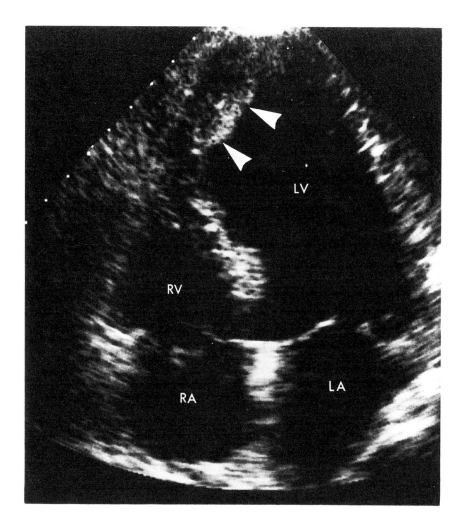

**Figure 10.4**
*Left ventricular throm-
bus. An apical four
chamber view using
transthoracic echocar-
diography in a patient
with an anterior myocar-
dial infarction. There is
a sessile thrombus
(arrowed) layered over
the akinetic segment.*

usually it detects a potential underlying cause
of thromboembolism, e.g. left ventricular
dysfunction or mitral stenosis. On balance, the
substrate for thromboembolism is more important than the presence or absence of overt
thrombus. Transthoracic echocardiography is
well known to be insensitive for atrial thrombus, and if a patient had mitral stenosis or a

large left atrium as a result of restrictive
myopathy, anticoagulation would be essential
even in the absence of thrombus. The same
applies to left ventricular thrombus. Although
transthoracic echocardiography is said to be
sensitive for the detection of left ventricular
thrombus,[56] the sensitivity for small thrombus,
<5 mm in diameter, or mural thrombus is less

secure. Cerebral infarction complicates about 6 per cent of acute anterior myocardial infarctions, usually within 2 weeks (Figure 10.4). The risk of embolism when thrombus is detected late, more than 1 month, after an anterior infarction is uncertain but probably around 5 per cent per year.[56,57] Protruding thrombus is more likely to embolize than mural thrombus.[58] If cerebral infarction occurs with clinical features suggesting embolism, the heart remains a likely source after infarction even if thrombus is not demonstrated. The thrombus might have embolized in its entirety or simply not have been detected. In patients with dilated cardiomyopathy, thrombus is found in about one-third of cases.[23] However, embolic stroke occurs with equal frequency in those with and without echocardiographic thrombus at a rate of about 5 per cent per year.[59,60]

Controversial causes of stroke, mitral prolapse, mitral annular calcification, interatrial aneurysm and aortic stenosis are discussed below.

# Transoesophageal echocardiography

Whilst transthoracic echocardiography is mostly unrewarding in patients with ischaemic stroke, the reverse is true of the transoesophageal approach, which is arguably oversensitive in the detection of a potential source for emboli. For example, Vandebogaerde et al[7] found abnormalities in a transoesophageal study in 83 per cent of 40 patients aged 65 (SD = 13) years with features suggesting an embolic stroke. The most common abnormality was left atrial spontaneous contrast, which was found in over one-half of cases, far higher than the 15 per cent or so proportion in all other studies (Table 10.2). It is possible that expertise and interest in diagnosing a particular abnormality affects reporting.

The transoesophageal approach is necessary for the diagnosis of aortic atheroma and dissection, and left atrial thrombus or spontaneous contrast, particularly in the presence of a mechanical prosthetic mitral valve. It is also much more sensitive than transthoracic echocardiography for detecting patent foramen ovale and atrial septal aneurysm. These diagnoses will be discussed in turn.

## Patent foramen ovale

After birth, the foramen ovale is closed as the flap valve formed by the septum primum is pressed against the limbus of the fossa ovalis formed from the septum secundum. This remains as a potential communication until fibrous adhesions develop during the first year of life. However, in about one-third of subjects aged under 30 years adhesions fail to develop. The patent foramen ovale tends to close with age and is only patent in about one-fourth of subjects aged between 30 and 79 and only about one-fifth aged over 80 years.[66,67] Thomson and Evans found that most patent foramina were only probe patent with a mean diameter of 0.1 cm, but Hagen et al more recently have shown that 58 per cent are 5 mm or more in diameter. On average, the diameter was 3.4 mm in the first decade and 5.8 mm in the tenth decade of life.

The potential size of the patent foramen ovale is important, since it is one factor determining the likelihood and size of a paradoxical embolism. Another factor is the magnitude and duration of a pressure difference between the right and left atria. A pressure difference may occur transiently in normal people at rest, but is exaggerated by the valsalva manoeuvre, coughing, crying or straining, or with the use of positive end expiratory pressure ventilation

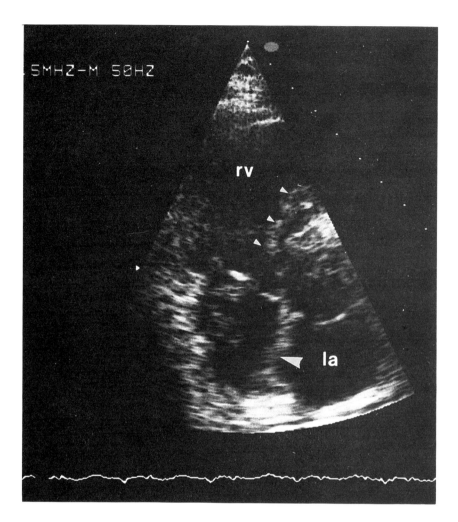

**Figure 10.5**
*Pulmonary embolism in evolution. A long mass (arrowed) is coiled within the right atrium and ventricle with its distal end in the pulmonary artery. At surgery its proximal end was found to be lodged in a patent foramen ovale (large arrow).*

or any process that increases right-sided pressure (e.g. pulmonary embolism, right ventricular infarction, pulmonary hypertension, pneumonectomy). Also necessary is a right-sided thrombus capable of passing through the patent foramen ovale. That this mechanism of stroke is possible is demonstrated by the finding of emboli straddling the patent foramen ovale in 1 per cent of patients with pulmonary emboli (Figure 10.5).

A patent foramen ovale is diagnosed by the passage of contrast from right to left atrium as follows. A 21-mm cannula is positioned in a large vein in the antecubital fossa and attached

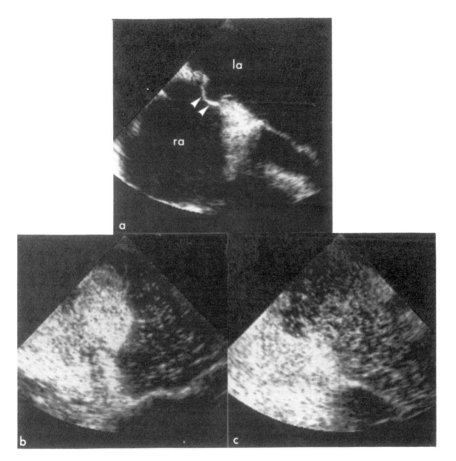

**Figure 10.6**
*Patent foramen ovale. These views are taken using transoesophageal echocardiography. In panel (a) there is an interatrial aneurysm (arrowed) which bulges both to left (panel b) and right (panels a and c). Contrast injection into an antecubital vein causes dense opacification of the right heart and passage of a large volume of contrast to the left.*

to a three-way tap with two 10-ml syringes. One millilitre of blood is drawn into one of the syringes, which has already been filled with 10 ml dextrose or water for injections and about 1 ml air. This mixture is pushed between the two syringes until it becomes frothy, any macroscopic air is expelled and the mixture is injected as fast as possible whilst images are recorded at atrial level (Figure 10.6). This is usually repeated as a valsalva manoeuvre is released, although this is impossible in a sedated patient. By analogy with transthoracic studies, the passage of more than five microbubbles is sometimes taken as the threshold above which to diagnose a patent foramen ovale. However, image quality is usually so good that false positives are unlikely and it seems reasonable to make the diagnosis if any left-sided bubbles appear. Accurate quantification of the shunt is not possible, but an approximate guide is given by the number of bubbles seen. A pulmonary arteriovenous communication can be suspected if the bubbles cross after a delay of two or three cardiac cycles and appear from the direction of the pulmonary veins rather than across the interatrial septum. The technique is safe. From experience with contrast injection using the transthoracic approach before the advent of Doppler ultrasound, we know that transient neurological symptoms, usually minor blurring of vision, are only ever reported in the presence of a large right-to-left shunt as found with an ASD and pulmonary hypertension.

Lechat et al[68] first reported a series of young patients with ischaemic stroke examined using the transthoracic approach. They showed a patent foramen ovale in 40 per cent of cases compared with only 10 per cent of control subjects. In the subgroup with clinical features favouring an embolic stroke, the incidence of patent foramen ovale was even higher, 54 per cent. However, using the more accurate transoesophageal approach the incidence of patent foramen ovale is only about 15–20 per cent (Table 10.2).[7,61–63,65] Unfortunately, most of these studies are uncontrolled. The only study with a control group is that of Vandeboegerde et al,[7] who used patients mostly with lacunar infarctions, vertebrobasilar insufficiency, ischaemic stroke as a result of hypotension or arterial dissection as control subjects. The authors acknowledged that the separation between the clinical groups may not have been perfect; for example, there were two cases with multiinfarction dementia in whom presumably cardiac emboli might have been causative. However, the incidence of patent foramen ovale was similar in each, 15 per cent in the embolic and 23 per cent in the control group. At first sight this finding is worrying for advocates of the importance of patent

foramen ovale, but it only serves to remind us that a patent foramen ovale alone is not a sufficient cause for stroke and there must also be a source of emboli on the right side of the heart. I believe that, where appropriate, venography or ultrasonography should always be used to look for venous thrombosis, and Lechat et al[68] also state this.

Most studies have assessed patent foramen ovale in young subjects. In older patients the incidence of patent foramen ovale is lower, but they tend to be a little larger. Of more importance is that elderly patients are more likely to have raised pulmonary artery pressures and venous thromboses. There is reasonable anecdotal evidence that patent foramina can occasionally cause stroke in the elderly,[69] although systematic studies in this group are still in progress.

## Thrombus and left atrial spontaneous contrast

There is probably a relationship between large left atria, spontaneous contrast, thrombus and peripheral embolism (Figures 10.7 and 10.8). Daniel et al[70] found spontaneous contrast in 61 of 122 patients with mitral valve disease or mitral prostheses and in 11 there was a thrombus and in 25 emboli to brain, kidney or limbs. No patient without spontaneous contrast had thrombus and only four had a history of embolism. Most authors have failed to confirm such a neat relationship and some have found thrombus without spontaneous contrast.[71] However, a number of studies (Table 10.4) in patients with ischaemic stroke have shown thrombus in about 10 per cent and left atrial spontaneous contrast in 10–20 per cent. By contrast, thrombus occurs in about 3 per cent and spontaneous contrast in about 5 per cent of controls.[7]

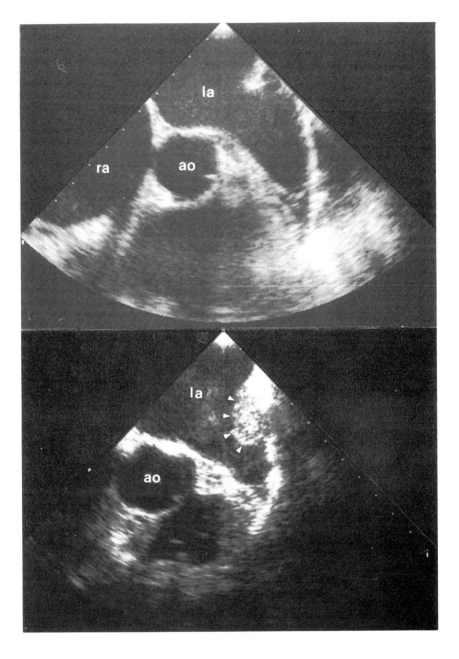

**Figure 10.7**
*Left atrial appendage thrombus. Transoesophageal views in a normal subject (upper panel) and in a patient after cerebral infarction. In the upper panel the appendage is clear although there are prominent pectinate muscles towards its tip. The lower panel shows a 2 cm long thrombus (arrowed) at the base of the appendage. There is also a little spontaneous contrast adjacent to the thrombus.*
*Abbreviations: ao aorta, la left atrium, ra right atrium.*

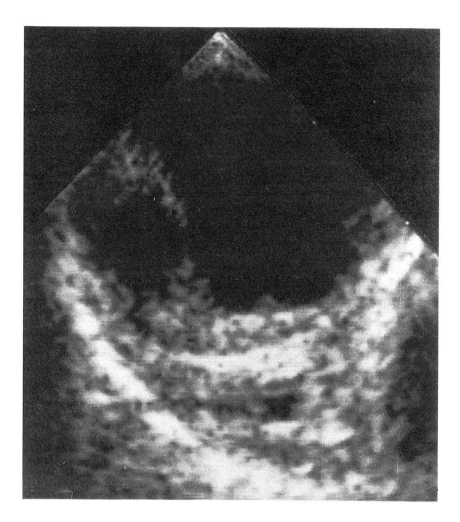

**Figure 10.8**
*Severe aortic atheroma. Transoesophageal view of the descending thoracic aorta just below the arch. There is an ulcerated atheroma protruding more than 5 mm into the lumen. Ulcerated or pedunculated atheroma is strongly associated with stroke or peripheral embolism.*

## Aortic atheroma

Atheroma of the thoracic aorta occurs in about 10 per cent of unselected transoesophageal studies, but in patients with a history consistent with embolic stroke, the prevalence is about 40 per cent.[64,72] Karalis et al[72] found that embolic events occurred in 31 per cent of those with atheroma compared with only 4 per cent of 100 age-matched control subjects.

The morphology of the atheroma affects embolic risk. Embolism occurred in 73 per cent of patients with mobile atheroma protruding more than 5 mm into the lumen compared with 12 per cent of those with simple atheroma (Figure 10.8). The risk of embolism is also increased after invasive procedures. Karalis et al[72] noted embolism in 4 of 15 (27 per cent) patients with atheroma undergoing such procedures as cardiac catheterization or placement of intra-aortic balloons. All the embolic events occurred in patients with complex pedunculated atheroma. In patients with a history suggesting cerebral or peripheral embolism, transoesophageal echocardiography is probably indicated before invasive procedures, since the finding of complex aortic atheroma may modify management. For example, brachial rather than femoral cardiac catheterization might be recommended or the site of aortotomy during coronary grafting might be changed.

## Controversial causes of stroke on echocardiography

### Mitral prolapse

Mitral prolapse has been reported in as many as 40 per cent of patients with ischaemic stroke.[73] However, most authors have found a much lower incidence. Caplan et al[1] found no cases in 127 patients with stroke, Vandenbogaerde et al[7] found an incidence of only 5 per cent, the same as in a control group, and in the SPAF study[21] mitral prolapse was no more common than in the general population. Furthermore, the incidence of stroke in follow-up studies of patients with mitral prolapse is low. Nishimura et al[74] followed 237 patients for a mean of 6.2 years. Ten patients suffered a stroke, but of these, six were in atrial fibrillation, one had bacterial endocarditis and one had a left ventricular aneurysm. Thus, only two

cases might have been asociated with the mitral prolapse alone. In another series, no strokes were reported.[24]

There is circumstantial evidence for a mechanism for embolic stroke in mitral prolapse because platelets and fibrin have been found on the atrial side of the prolapsing segment or at the junction of the left atrial wall and the posterior leaflet in myxomatous mitral valves.[73,75] The echocardiographic diagnosis of prolapse is, however, distinct from, although overlapping with, the diagnosis of myxomatous mitral valve. It relies upon criteria which to some extent are arbitrary and have evolved over the last few years. For example, a prevalence of 35 per cent in normal schoolchildren aged 10–18 years was reduced to less than 1 per cent by the adoption of more stringent criteria.[76] Some authors have reported being able to induce the appearance of prolapse in any subject by tilting the probe to slice obliquely across the leaflet.[77] Mitral prolapse is diagnosed 1½ times more frequently by transoesophageal than by transthoracic echocardiography and this may be artefactual rather than a result of greater sensitivity. One transoesophageal study has found a 60 per cent prevalence in young patients with cerebral infarctions compared with 17 per cent in a control group.[78] The mean age of this group was 35 years. In another study, with a mean age 60 years, mitral prolapse was diagnosed in only two cases (3 per cent).[64] It is easy to overdiagnose mitral prolapse and I believe that reporting bias rather than differences in population demographics explain these major discrepancies between studies in the frequency of mitral prolapse.

Another possible confounding factor is the association between mitral prolapse and other possible sources of embolism, particularly patent foramen ovale. Lechat et al[68] found a higher incidence of mitral prolapse in patients with stroke than in control subjects. However, when they controlled for the presence of patent foramen ovale, this difference disappeared. Mitral prolapse should not be assumed to be the cause of stroke or TIA.

## Mitral annulus calcification

Korn et al[79] noted a few cases of stroke in their original description of massive mitral annular calcification. However, Debono and Warlow[80] suggested an association after noting calcification in 8 of 151 patients with stroke, but in no age- and sex-matched controls. Other authors have reported annular calcification in their series,[1] and in the Boston trial of warfarin in non-rheumatic atrial fibrillation, 67 per cent of those patients who developed stroke had mitral annulus calcification compared with only 119 of 404 (29 per cent) without stroke. There was no associated left atrial enlargement in this study.

Extrusion of material to the surface of the leaflet has been reported and it is conceivable that this might then embolize. Occasionally, thrombosis or endocarditis may develop on the calcific deposit.[81] These mechanisms seem intuitively unlikely and other authors have suggested an association between mitral annulus calcification and aortic atheroma. However, this association has never been tested experimentally. In practical terms it is certainly not safe to assume that annular calcification is the cause of stroke.

## Interatrial aneurysm

An atrial septal aneurysm (Figure 10.6) is an outpouching of the region around the fossa ovalis and is found in about 1 per cent of autopsies.[82] It may be diagnosed by transthoracic echocardiography but transoesophageal echocardiography is more sensitive. The aneurysm may bulge to the left or right or move either way with the cardiac or respiratory cycle. About 15 per cent of patients with ischaemic stroke and 1–3 per cent of control subjects have interatrial aneurysms shown by transoesophageal echocardiography.[61,62,83]

There are two possible mechanisms of stroke in the presence of an interatrial aneurysm. The most likely is by paradoxical embolism since over three-quarters are associated with a patent foramen ovale.[61,62,83,84] Secondly, it is possible that thrombus may occasionally form at the apex of the aneurysm as has been noted at autopsy[82] and on transoesophageal echocardiography.[61,62,83] Care must be taken not to overdiagnose thrombus by misinterpreting tangential cuts across the aneurysm.

## Aortic stenosis

Aortic stenosis is usually included in the list of possible causes of embolic stroke although its prevalence is no higher in patients with stroke than in the general population. Holley et al[85] examined 165 post-mortem cases with aortic stenosis over a 21-year period and found calcareous emboli up to 3 mm in diameter, mainly in the coronary arteries. There was one cerebral embolus. No cases had antemortem evidence of stroke or myocardial infarction and the authors concluded that the emboli were usually silent and of doubtful clinical significance.

# Does echocardiography help?

The major cardiovascular risk factors for stroke are determined clinically: hypertension, heart failure, ischaemic disease and atrial fibrillation. Does echocardiography contribute?

Transthoracic echocardiography is not indicated in patients without clinical evidence of heart disease because the yield is virtually zero. Most people would accept that echocardiography is indicated if there is any abnormality on clinical examination or on the electrocardiogram or chest X-ray. It can then confirm and refine the clinical diagnosis, although, of course, not all abnormalities detected will be relevant (e.g. aortic stenosis, mitral annular calcification). Mitral stenosis is the most important diagnosis linked with stroke, but others are listed in Table 10.2. There is also some evidence that transthoracic measurements such as left atrial diameter or left ventricular systolic function may stratify risk of stroke in patients with non-rheumatic atrial fibrillation.

However, I believe that, for the moment, transoesophageal echocardiography should be regarded as a research technique. In practical terms, patients with large left atria, thrombus or spontaneous contrast shown on transoesophageal echocardiography tend to have mitral valve disease or atrial fibrillation. Lee et al[63] showed that 94 per cent of abnormal transoesophageal scans could be predicted by the presence of atrial fibrillation, a large left atrium or mitral valve thickening on transthoracic echocardiography. Furthermore, a number of abnormalities detected are likely to be spurious or uncommon as a genuine cause (mitral prolapse, isolated interatrial aneurysm). It is not even certain that patent foramen ovale is a genuine cause of stroke.

Even if thrombus or a patent foramen ovale found on transoesophageal echocardiography are causative, there is no proof yet that anticoagulation works as secondary prevention. Although some authors advocate surgical closure of patent foramen ovale in patients after stroke, there is certainly no agreement that this is a reasonable treatment. If proof that anticoagulation is effective as secondary prophylaxis emerges from current trials, it may be that transoesophageal echocardiography will become important in stratifying risk of recurrence. This will be of particular importance in elderly patients or others at high risk of bleeding from warfarin, where the balance between benefit and risk during anticoagulation must be weighed carefully. I think that there should be a trial of warfarin based not on the presence of atrial fibrillation alone but also on the presence of abnormalities on transoesophageal echocardiography.

## Other investigation

There is a little work on the ability of magnetic resonance imaging (MRI) and computerized tomography (CT) scanning to detect intracardiac masses, notably thrombus. Both are better than transthoracic echocardiography at detecting left atrial thrombus, although a comparison with multiplane transoesophageal echocardiography has not been performed.[86,87] Transthoracic echocardiography is said to be 92 per cent sensitive and 88 per cent specific for left ventricular thrombus,[56] although it is less effective for small thrombus, less than 5 mm in diameter. Foster et al[87] found thrombus in 13 patients by CT scanning compared with only 5 by transthoracic echocardiography, although CT scanning may also be troubled by the problem of artefacts.[88]

However, the detection of overt thrombus is usually of secondary importance to establishing a thromboembolic risk as a result of an underlying abnormality. This comparison between techniques, therefore, is not of major practical importance. Both CT scanning and MRI are better than echocardiography for

- **Platelet function**
  Platelet count                    Beta thromboglobulin

- **Coagulation**
  Prothrombin time                  Partial thromboplastin time
  Factor VIII:C                     von Willebrand factor
  Protein S                         Protein C
  Fibrinogen                        Fibrinopeptide A
  Antithrombin

- **General haematology**
  Haematocrit                       ESR

- **Antibodies**
  Lupus anticoagulant               WR
  Anticardiolipin antibody

- **General biochemistry**
  Renal function                    Hepatic function
  Fasting cholesterol               Blood glucose
  Protein electrophoresis

*Source:* Sacco et al[89]; Gustaffson et al.[15]

*General investigation in stroke/TIA.*

tissue characterization. This may be of use, for example, to diagnose myocardial invasion by a tumour or to differentiate thrombus from tumour.

# If I had ...

If I was very young (say under 40!), and had no obvious risk factors for cerebrovascular disease like chronic severe hypertension, I would accept wide investigation. This would include neurological investigation, general investigation and a 12-lead electrocardiogram and transoesophageal echocardiography. If a patent foramen ovale were found I would want a venogram or ultrasound scanning of the deep veins of my leg.

If I was young (under 60), I would want transthoracic echocardiography only if there was clinical evidence of heart disease. I would want transoesophageal echocardiography if there was no evidence of cerebrovascular disease on neurological investigation. I would have myself anticoagulated if a patent foramen ovale with deep vein thrombosis or left atrial thrombus or spontaneous contrast were found. There is no proof that this would be effective, but I think that in the absence of significant contraindications to warfarin, there is obvious common sense in this approach. I would certainly not rush to have a patent foramen ovale closed[90] or have my ascending aorta replaced if there was severe atheroma.[91]

If I was aged over 60 years, I would be less inclined to be investigated aggressively unless there were clinical signs of cardiac disease or unless the trials of therapy guided by transoesophageal echocardiography showed that there was good reason to do so.

# References

1 Caplan LR, Hier DB, D'Cruz I, Cerebral embolism in the Michael Reece Stroke Registry, *Stroke* (1982) **14**:530–7.

2 Ramirez-Lassepas M et al, Can embolic stroke be recognised on the basis of neurologic clinical criteria? *Arch Neurol* (1987) **44**:87–9.

3 Asinger RW et al, Cardiogenic brain embolism: the second report of the Cerebral Embolism Task Force, *Arch Neurol* (1989) **46**:727–43.

4 D'Olhaberriague L et al, A prospective study of atrial fibrillation and stroke, *Stroke* (1989) 20:1648–52.

5 Wolf PA et al, Epidemiological assessment of chronic atrial fibrillation and the risk of stroke, *Neurology* (1978) **28**:973–7.

6 Yamanouchi H et al, Nonvalvular atrial fibrillation as a cause of fatal massive cerebral infarction in the elderly, *Stroke* (1989) 20:1653–6.

7 Vandenbogaerde J et al, Transoesophageal echo-Doppler in patients suspected of a cardiac source of peripheral emboli, *Eur Heart J* (1992) **13**:88–94.

8 Bogousslavsky et al, Cardiac and arterial lesions in carotid transient ischaemic attacks, *Arch Neurol* (1986) **43**:223–8.

9 Good DC et al, Cardiac abnormalities in stroke patients with negative arteriograms, *Stroke* (1986) **17**:6–11.

10 Friedman GD, Loveland DR, Ehrlich SP, Relationship of stroke to other disease, *Circulation* (1968) **38**:533–41.

11 Chesebro JH, Fuster V, Halperin JL, Atrial fibrillation—risk marker for stroke, *N Engl J Med* (1990) **323**:1556–8.

12 Lake FR et al, Atrial fibrillation and mortality in an elderly population, *Aust NZ J Med* (1989) **19**:321–6.

13 Sage JI, van Uitert RL, Risk of recurrent stroke in patients with atrial fibrillation and nonvalvular heart disease, *Stroke* (1983) **14**:537–40.

14 Sandercock P et al, Atrial fibrillation and stroke: prevalence in different types of stroke and influence on early and long term progno-sis (Oxfordshire Community Stroke Project), *BMJ* (1992) **305**:1460–5.

15 Gustaffson C et al, Coagulation factors and the increased risk of stroke in patients with atrial fibrillation, *Stroke* (1990) **21**:47–51.

16 Hart RG, Coull BM, Hart D, Early recurrent embolism associated with nonvalvular atrial fibrillation: a retrospective study, *Stroke* (1983) **14**:688–93.

17 Wolf PA, Abbott RD, Kannel WB, Atrial fibrillation as an independent risk factor for stroke: the Framingham study, *Stroke* (1991) **22**:983–8.

18 Kopecky SL et al, The natural history of lone atrial fibrillation: a population-based study over three decades, *N Engl J Med* (1987) **317**:669–74.

19 Petersen P, Godtfredsen J, Embolic complications in paroxysmal atrial fibrillation, *Stroke* (1986) **17**:622–5.

20 Kagure S et al, High risk of systemic embolism in hypertrophic cardiomyopathy, *Jpn Heart J* (1986) **27**:475–80.

21 Stroke Prevention in Atrial Fibrillation Study Group Investigators, Predictors of thrombo-embolism in atrial fibrillation, II Echo-cardiographic features of patients at risk, *Ann Int Med* (1992) **116**:6–12.

22 Fairfax A, Lambert C, Leatham A, Systemic embolism in chronic siuatrial disorder, *N Engl J Med* (1976) **295**:190–2.

23 Roberts WC, Siegel RJ, McManus BM, Idiopathic dilated cardiomyopathy: analysis of 152 necropsy patients, *Am J Cardiol* (1987) **60**:1340–55.

24 Mills P et al, Long term prognosis of mitral valve prolapse, *N Engl J Med* (1977) **297**:13–18.

25 Brand FN et al, Characteristics and prognosis of lone atrial fibrillation: 30 year follow-up in the Framingham study, *JAMA* (1985) **254**:3449–53.

26 Kannel WB et al, Coronary heart disease and atrial fibrillation: the Framingham Study, *Am Heart J* (1983) **106**:389–96.

27  Dunn M et al, Antithrombotic therapy in atrial fibrillation, *Chest* (1986) **89**(suppl): 68S–74S.

28  Arnold AZ et al, Role of prophylactic anticoagulation for direct current cardioversion in patients with atrial fibrillation or atrial flutter, *JACC* (1992) **19**:851–5.

29  Petersen P et al, Placebo-controlled randomized trial of warfarin and aspirin for prevention of thromboembolic complications in chronic atrial fibrillation. The Copenhagen AFASAK Study, *Lancet* (1989) **1**:175–9.

30  Boston Area Anticoagulation Trial for Atrial Fibrillation Investigators, The effect of low-dose warfarin on the risk of stroke in patients with nonrheumatic atrial fibrillation, *N Engl J Med* (1990) **323**:1505–11.

31  Connolly SJ et al, Canadian atrial fibrillation (CAFA) study, *JACC* (1991) **18**:349–55.

32  Stroke Prevention in Atrial Fibrillation Study Group Investigators, Report of the Stroke Prevention in Atrial Fibrillation Study, *Circulation* (1991) **84**:527–39.

33  Ezekowitz MD et al, Warfarin in the prevention of stroke associated with nonrheumatic atrial fibrillation, *N Engl J Med* (1992) **327**:1406–12.

34  Easton JF, Sherman DG, Management of cerebral embolism of cardiac origin, *Stroke* (1980) **11**:433–42.

35  Wolf PA et al, Duration of atrial fibrillation and imminence of stroke: the Framingham study, *Stroke* (1983) **14**:664–7.

36  Koller RL, Recurrent embolic cerebral infarction and anticoagulation, *Neurology* (1982) **32**:283–5.

37  Landefeld CS, Goldman L, Major bleeding in outpatients treated with warfarin: incidence and prediction by factors known at the time of outpatient therapy, *Am J Med* (1989) **87**:144–52.

38  Lundström T, Ryge'n L, Haemorrhagic and thrombotic complications in patients with atrial fibrillation on anticoagulant prophylaxis, *J Int Med* (1989) **225**:137–42.

39  Caplan LR et al, Atrial size, atrial fibrillation and stroke, *Ann Neurol* (1986) **19**:158–61.

40  Rem JA et al, Value of cardiac monitoring and echocardiography in TIA and stroke patients, *Stroke* (1985) **16**:950–6.

41  Come PC, Riley MF, Bivas NK, Role of echocardiography and arrhythmia monitoring in the evaluation of patients with suspected systemic embolism, *Ann Neurol* (1983) **13**:527–31.

42  Koudstaal PJ et al, Risk of cardiac events in atypical transient ischaemic attack or minor stroke, *Lancet* (1992) **340**:630–3.

43  Nishide M et al, Cardiac abnormalities in ischaemic cerebrovascular disease studied by two-dimensional echocardiography, *Stroke* (1983) **14**:541–5.

44  Knopman DS et al, Indications for echocardiography in patients with ischaemic stroke, *Neurology* (1982) **32**:1005–11.

45  Bergerson G, Shah P, Echocardiography unwarranted in patients with cerebral ischaemic events, *N Engl J Med* (1981) **304**:489.

46  Burnett PJ et al, The role of echocardiography in the investigation of focal cerebral ischaemia, *Postgrad Med J* (1984) **60**:116–9.

47  Shapiro LM et al, Is cardiac ultrasound mandatory in patients with transient ischaemic attacks? *Br Med J* (1985) **291**:786–7.

48  Robbins JA et al, Influence of echocardiography on management of patients with systemic emboli, *Stroke* (1983) **14**:546–9.

49  Cujek B et al, Transesophagal echocardiography in the detection of potential cardiac source of embolism in stroke patients, *Stroke* (1991) **22**:727–33.

50  Pruitt AA et al, Neurologic complications of bacterial endocarditis, *Medicine (Baltimore)* (1978) **57**:329–43.

51  Graus F, Rogers LR, Posner JB, Cerebrovascular complications in patients with cancer, *Medicine* (1985) **64**:16–35.

52  Lopez JA et al, Nonbacterial thrombotic endocarditis: a review, *Am Heart J* (1987) **113**:773–84.

53  Cooke RA, Chambers JB, The role of echocardiography in the diagnosis and management of infective endocarditis, *Brit J Clin Prac* (1992) **46**:111–5.

54  Hart RG, Miller VT, Cerebral infarction in young adults: a practical approach, *Stroke* (1983) **14**:110–4.

55  Jordan RA et al, Thromboembolism in acute and in healed myocardial infarction. I

Intracardiac mural thrombosis. II Systemic and pulmonary artery occlusion, *Circulation* (1952) **6**:1–6, 7–15.

56 Visser CA et al, Two-dimensional echo in the diagnosis of left ventricular thrombus, *Chest* (1983) **83**:228–32.

57 Stratton JR, Resnick JL, Increased embolic risk in patients with left ventricular thrombi, *Circulation* (1987) **75**:1004–11.

58 Lloret RL et al, Classification of left ventricular thrombi by their history of systemic embolization using pattern recognition of two-dimensional echocardiograms, *Am Heart J* (1985) **110**:761–5.

59 Fuster V et al, The natural history of idiopathic dilated cardiomyopathy, *Am J Cardiol* (1981) **47**:525–30.

60 Gottdiener JS et al, Frequency and embolic potential of left ventricular thrombus in dilated cardiomyopathy: assessment by 2-dimensional echocardiography, *Am J Cardiol* (1983) **52**:1281–5.

61 Pearson AC et al, Superiority of transoesophageal echocardiography in detecting cardiac source of embolism in patients with cerebral ischaemia of uncertain etiology, *JACC* (1991) **17**:66–72.

62 Pearson AC et al, Atrial septal aneurysm and stroke: a transoesophageal echocardiographic study, *JACC* (1991) **18**:1223–9.

63 Lee RJ et al, Enhanced detection of sources of cerebral emboli by transesophageal echocardiography, *Stroke* (1991) **22**:734–9.

64 Pop G et al, Transoesophageal echocardiography in the detection of intracranial embolic sources in patients with transient ischaemic attacks, *Stroke* (1990) **21**:560–5.

65 DeBelder MA et al, Limitations of transoesophageal echocardiography in patients with focal cerebral ischaemic events, *Br Heart J* (1992) **67**:297–303.

66 Thompson T, Evans, W, Paradoxical embolism, *Q J Med* (1930) **23**:135–50.

67 Hagen PT, Scholz DG, Edwards WD, Incidence and size of patent foramen ovale during the first 10 decades of life: an autopsy study of 965 normal hearts, *Mayo Clin Proc* (1984) **59**:17–20.

68 Lechat P et al, Prevalence of patent foramen ovale in patients with stroke, *N Engl J Med* (1988) **318**:1148–52.

69 Vella M et al, Paradoxical emboli in elderly patients, *Br J Clin Prac* (1992) **46**:65–6.

70 Daniel WG et al, Left atrial spontaneous contrast in mitral valve disease: an indicator for an increased thromboembolic risk, *JACC* (1988) **11**:1204–11.

71 Castello R et al, Atrial spontaneous contrast in patients undergoing transoesophageal echocardiography: prevalence and clinical implications, *Am J Cardiol* (1990) **65**:1149–53.

72 Karalis DG et al, Recognition and embolic potential of intraaortic atherosclerotic debris, *JACC* (1991) **17**:73–8.

73 Barnett HJM et al, Further evidence relating mitral valve prolapse to cerebral ischaemic events, *N Engl J Med* (1980) **307**:369–70.

74 Nishimura RA et al, Echocardiographically documented mitral valve prolapse. Long-term follow-up of 237 patients, *N Engl J Med* (1985) **313**:1305–9.

75 Shrivastava S, Guthrie RB, Edwards JE, Prolapse of the mitral valve, *Mod Concepts Cardiovasc Dis* (1977) **46**:57–61.

76 Warth DC et al, Prevalence of mitral prolapse in normal children. *JACC* (1985) **5**:1173–7.

77 Sahn DJ et al, Echocardiographic spectrum of mitral valve motion in children with and without mitral valve prolapse: the nature of false positive diagnosis, *Am J Cardiol* (1977) **38**:422–431.

78 Zenker G et al, Transesophageal two-dimensional echocardiography in young patients with cerebral ischaemic events, *Stroke* (1988) **19**:345–8.

79 Korn D, DeSanctis RW, Sell S, Massive calcification of the mitral annulus. A clinicopathological study of 14 cases, *N Engl J Med* (1962) **267**:900–9.

80 DeBono DP, Warlow CP, Mitral-annular calcification and cerebral or retinal ischaemia, *Lancet* (1979) **2**:383–5.

81 D'Cruz IA et al, Clinical manifestations of mitral annulus calcification with emphasis on its echocardiographic features, *Am Heart J* (1977) **94**:367–77.

82 Silver MD, Dorsey JS, Aneurysm of the septum primum in adults, *Arch Pathol Lab Med* (1978) **102**:62–5.

83 Schneider B et al, Improved morphologic characterization of atrial septal aneurysm by transoesophageal echocardiography: relation to

cerebrovascular events, *JACC* (1990) **16**:1000–9.

84 Zabalgoitia-Reyes M et al, A possible mechanism for neurologic ischaemic events in patients with atrial septal aneurysm, *Am J Cardiol* (1990) **66**:761–4.

85 Holley KE et al, Spontaneous calcific embolization associated with calcific aortic stenosis, *Circulation* (1963) **27**:197–202.

86 Gomes AS et al, Cardiac tumors and thrombus: evaluation with MR imaging, *Am J Radiol* (1987) **149**:895–9.

87 Foster CJ et al, Identification of intracardiac thrombus: comparison of computed tomography and cross-sectional echocardiography, *Br J Radiol* (1987) **60**:327–31.

88 Goldstein JA et al, Evaluation of left ventricular thrombi by contrast-enhanced computed tomography and two-dimensional echocardiography, *Am J Cardiol* (1986) **57**:757–60.

89 Sacco RL et al, Free protein S deficiency: a possible association with cerebrovascular occlusion, *Stroke* (1989) **20**:1657–61.

90 Harvey JR et al, Clinically silent atrial septal defects with evidence of cerebral embolization, *Ann Int Med* (1986) **805**:695–7.

91 Culliford AT et al, The atherosclerotic ascending aorta and transverse arch: a new technique to prevent cerebral injury during bypass: experience with 13 patients, *Ann Thorac Surg* (1986) **41**:28–35.

# 11

# Aortic dissection

*Tom Treasure and Iain A Simpson*

Aortic dissection is said to occur with an incidence of 5–10 cases per million per annum in Western society. It is twice as common in males as in females with a peak incidence between the ages of 50 and 70. In St George's we see about 15 cases per annum, mainly from the South West Thames Region, which would suggest, if these estimates are correct, that more than half of all cases reach us.

Nationally there might be up to 500 cases per annum. According to the UK Cardiac Surgical Register, in very round figures, about 200 operations are performed to replace the ascending aorta each year, and in British practice, dissection will be the commonest indication (Figure 11.1). In terms of surgical availability, therefore, these figures would suggest that our ability to offer surgery for this condition is, in proportional terms, much better than for interventions for ischaemic heart disease.

Italian authors have claimed that there is an increasing incidence[1,2] but these estimates depend on the relative numbers being examined post mortem and the diagnostic certainty. On the evidence available it seems to be no more than an impression.

## Presentation

Clinical suspicion is the most important factor in identifying aortic dissection and since the vast majority present outside cardiac surgical centres it is important for those physicians and surgeons who provide an acute admissions service to be aware of its presentation. Having reviewed many cases of aortic dissection after the diagnosis has been made, our impression is that more careful attention to the history might saved diagnostic difficulty in at least some cases. The presentation is variable but the most common clinical symptom by far is the onset of severe chest pain.

The patient with aortic dissection had an intact aorta at a point in time and then, a second or so later, a dissection. The suddenness of onset is typical. Patients really do talk about spears between the shoulders, being torn apart from top to bottom etc. In marked contrast the symptoms of myocardial ischaemia build up over at least minutes, may come and go, and the associated sensations of nausea and apprehension are on a similar time base.

The location of pain may be helpful. Those patients with ascending aortic dissection more often have anterior chest pain while those with dissection originating in the descending aorta describe interscapular pain. Indeed, the onset of anterior chest pain which subsequently radiates through to the interscapular region is often indicative of a type I aortic dissection originating in the ascending aorta and extending over the arch to involve the descending portion. Associated symptoms of nausea,

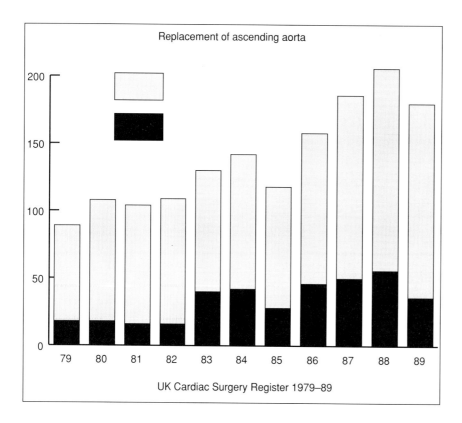

**Figure 11.1**
*Data from the UK Cardiac Surgery Register 1979–89 recording all operations categorized as replacement of the ascending aorta. It is impossible to be sure how many of these are for dissection, but that is the commonest indication for aortic surgery in British practice. The mortality is indicated in the bar chart for each year.*

vomiting and sweating are usually related to vasovagal effects.

Other presentations are less common but important to recognize and can be related to the patho-physiological manifestations of the condition. The dissection may involve the head and neck vessels and so a presentation with syncope or a cerebral vascular event may occur and dissection in the critical area of the lower thoracic aorta may interrupt the spinal blood supply and cause paraplegia. When dissection extends retrogradely, typically into the non-coronary sinus, the aortic valve becomes regurgitant and result in pulmonary oedema. Presentation may be with acute myocardial infarction if there is coronary ostial involvement. Rupture into the pericardium, or rather slower seepage through thinned aortic adventitia, results in tamponade.

With ascending aortic dissection are are usually very unwell and peripherally vasoconstricted but the arterial pressure is often elevated. If a proximal dissection involves the arch vessels then different blood pressures may be recorded in the right and left arms or between the arms and legs. This is an important clinical sign as it almost always indicates a dissection originating in the ascending aorta. Note that subclavian stenosis will also produce a differential blood pressure recording so, as with all clinical signs in medicine, it is not absolute. Aortic regurgitation will be present on auscultation in around half of the patients with a dissection of the ascending aorta. Extension of the dissection into the abdominal aorta may produce ischaemic bowel or anuria, which are important prognostic features, as are neurological sequelae. Pyrexia is common, presumably as a response to the presence of intraluminal haematoma. Overt 'heart failure' is usually a result of acute severe aortic regurgitation, and haemodynamic collapse is likely to indicate aortic rupture, often into the pericardium, or less commonly the left pleural space.

## Management

Control of hypertension is essential and must not be overlooked in the course of striving for a diagnosis. Arterial pressure monitoring is ideal but not absolutely essential.

Nitroprusside is an extremely useful first-line drug. Some are afraid of it because of the need to use it intravenously and its rapidity of action. In fact it is its rapid onset and the short half-life of its vascular effect (2–3 min) which make it a safe drug to use. The great advantage of nitroprusside is that if hypotension is accidentally induced it will go away in a few minutes. Elevation of the legs meanwhile may be all that is required. The mistake is to panic,

initiate massage, and inject calcium and adrenaline, all of which are bad for the patient with dissection.

The algorithms developed for automatic computer-driven systems to administer nitroprusside have taught us the rules for its administration:

- Start at a modest dose, at the lower end of the therapeutic range.
- Revise the dose at 3–5-min intervals.
- Always make conservative alterations aimed at no more than half correction of the perceived hyper- or hypotension.
- Avoid 'all-or-none' panic responses such as turning the infusion full on or off.
- Leave it in the hands of a properly trained intensive care nurse whenever possible because the doctors, especially cardiologists and surgeons, will go away to do other things and fail to obey the algorithm in the slavish way that a computer does. While the algorithm may bring the pressure down smoothly to the required asymptote, the doctor produces a blood pressure chart like a Himalayan mountain range.

Nitroglycerine has potent venodilating effects and a longer half-life and is not appropriate for this use.

Beta-blockade is logical and attractive as it reduces not only the systolic pressure but also the rate of rise of pressure, which may be important in preventing extension of the dissection. Duration of action is a consideration and has led to the underuse of beta-blockade in the acute case quite frequently, but labetolol by infusion has been useful and now esmolol is probably a good choice. It has an elimination half-life of 9 min and is metabolized by esterases in red blood cells. Renal and hepatic clearance may be in doubt in aortic dissection but red blood cells remain readily available.

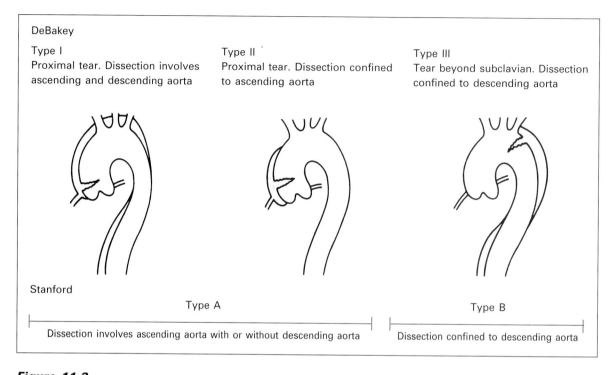

DeBakey

Type I
Proximal tear. Dissection involves
ascending and descending aorta

Type II
Proximal tear. Dissection confined
to ascending aorta

Type III
Tear beyond subclavian. Dissection
confined to descending aorta

Stanford

Type A

Dissection involves ascending aorta with or without descending aorta

Type B

Dissection confined to descending aorta

**Figure 11.2**
*Classification of aortic dissection. This illustrates the characteristic types according to the De Bakey
and Stanford classifications. Other combinations of unusually sited tears and extensive dissection
occur, and are best grouped according to whether they involve (type A) or do not involve (type B) the
ascending aorta. Adapted from* Surgery (Oxford) *1989; **74**: 1765–70, with permission.*

Simple but effective immediate management
such as oxygen administration, analgesia and
volume replacement should not be forgotten,
but once the immediate management and blood
pressure control has been rapidly but smoothly
achieved, diagnostic confirmation and identification of the site and extent of the dissection
is of paramount importance so that effective
surgical management can be instituted if necessary.

## Classification of aortic dissection

The terminology used to classify aortic dissection seems to cause some difficulty (Figure
11.2). The fact that, in the DeBakey classification, a patient with a type I dissection has what
amounts to a combination of type II and type
III seems to create some confusion for numer-
ically orderly minds.

The much simpler division of aortic dissection into those that involve the ascending (or anterior) aorta (type A) and those that spare it (type B) also the merit of dividing the cases into those in which we feel compelled to operate (A) and those which we would prefer to manage conservatively (B).

This simple division has much to recommend it in the early decision-making stage of management. As far as subsequent analysis of results is concerned, it is less satisfactory. The rather uncommon type II dissections are technically easier to handle, and surgery to the ascending aorta has the potential for excluding all the dissected part of the aorta. On the other hand, type I, with which it is grouped in the simpler dichotomous classification, is only palliated. Only the ascending aortic component is dealt with and the aorta may remain double-barrelled with branches coming off the false or true lumen.

When long-term results are being quoted the relative contribution of types I and II to the series is of importance.

# Pathology, aetiology and some misconceptions

## Pathology

Aortic dissection has two components, the intimal tear and cleavage of the aortic media over some of its length. For dissection to occur there has to be some degeneration in the media, with a histological appearance also known as cystic medial necrosis. This is a non-specific appearance of the aorta, not a discrete pathological entity. However, it is, it would appear, a necessary component of the problem because a healthy aorta cannot be made to cleave along its length in this way.

The tear can be anywhere in the aorta, varies in length, and varies in orientation. It tends to be more transverse than longitudinal. Typically, it runs 60–70 per cent round the circumference. The commonest site is at the level of the commissures of the aortic valve, and the second is just beyond the left subclavian artery.

In types I and II, retrograde dissection the short distance back to the aortic annulus, particularly in the non-coronary sinus, is almost invariable with a varying degree of coronary ostial involvement, right more than left. Antegrade dissection may involve the whole aorta to its bifurcation, frequently extends into the branches of the aorta and is not infrequently seen in the femoral artery exposed for cannulation at operation. By definition, in type II, antegrade dissection is not beyond the brachiocephalic (innominate) artery.

Interestingly, retrograde extension when the tear is beyond the left subclavian artery is relatively unusual. When it does occur and involves the ascending aorta it creates some difficulties in classification. It has to be called type A in the dichotomous classification. If we let the site of the tear determine classification in the DeBakey terminology it is type III with retrograde extension (or type IIIa, as some call it) but in its hazard it more resembles type I. It also creates some difficulties with operative decision-making.

Any combination of arterial branches can temporarily or permanently be occluded with appropriate patterns of regional ischaemia, including stroke, paraplegia, renal failure, mesenteric ischaemia and cold, pulseless limbs.

## Aetiology

The commonest aetiological factor is hypertension. The aorta has presumably suffered degeneration of its media over years. Why the intima should give way is not clear but once the intima is breached, dissection propagates. There is often hypertension at presentation.

Occasionally there is a history of exertion, particularly an isometric, straining-type of effort. The commonest patterns associated with hypertension are type I and type III.

The Marfan syndrome is a well-known cause of both dissection and proximal aortic aneurysmal dilatation. An individual may have one, or the other, or both. Dissection is more likely in a dilated aorta but dilatation is not a prerequisite.

Congenital abnormalities of the aortic valve, i.e. specifically bicuspid or unicommissural valves, increase the likelihood of aortic dissection starting in the ascending aorta, with the tear occurring where the eccentric jet impinged on the convexity of the aorta. The risk for an individual with such a valve is very small but in series of cases of dissection, bicuspid aortic valve is seen 10 times more frequently than in the general population. Type III dissection is not associated with aortic valve abnormalities.

The risk of dissection in pregnancy is of course minute but if a young woman dissects she is either pregnant, or marfanoid, or both. If she is both, the risk of dissection occurring in that pregnancy may be as high as 20 per cent.

## Some misconceptions

It is commonly and perhaps loosely said that atherosclerosis is an aetiological factor. Atherosclerosis is common and is associated with hypertension but in fact when we operate on the ascending aorta there is rarely atheromatous disease of the intima. Similarly it is commonly said that a pre-existing aneurysm may dissect. They may expand and leak, which is not the same.

One question that arises is which comes first, the intimal tear permitting entry of blood which then dissects the aorta along its length, or bleeding into the media, which in due course ruptures through, creating an intimal tear.

Some pathologists have argued for the latter. A pathologist (not a cardiac specialist) once triumphantly produced an aorta to show me (TT) a dissection with no intimal tear. With a fairly brief inspection of the aortic lumen I was able to point out the tear, to the satisfaction of all present, albeit not in the commonest site, but in one of the typical positions in the arch of the aorta. Not only did that fail to persuade me of the argument for dissection before tear but it made me circumspect about similar claims. The sudden tearing pain that is typical of dissection also suggests the sudden entry of blood from the aortic lumen rather than the much slower accumulation of blood from an intramural bleed.

Sometimes when the inside of the Marfan aorta is inspected, rather flat, fibrosed scars are seen in the intima. These have been called 'healed dissections'. They may be healed intimal tears but there is no evidence whatever that they were ever dissections in the sense that they had length. This is important because it has led to a notion that Marfan dissections can heal spontaneously, which may be dangerous for the Marfan patient with a dissection who is then managed conservatively in the hope that his florid type I dissection will marvellously heal back to such an innocent-looking intimal split. Unlikely!

Traumatic aortic transection or rupture, which most commonly occurs beyond the left subclavian, does not propagate as a dissection but is contained within the aortic adventitia and the pleura as a localized haematoma.

## Imaging the aorta in suspected dissection

As new diagnostic methods have arrived, and older methods have been refined, clinical papers have appeared evaluating new imaging methods, measuring their performance against older ones. More recently these papers have become cluttered with the terminology of Bayesian statistics, such as sensitivity, specificity and predictive value. While these evaluations are valuable, and perhaps even essential, there is a tendency for the authors to create an aura of difficulty, sometimes emphasizing imagined inadequacies of the old technique, in order to justify their study and their expensive equipment. Words like 'gold standard' are in the lingua franca of such studies.[3,4]

Bayesian statistics are a valuable method for assessing the cost-effectiveness of a test and exploring its value as either a diagnostic or, on the other hand, a mass screening test, but while they are valuable in the hands of epidemiologists and actuaries, they appear to have created one of the 'difficulties' in the diagnosis of aortic dissection. In order to make a statistical evaluation the authors may have been constrained by two fundamentally false premises. The first is that the result has to be either 'positive' or 'negative'. This permits the construction of tidy $2 \times 2$ contingency tables and the analysis of diagnostic accuracy. It then results in a paper in which claims for relative superiority of one technique over another are made and, in no time, common sense is lost amongst claims and counterclaims. This simple sorting of tests into positive and negative overlooks the variable reliability of the tests according to the skill of the operator, the quality of the equipment available, the suitability of the subject and the many subtle clues that the experienced clinical team pick up as they discuss the investigations of an acutely ill patient.

In a typical DeBakey type I dissection with a typical history, physical signs and chest X-ray, it is highly likely that any investigation—contrast aortography, computerized tomography or oesophageal ultrasound—will confirm unequivocally that some part of the aorta is dissected. Transthoracic ultrasound may well be adequate. At the other extreme, if a patient has a limited dissection and the false lumen has thrombosed because there is no re-entry and therefore no flow, some tests may be suggestive to the highly critical observer but none totally convincing.

The second false premise is that they are equally available or equally applicable. They are not. The following scenarios illustrate the illogicality of the $2 \times 2$ contingency table approach to the problem.

- In a stable patient in a district hospital with good CT but no angiography suite, a diagnostic CT to decide about transfer is not only appropriate, but ideal.
- In a critical patient in a cardiac surgical unit, we would prefer transoesophageal ultrasound, in the operating theatre, with the patient anaesthetized and monitored (Figure 11.3). A trip to the basement of the hospital to the CT scanner would not be appropriate.
- In a patient with a chronic stable dissection being electively evaluated in a cardiac unit, aortography would be best, to determine the exact relationship of the arch vessels to the two lumens, for example, and to provide a surgeon with the longitudinal image of the aorta with which he feels comfortable.
- A chronic patient with a decision to be made about the state of the descending aorta might be referred on for magnetic resonance imaging.

A cautionary note should be sounded. The ideal imaging technique for all cases of suspected dissection does not exist. Each has its own merits and disadvantages. In an acute dissection, the rapidity of diagnosis is important and echocardiography, both transthoracic

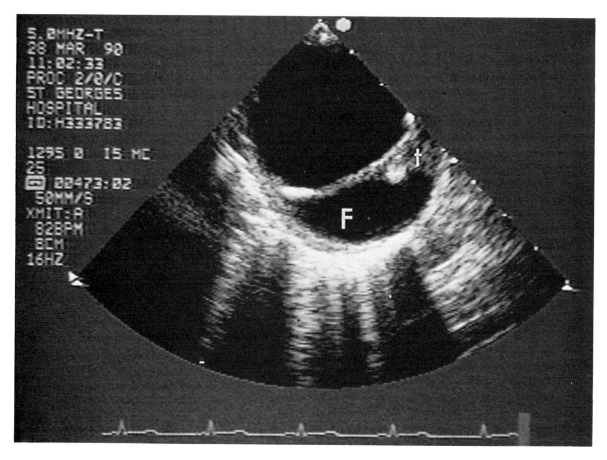

**Figure 11.3**
Transoesophageal echo in a patient with aortic dissection. The aorta is seen in cross-section divided by an intimal flap. The false lumen (F) is seen to contain an area of thrombus (t)

and transoesophageal, fulfils the role of an imaging technique applicable within the intensive care unit. As already stated, when there is a chronic dissection, or echocardiography has provided incomplete information, a variety of alternative investigations are potentially available. Sometimes a number of different imaging modalities are required before a complicated picture is clarified. Transoesophageal echo-

cardiography may indicate a dissection confined to the descending aorta but angiography or magnetic resonance imaging is required to determine the extent of dissection and the involvement of the abdominal viscera.

A good CT scan at the time of presentation in a district hospital to determine the need for referral is desirable but only if two criteria are achieved:

1 The imaging technology must be readily available and with a 24-h on-call service.
2 A clinician with appropriate training must be available to interpret the images.

One might naïvely expect that one naturally goes with the other. This is not always the case. We have seen the situation where an adequate CT scan had been reported as normal, yet, when the patient was eventually referred to a regional cardiac centre, the diagnosis of aortic dissection was apparent. The reverse situation has also been encountered! This is not to cast scorn on radiologists in district hospitals but to highlight the fact that aortic dissection is an uncommon presentation to a district hospital and is therefore easily misinterpreted. A large regional centre will see many more dissections and is therefore more experienced in diagnosis. Availability of high-resolution cardiac imaging equipment is only part of the solution. Adequate training to use such facilities is also important. Transoesophageal echocardiography is a classic example. Many such probes are being sold to echocardiography departments, yet very few have the training and expertise to use them properly. It is only natural and proper that different departments will place different emphasis on the various imaging techniques available to them for the investigation of suspected aortic dissection, trusting those in which they have the most experience and confidence.

## *What is the purpose of the investigation[5]?*

In medicine, diagnosis is of paramount importance. Without it we cannot make rational decisions about management or give any useful indication of prognosis, and yet it is a good discipline to ask ourselves 'How will it influence management?' before embarking on each diagnostic investigation.

There are three components to the diagnosis of aortic dissection:

1 Is there a dissection of the aorta?
2 Does it involve the ascending aorta?
3 What is its full extent and what does it involve?

They form a logical progression although they do not always come out so neatly and all or some may be answered by any given test on any particular occasion. If the answer to the first is 'no', then the second two are obviated. The anxiety about dissection can be set to one side. The possibilities of emergency aortic surgery or transfer to a specialist unit for this to be considered are no longer applicable.

What is available on site usually overrides all other considerations for which is more important, sensitivity or specificity? In this instance a false positive is considered safer than a false negative by the district physician because he can transfer the patient on to a specialist unit and not have the embarrassment of having missed a dissection. He is interested in high sensitivity, to use Bayesian terminology. Transthoracic echo is unsatisfactory because while visualization of a flap in expert hands is reliable, failure to see a flap is not. The other standard methods, CT, angiography and transoesophageal ultrasound, will all provide the answer to this question.

If the answer to the second question is that the dissection does *not* involve the ascending aorta, then emergency surgery drops from being first-line treatment to something which most experts would strive to avoid. If the ascending aorta is involved, surgery is the preferred treatment. The surgeon, unlike the district physician, does not want any false positives. To open the aorta on cardiopulmonary bypass and find no dissection leaves him in an awkward position which he may wish to share with the referring physician. He is therefore interested in specificity.

The third question becomes relevant only if an operation is to be undertaken, and then only if the circumstances are such that the surgeon places a high priority on this information, and believes it will help.

# Surgery of aortic dissection

## The decision to operate

A patient in immediate danger of death from aortic dissection is a challenge from the surgeon's point of view. The aorta is amenable to replacement with a synthetic graft and patients that do well leave the intensive care unit promptly, much as routine cases do, and are restored to good health. The risk–benefit equation is attractive—near-certain death against a reasonable prospect of success. However, this simplistic view of the equation merits closer examination.

The probability of death without surgery in ascending aortic dissection is high but we know that it is not 100 per cent because from time to time we see patients referred electively with aortic regurgitation in whom the aetiology proves to be aortic dissection. On questioning, one can elicit a history of a sudden event months or years ago. The pain may even have been typical (as we retake the history with the diagnosis known). The patients may even know that the doctors were worried about why the blood pressure was high. If these few patients come to elective investigation having survived, we ask ourselves, as Wheat did in the 1960s, is there a place for non-operative management? We do not believe there is.

Over a 10-year period we have known a number of patients with ascending aortic

dissection who, for various reasons, were not operated on acutely (some because the surgeon in charge followed Wheat's philosophy, some because there were other reasons to make us wish to avoid surgery) but all were followed. They all died in hospital. Statistically, that should not convince us that conservative management leads to 100 per cent mortality because the 95 per cent confidence limits of 0/8 includes 0–37 per cent, but eight consecutive deaths with no survivors has not encouraged us to offer conservative management to any more patients with ascending aortic dissection as the preferred course of action. We decline to operate on some patients but it is because we do not expect them to survive surgery or get any useful benefit for other reasons. On the other hand, the majority of patients who have been managed conservatively with descending aortic dissection have survived to leave hospital. This experience is in line with published series.

## Contraindications to operation in ascending aortic dissection

Established stroke, paraplegia, renal failure and proven mesenteric ischaemia are good reasons to believe that even if the ascending aorta can be repaired, the prospect of return to health is so remote that we should not operate. We have operated on patients after transient ischaemic attacks and restored the anatomy of the cerebral blood supply successfully. We have also operated in the presence of deteriorating renal function and had it improved. Each case must be judged on its merits but we do not subscribe to the view, sometimes expressed, that the patient is bound to die without surgery so we might as well 'have a go'. There has to be some realistic prospect of useful benefit to justify putting a patient, the family, our clinical team and ourselves through what can be a very grim experience. Old age and co-morbidity are relative contraindications.

## *The objectives of operation for acute ascending aortic dissection*

The primary purpose of operating is to save the patient's life. In the majority of cases, death results from rupture into the pericardium. Aortic regurgitation and coronary obstruction are also fatal complications of dissection in this part of the aorta. Reconstitution of the ascending aorta can prevent these cardiac causes of death.

In type II dissection the repair is complete. In type I dissection the surgeon only controls the component involving the ascending aorta, and possibly the arch, and death from other causes is still a risk. In a way, the condition has been converted to type III, and the patient faces the residual risk which might be expected with conservative management of that type of dissection.

The causes of death associated with dissection beyond the surgically correctable ascending aortic component are rupture of the false lumen in the mediastinum, left chest or the abdomen, or ischaemia of the brain, kidney or viscera. If the whole of the dissection is not excluded, these cannot be reliably controlled. If the primary tear is not excluded, the false lumen will continue to fill under pressure, and even if the primary tear is repaired we know that there are often multiple re-entries at various levels. The results then are unpredictable. Usually the condition stabilizes and the residual dissection is compatible with survival and reasonable long-term recovery. Occasionally an organ not previously ischaemic, the brain or the kidney, becomes ischaemic after the repair, presumably because

it was relying on its blood supply from the false lumen. In the acute case, this is largely the luck of the lottery. It is a more legitimate surgical anxiety in the chronic case, where abnormal flow has become established, the diagnosis should be more complete, the operation can be planned more carefully, and a technically more precise procedure may be possible.

## *The operation for aortic dissection*

Aortic dissection is viewed as a surgical emergency, and operation is usually undertaken as soon as the diagnosis is made. It is a dramatic cause of sudden death but sudden, dramatic operations may also result in death. In the much cited study of natural history by Anagnostopoulos of 963 cases collected from six reported series,[6] 20 per cent had died within 6 h. But of those still alive at 6 h (which would be representative of the time to reach a definitive diagnosis in a cardiac surgical unit for an immediately referred acute dissection), 80 per cent were alive at 24 h, and that without any selection or sophisticated management. At the Middlesex Hospital we formed a joint surgical and anaesthetic policy to avoid precipitate unscheduled surgery and to plan to operate within 24 h using a well-rehearsed anaesthetic and surgical protocol.[7] In practice this meant that the patient would be taken to theatre at the beginning of the following morning. No patients died in the interim.

This policy was not just for the sake of the operating theatre team, although if it is as safe for the patient to wait until morning as for us to be operating all night, why should we not be considered? In fact, it is probably safer. In an operation beginning in the late evening it is in the early hours of the morning an exhausted

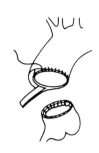 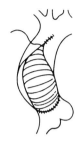 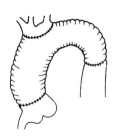 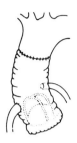

(a) If the tissues will take sutures, and the tear is localised, the dissection can be repaired locally

(b) More commonly, a length of the fragile aorta must be replaced, and an inclusion technique is the safest and simplest method

(c) Occasionally, more extensive replacement may be necessary

(d) In Marfan's disease, the valve must also be replaced and the coronary arteries reimplanted (Bentall's operation)

**Figure 11.4**

*Surgical options in the repair of ascending aortic dissection. The actual operation will employ a range of individual options according to the preference of the surgeon and the demands of the case. Protecting the aortic valve, coronary orifices and intrapericardial portion of the aorta is paramount. Controlling the aortic tear is preferable. Complete exclusion of the dissected segment is not always achievable.*

team which worked all the previous day, selected not for experience but for availability, is tries to stop bleeding from a fragile aorta. Meanwhile, platelets, fresh frozen plasma and cryoprecipitate are being demanded from a haematology service which is not running at its best at 3.00 a.m.

## Preparation for theatre

By the time the patient with acute dissection arrives in the operating theatre we would expect to have control of the blood pressure with intravenous agents (see above) and monitoring with a radial artery cannula, in the most representative side if there is a discrepancy. One of the groins should be left for the surgeon if at all possible and most commonly that is the left if an aortogram has been performed through the right side.

## Operating on the ascending aorta

### General strategies

In acute dissection, cardiopulmonary bypass is always required, and in our practice, periods of profoundly hypothermic circulatory arrest are commonly used. The ascending aorta is the usual site of arterial cannulation for bypass but is not appropriate in this condition. Therefore, as a policy we start the operation by dissecting the left femoral artery and, unless there is any reason to wait until we have seen the aorta, heparinize and cannulate the aorta before opening the chest. Some surgeons, nervous that the dissection will rupture and they will lose control when they open the chest, obtain venous drainage through one or more long cannulae introduced through the femoral vein. Venous access through this route can be awkward to obtain, provides suboptimal control over the venous drainage and creates an unnecessary interference with the deep veins. We prefer to open the chest at this point and cannulate the right atrium in the usual way.

At this stage the dissection is usually evident as a haematoma extending into the mediastinum, there is usually heavily blood-stained pericardial fluid, and sometimes the outer layer of the dissection is so thin that one can see the blood swirling in the false lumen through the transparently thin aortic adventitia.

On bypass, with a clamp across the ascending aorta (across tissue which is to be replaced), the proximal part can be dealt with. This is conveniently done while the patient is being cooled down, and later, while the patient is being rewarmed. With the body, including the brain, profoundly hypothermic at 18°C, and, in our practice, the EEG activity suppressed with intravenous barbiturates administered on bypass, a period of time of up to 30 min of total circulatory arrest is available with safety for the brain. The rules for this have been carefully studied.[8,9] By 40 min at 18°C there is functional, chemical and structural evidence that neuronal damage is occurring. Sixty minutes of arrest under these circumstances is compatible with gross functional recovery, which led to the belief that this length of time was available to the surgeon. Good clinical results are obtainable but there can be no remaining doubt that it is at the price of some neurones. We prefer to organize the operation so that the critical distal surgery can be performed in 20–30 min.

An alternative which we have employed when it is clear that, because of the complexity of the dissection requires in the arch, is to cannulate one or both of the brachiocephalic and left common carotid arteries for part of the time. This is done from within the lumen of the aorta with a tape snugging the cannula passed around the vessel outside the aortic arch.

Embolization of air, thrombus or debris into the head vessels are hazards to be avoided.

Meticulous care of the myocardium is well worthwhile, with cold blood hyperkalaemic arrest and further topical cooling. The hypertensive ventricle is particularly vulnerable to subendocardial ischaemia. It is surprising that surgeons can be anything short of obsessional about this because there are enough problems which can be 'hit and miss' in aortic dissection. There is no need to leave postoperative myocardial performance to chance when there are reliable means at our disposal to protect it.

## Specific operative decisions

### The aortic valve

In the majority of cases the aortic valve is an anatomically normal tricuspid valve which functioned satisfactorily until the aorta dissected. If the configuration of the aorta at the level of the commissures is restored, the valve will function again. This is rather loosely termed 'resuspension' of the valve but the technique requires similar considerations to making a homograft function, although in the case of dissection the aortic wall has to be restored to a stable cylinder in which the valve can function. We have never had aortic regurgitation as a remaining problem in a patient who has survived surgically repaired aortic dissection. Aortic competence can be confirmed on the operating table before the aorta is closed and again immediately on discontinuing bypass.

There are specific circumstances when we would replace the aortic valve. If there is a bicuspid valve, even if it had been neither stenotic or regurgitant, I have always changed it. In the course of surgery for dissection the access is good and the tissues of the annulus are uncalcified. The valve can be inserted with a continuous suture with great rapidity. In any case, there is often time spent standing waiting for cooling or rewarming. In the Marfan syndrome, the valve will need to be replaced along with the ascending aorta.

Under any of these circumstances we use a mechanical valve. Some argue that the patient at risk from further dissection (as they all are) should be spared anticoagulation. On the other hand, other factors play a greater part than the integrity of clotting mechanisms in determining survival after a second aortic dissection. We and others[10] have had to reoperate to replace a failing tissue valve within a conduit and, while it is an interesting technical challenge, it is best avoided.

### The coronary arteries

There is not usually information available about disease of the coronary arteries in a case of acute dissection. It is probably dangerous to try to obtain it at catheterization and unrealistic for the surgeon to ask for it.[11] The left coronary artery has not been a surgical problem. Perhaps in those dissections where the left coronary orifice is significantly involved, it is the pathologist, not the surgeon, who inspects it. So if the patient survives to be operated on, the surgeon's only responsibility is to ensure that he protects it if he sutures close to it to make a proximal repair.

The right coronary artery is sometimes completely severed by the aortic dissection. If it is filling from the false lumen it may have to be grafted and this can be done most conveniently with a length of saphenous vein from the thigh adjacent to the arterial cannulation site. Otherwise, careful reconstruction in this area is required.

### The Marfan syndrome

In the Marfan syndrome there is typically expansion of the aortic segment between the annulus and the origin of the coronary arteries. This is a major hazard for further dissection. Under these circumstances the whole root should be replaced, including reimplanting the coronary arteries into the graft. We employ the Bentall operation very much as he described it for this condition.[12,13] There are surgical debates about the exact technique for handling the coronaries, whether or not to wrap the graft, and how to cope with haemorrhage from the perigraft space, which are technical, lengthy, unresolved and can be read elsewhere by those with a special need to know.

### The tear

If the tear is in the low ascending aorta, as it usually is, it is included in the repair. If it is more distal in the ascending aorta, or in the arch, it can be reached, but only after the cross-clamp has been removed during circulatory arrest. If it is in the descending aorta, it cannot be reached on this occasion.

It is not absolutely essential to reach the tear and repair it. The philosophy then is that the

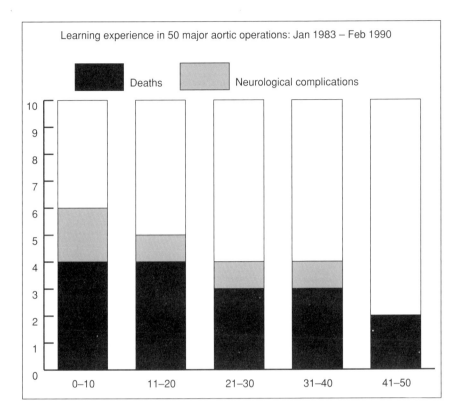

Learning experience in 50 major aortic operations: Jan 1983 – Feb 1990

■ Deaths    ▨ Neurological complications

**Figure 11.5**
*An analysis of a personal series of the first 50 major aortic operations undertaken between 1983 and 1990. There is a heterogeneous mixture of cases and selection may not be even throughout. However, it is difficult to escape the conclusion that there is a practice effect or what we now call a 'learning curve'.*

dissection is being converted to a type III with its lower hazard. Most surgeons who feel confident in operating on the aorta do try to reach and repair the tear whenever possible.

### The aortic repair itself (Figure 11.4)
In the simplest option, with a tear in the ascending aorta, the aorta can be transected at this level, the ends reconstituted with buttressing and the aorta reanastomosed. In the ideal case this may be quick, simple and highly successful.

More often, even in the relatively localized case, a length of graft is used to exclude the most fragile and damaged part of the aorta. In Britain we have had the luxury of biologically sealed waterproof grafts. Initially these were sealed with collagen and more recently gelatin. This permits us to use soft, flexible, surgically friendly knitted Dacron grafts. The alternatives are to use low-porosity woven grafts which are hard to sew and relatively unyielding to the tissues, and/or to engage in one or other of the preclotting techniques.

French surgeons have been promulgating the use of tissue glues[14] and others have described the use of tie-in grafts[15,16] and these may be adjuncts to conventional surgery but do not replace it.

At St George's Hospital all four surgeons undertake these operations and we replace aorta, up to and including the arch, with gelatin-impregnated Dacron, and make *ad hoc* judgements, based on purely technical considerations, about use of buttressing, glue and other adjuncts to operative technique.

## Descending aortic dissection

If dissection is confined to the descending aorta, the first choice of treatment is conservative,[17] with meticulous control of the blood pressure with vasodilators and beta-blockers.

The medium- and long-term management of a dissection involving the descending aorta should be primarily medical; surgical intervention should only be considered for the reasons described. The immediate medical management is identical to that of ascending dissection, with rapid and smooth control of arterial blood pressure. Once this has been achieved and the patient's symptoms have resolved, it is safe to change to oral medication for long-term treatment of hypertension. This should always include a beta-blocker unless absolutely contraindicated, and often additional vasodilator therapy will be necessary; both calcium channel blockers and ACE inhibitors are appropriate combination therapy with a beta-blocker. Careful follow-up and regular monitoring of blood pressure is essential but it is also important to recognize the need for serial imaging of the descending aorta. The appropriate baseline investigation, CT, MRI or transoesophageal echocardiography, should have been completed before the patient leaves hospital.

### Indications for departing from conservative management in type IIIb dissection in the acute phase

If there is progressive collection of blood in the left chest and exsanguination seems imminent, conservative management may be abandoned in favour of immediate surgery. If there is progressive enlargement of the descending aorta, surgery might be the only chance of survival.

If there is deteriorating renal function, surgery offers the chance of restoring blood-flow to the kidney. This can be achieved by reconstituting the dissected layers, but is unpredictable.

### Longer term management of type IIIb aortic dissection

Patients can be managed indefinitely with control of the blood pressure and return to good health. The prospects are at least as good with conservative management as with attempts at urgent surgery.[17] Our results with conservative management have been so satisfactory in the majority of patients that we have continued with this policy.

Our preference would be that these patients are kept under review by the surgeon himself. They are relatively uncommon and do not represent a large commitment in the surgical outpatients. On the other hand, in a busy medical clinic, they may be lost amongst other cases and the exact reason for review may be overlooked.

The reason for review is to watch the size of the aorta. At some point in the post-acute phase, before the patient leaves hospital, we obtain a good quality contrast CT. This is widely available, harmless and definitive, but MRI and transoesophageal echocardiography (TOE) would serve as well. At the same time we obtain a plan PA chest film, standard in every way but for its penetration. The aortic dimensions are measured and recorded in the notes with references to specific landmarks so that subsequent measurements can be compared. If the patient comes from any distance, is likely to travel, or is being seen by other doctors, we give them their set of X-rays to keep with them. At subsequent visits we perform only the penetrated X-ray, and only if we need more specific information, say to plan an operation, would we ask for more images.

### Surgery on the descending aorta

The number of patients coming to surgery for descending aortic dissection is relatively few. The particular hazard is paraplegia, a dreaded complication of surgery on the descending thoracic aorta. The patient should always be specifically forewarned. It may occur during surgery for coarctation, descending aortic aneurysm, aortic dissection and aortic trauma. It may occur in these last three spontaneously, without surgical intervention. It can even occur with introduction of a needle into the aorta to perform an angiogram, or by dislodging a plaque in retrograde aortography, and has been documented after insertion of the balloon pump. It is sporadic in its occurrence. The exact blood supply to the spinal cord is variable and unpredictable. The problem of paraplegia in this context is reviewed by Keen.[18]

The techniques to minimize the risk include use of partial left heart bypass and shunts from above to below the clamped segment. The objective is to exclude the tear and restore flow in the true lumen and thus decompress the thin-walled false lumen.

## Operations on chronic aortic dissection

Once some months have elapsed, the aortic tissues are strong and take sutures well. Surgery can be planned carefully, with detailed imaging and reconstruction of the aorta performed with more technical confidence. Ideally, all dissected tissue should be replaced to minimize the risk of late expansion. On the other hand, if there is a stable length of double-barrel aorta it may be safer to leave it than risk paraplegia. The surgeon should be aware of the possibility that critical mesenteric, renal, spinal or lower limb vessels are arising from the false lumen, and if the aorta is reconstructed, the situation may be made worse rather than better.

## Conclusions

Aortic dissection is a life-threatening condition, particularly if it involves the ascending aorta. A high level of clinical suspicion, prompt recognition and confirmation by the appropriate imaging technique, followed by immediate referral to a cardiac surgical centre, will allow effective management to be instituted and provide the patient with the highest possibility of a successful outcome.

## If I had ...

Perhaps the swings of blood pressure induced by a busy and understaffed outpatient clinic, or the frustrations of getting our patients into the operating theatre or intensive care unit, puts us at risk of aortic dissection! The management guidelines above are what we would wish for ourselves.

It is in the nature of the condition that there is not much room for choice about hospital, surgeon or treatment. If the admitting doctor had not thought about dissection we might tactfully mention the possibility to raise the level of clinical suspicion. If the pain was as described we might push the syringe of thrombolytic aside and drop the name of the keenest imaging cardiologist in the area. While a quick transthoracic echo was being organized to look for aortic regurgitation or pericardial fluid, either of which would put up the diagnostic probability, we would have sent an ally to the telephone to check which surgeons were in town and then, having formed the shortlist, think of who had the best hands, and the best track record, in this unforgiving area. We would unashamedly use influence, bribery and blackmail. IAS would eschew the arterial line, but TT would send for a cardiac anaesthetist to start work and ask her or him to stay close by and help monitor and provide analgesia. Next would be transoesophageal echo, but ideally near theatre with the anaesthetist already at work and the surgeon identified. We would prefer not to travel to the bowels of the hospital on a trolley to have a CT scan, for fear of dying alone in the basement. Unless things were desperate, we would prefer to be sedated, with blood pressure controlled, until the 'A' team assembled at the start of the operating day. Before losing control of cerebration we would talk to the haematologists and ask that, just this once, the platelets and fresh frozen plasma were available ahead of time rather than have to beg for them in desperation after the initiative was lost!

# References

1 Chirillo F et al, Outcome of 290 patients with aortic dissection. At 12 year multicentre experience, *Eur Heart J* (1990) **11**:311–19.

2 Mollo F, Comino A, Passarino G, Incidence of acute aortic dissection at autopsy, *Chest* (1983) **83**:712.

3 Erbel R et al, Echocardiography in diagnosis of aortic dissection, *Lancet* (1989) **i**:457–61.

4 Nienaber CA, Spielmann RP, von Kodolitsch Y, Diagnosis of thoracic aortic aneurysm. Magnetic resonance imaging versus trans-esophageal echocardiography, *Circulation* (1992) **85**:434–7.

5 Treasure T, Raphael MJ, Investigation of suspected dissection of the thoracic aorta, *Lancet* (1991) **338**:490–5.

6 Anagnostopoulos CE, Prabhakar MJS, Kittloe CF, Aortic dissections and aortic aneurysms, *Am J Cardiol* (1972) **30**:263–73.

7 Tan PSK et al, Experience with circulatory arrest and hypothermia to facilitate thoracic aortic surgery, *Ann R Coll Surg Engl* (1989) **71**:81–6.

8 Treasure T et al, The effect of hypothermic circulatory arrest time on cerebral function, morphology, and biochemistry: an experimental study, *J Thorac Cardiovasc Surg* (1983) **86**:761–70.

9 Treasure T, The safe duration of total circulatory arrest with profound hypothermia, *Ann R Coll Surg Engl* (1984) **66**:235–40.

10 Shawkat S, Sarangi PP, Firmin RK, A technique for replacing a prosthetic valve after total aortic root replacement, *Br Heart J* (1990) **63**:260–1.

11 Kern MJ et al, Use of coronary arteriography in the preoperative management of patients undergoing urgent repair of the thoracic aorta, *Am Heart J* (1990) **119**:143–48.

12 Bentall HH, De Bono A, A technique for complete replacement of the ascending aorta, *Thorax* (1968) **23**:338–9.

13 Treasure T, Elective replacement of the aortic root in Marfan's syndrome, *Br Heart J* (1993) **69**:101–3.

14 Carpentier A, Glue aortoplasty as an alternative to resection and grafting for the treatment of aortic dissection, *Semin Thorac Cardiovasc Surg* (1991) **3**:213–14.

15 Lansman SL et al, Intraluminal graft repair of ascending, arch, descending and thoraco-abdominal aortic segments for dissecting and aneurysmal disease: long term follow up, *Semin Thorac Cardiovasc Surg* (1991) **3**:180–2.

16 Lemole GM et al, Improved results for dissecting aneurysms. Intraluminal sutureless prosthesis, *J Thorac Cardiovasc Surg* (1982) **83**:249–55.

17 Neya K et al, Outcome of Stanford Type B acute aortic dissection, *Circulation* (1992) **86**:II-1–7.

18 Keen F, Spinal cord damage associated with surgery of the descending aorta. In: Hadfield J, Hobsley M, Treasure T, eds. *Current Surgical Practice* vol 5 (Edward Arnold: London, 1990) 260–69.

# Further reading

*Seminars in Cardiovascular Surgery* (1991) **3**(3) July.
*Seminars in Cardiovascular Surgery* (1991) **3**(4) October.

These two issues of *Seminars in Cardiovascular Surgery* are devoted to the subject of aortic surgery and provide the most up-to-date and authoritative collection of articles available.

# 12

# Peripheral vascular disease

*Peter R Taylor*

The term peripheral vascular disease is really a misnomer, for atherosclerosis is a generalized disease affecting central as well as peripheral arteries. The term is applied to differentiate cardiac disease from that of other arteries. However, as is well known, if clinically apparent atherosclerosis presents in one territory, the disease will be present (albeit silently) elsewhere.[1] For this reason it is important that cardiologists who deal with patients with ischaemic heart disease can also detect and understand the importance of symptoms and signs related to peripheral vascular disease.

For the purposes of clarity I shall divide this chapter into various sections:

1 Carotid arterial disease
2 Aneurysms
3 Stenosing disease of lower limb arteries
4 Iatrogenic peripheral arterial disease

## Carotid arterial disease

Carotid endarterectomy is performed much more frequently in the USA than in the UK, and many learned words have been written on why this should be so. Surgeons from many disciplines consider the carotid artery as part of their remit. These include general, vascular, cardiothoracic and ENT surgeons and neurosurgeons. In the UK most of the patients who need a carotid endarterectomy are referred initially to neurologists. Many neurologists believe that carotid endarterectomy is an enormous insult for the patient, only to be undertaken as a last resort. Although this view is still prevalent, more enlightened colleagues have been impressed by the results of two huge trials conducted in the USA and in Europe on symptomatic carotid arterial disease.[2]

Centres which had low morbidity and mortality rates for carotid endarterectomy were encouraged to randomize patients who had amaurosis fugax, transient ischaemic attacks or non-disabling strokes into two groups. The first group continued with best medical therapy. The second group were treated with best medical therapy and surgery in the form of carotid endarterectomy. Only those patients who were considered to be in a grey area were put into the trial. All patients had an assessment of the degree of stenosis of the internal carotid artery, by angiography and/or duplex scanning. On the basis of the degree of stenosis, patients were allocated to one of three groups: 0–29 per cent; 30–69 per cent; 70–99 per cent. The results of the two trials showed that surgery was associated with a 2–3 per cent increase in the rate of death or stroke within the first 30 days, compared with conservative treatment. Thereafter in the very tight stenosis group (>70 per cent), those patients undergoing surgery had a much lower rate of death and/or stroke by a factor of six- to ten-fold over an 18–24-month period. This difference was so great that the American arm of the trial

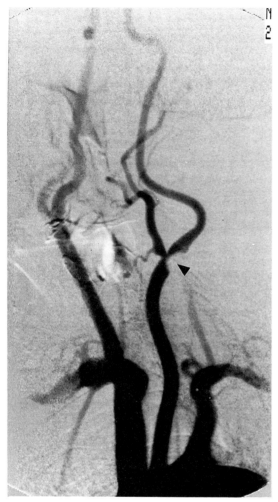

**Figure 12.1**
A DSA of the carotid arteries. The arrow
indicates a large plaque which is causing a
stenosis of the internal carotid artery on the left
side.

was stopped prematurely because it was deemed to be unethical to continue allocating patients to the medical group. There was no benefit of surgery compared to medical treatment if the stenosis was less than 29 per cent. The trials are continuing with the intermediate group of 30–69 per cent.

## Which is the best method to detect carotid artery disease?

The finding of a bruit in the neck should not be used as a reliable sign of carotid arterial disease. The loudness of a bruit is related to the amount of turbulence caused by the stenosis. Very tight stenoses which decrease the amount of flow within the vessel are not associated with bruits, and bruits may originate from the external carotid artery and therefore have little relevance to the cerebral circulation.

Duplex scanning has revolutionized the detection of carotid stenosis.[3] It is quick, non-invasive and in experienced hands is accurate. As with all ultrasound techniques, the skill of the operator is paramount in the detection of carotid artery stenosis, and there is little place for the occasional dabbler. Some centres now perform only duplex scans of the carotid arteries before surgery although the majority of surgeons would still ask for some form of angiography before operative intervention. Digital subtraction angiography (DSA) can be performed by intravenous or intra-arterial injection of contrast medium (Figure 12.1). Neurological complications are very rare with intravenous injection, but some of the images are of dubious quality. Intra-arterial injection is usually performed via the femoral route. The catheter can be positioned in either the aortic arch or in the origins of the carotid arteries to give selective views. The complication rate is higher than that of intravenous angiography but the quality of the image is better.

## Who should perform carotid endarterectomy?

This vexed question is answered quite easily: the person who is doing them most frequently and who performs an ongoing audit into the results. The days of anecdotal audit are long gone, and most good units run regular neurovascular meetings where the results of carotid endarterectomy are regularly reviewed jointly by surgeons and neurologists. It has been suggested that a minimum of 20 operations a year is necessary to ensure adequate experience. The 30-day joint morbidity and mortality should be less than 2–3 per cent.

Although only surgery has been mentioned as an interventional treatment for carotid arterial stenosis, there is interest in the application of balloon dilatation to these arteries. At present, this form of treatment is being carried out in only a few centres by enthusiasts, but, if it can be shown that the morbidity and mortality is equal to or lower than that of surgical endarterectomy, then this may become the treatment of choice in the future. Duplex scanning, which gives information on the type of plaque causing the carotid narrowing, may be able to select which patients will benefit from balloon dilatation. Those plaques which consist of heterogeneous friable pultaceous debris may do better with surgery, while those which are homogeneous may be suitable for balloon dilatation.

## What are the indications for carotid endarterectomy when coronary arterial bypass grafts are planned and what is the optimum timing for the two procedures?

At present the only definite indication for carotid endarterectomy is when there is a symptomatic tight stenosis of the order of 70–99 per cent. However, there has been much interest in asymptomatic stenoses, and some authorities suggest that an asymptomatic stenosis should be treated if there is an occluded internal carotid artery on one side and an asymptomatic stenosis of 70–99 per cent on the other. This must remain a matter for conjecture until a randomized trial has been undertaken. Regarding the optimum timing of the two procedures, conventional wisdom suggests that the carotid endarterectomy should be performed first, probably as a separate procedure, followed after approximately 7 days by the coronary artery bypass graft.[4] If the patient, however, has unstable angina, a joint procedure can be undertaken. Although this is often inconvenient for the surgeons, it means that the patient has only one general anaesthetic and this must cause less psychological trauma than that related to two major procedures carried out within a short time of each other. The carotid operation may well be reducing the chances of the patient having a stroke within the next few years rather than diminishing the risk of a neurological deficit during surgery. If a decision is taken to go ahead with cardiac surgery in a patient with carotid artery stenoses, then the bloodflow during bypass should be pulsatile and the pressure maintained at high levels.

## Point 1

Any patient, fit enough for surgery, who presents to a cardiology clinic with a history of amaurosis fugax, transient ischaemic attack or non-disabling stroke should have a carotid duplex scan to define the extent of any carotid arterial stenosis. If this is greater than 70 per cent the patient may well benefit from carotid endarterectomy.

# Aneurysms

## Aortic aneurysms

A vessel is ectatic up to twice its normal diameter, and thereafter it is said to be aneurysmal. Of course, the normal diameter depends upon the age and sex of the patient. In practice, any infrarenal aorta which measures more than 3 cm in transverse or anterior–posterior diameter should be regarded as significant. Many aortic aneurysms are asymptomatic and therefore an attempt should be made to diagnose these in all patients presenting to a cardiology clinic. Patients particularly at risk are men over the age of 60, and those with a history of hypertension. The aorta is palpable in most people, and by placing a hand on each side of the aorta in the epigastric region, an attempt can be made to size the transverse diameter of the vessel by estimating the distance between the hands (skin and subcutaneous tissues usually account for 1 cm). The examiner should pause for pulsation to ensure that the mass has an expansile pulsation. If the aorta cannot be easily palpated (because the patient is obese) or if it is greater than 3 cm, an ultrasound examination should be requested. If the aneurysm is symptomatic, i.e. causing back or abdominal pain, or if pressure on the aneurysm reproduces or provokes back or abdominal pain, the patient should not be allowed to go home, and must be referred to a vascular surgeon as a matter of urgency. Symptomatic aneurysms may have already ruptured, or be very close to it. Such patients, if haemodynamically stable, should have either an ultrasound or a CT scan (Figure 12.2). If the aneurysm is found to be intact, the patient should be placed upon the next available elective list for surgical repair. Any evidence of a leak should be treated by immediate surgery. If the patient with a tender aneurysm is haemodynamically unstable, they should be transferred immediately to theatre for laparotomy with no delay for any investigations. Two large-bore peripheral cannulae should be inserted and 20 ml of blood taken for emergency crossmatch.

The reasons for making every effort to diagnose aortic aneurysms in patients are clear from the results of surgical repair.[5] If a patient ruptures their aneurysm at home, the mortality approaches 100 per cent. Even if the patient survives to arrive at the operating table, the mortality is still 30–50 per cent, and this figure has not improved over the last two to three decades. In contrast, the mortality of elective aneurysm repair has fallen dramatically over the same time period to below 10 per cent. Mortality figures of 2–5 per cent have been reported from specialist units. Interestingly, this is because of the realization that the major cause of death during aneurysm surgery is from myocardial infarction. Most vascular surgeons will undertake some form of assessment of cardiac function before embarking upon operative repair, especially if there is a history of previous myocardial infarction or angina. However, silent myocardial disease may only be uncovered by investigations other than a chest X-ray and electrocardiogram. All of my patients having elective aortic surgery have both a cardiology opinion and a cardiac echo before surgery. At present the mortality of elective repair is 1.7 per cent, and I have turned down three patients in the last year who had very poor left ventricular function, one of whom gave no history consistent with such severe myocardial disease.

The much better mortality associated with elective surgery has also been associated with a willingness on the part of the vascular surgeon to repair aneurysms which were previously thought to be too small to treat. There is a multicentre trial currently being performed in the UK on the treatment of small aneurysms.

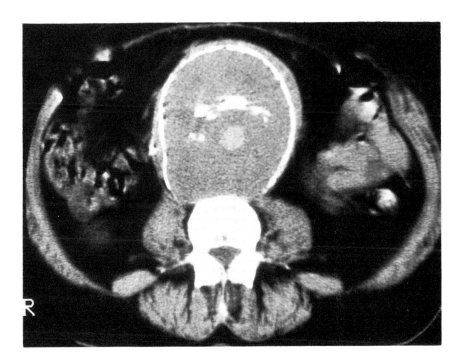

**Figure 12.2**
*A very large abdominal aortic aneurysm which measures more than 10 cm in diameter. The thickened wall anteriorly represents an inflammatory component suggesting that this aneurysm has already leaked.*

The small aneurysm study takes patients aged from 60 to 76. An infrarenal aortic diameter of 3–4 cm is managed conservatively with regular ultrasound examinations initially every 3 months. Those measuring 4–5.5 cm in diameter are randomized into two groups. The first group is treated conservatively with regular ultrasound examinations. If the diameter increases by more than 1 cm in a year, or if the aneurysm becomes symptomatic, then surgery is offered to the patient. The second group is surgically repaired. The results of this study should not only increase our knowledge of the natural history of aortic aneurysms, but should show us whether surgery is justified in these small aneurysms. At present surgery offers the only way of treating aortic aneurysms, but this may not always be so. In the USA, radiologists have successfully treated infrarenal aortic aneurysms by placing an expanding metal stent with Dacron attached at the neck of the aneurysm, and then introducing a second stent at the distal end of the aneurysm.

## Thoracoabdominal aneurysms

All aortic aneurysms affecting the aortic arch should be referred to cardiothoracic surgeons. However, aneurysms which commence distal to the origin of the left subclavian artery may be treated by either cardiothoracic or vascular surgeons. At present these are only performed by a few centres in the UK. The morbidity and mortality is much higher than that of infrarenal aneurysms and is related to the extent of the aneurysm. Those associated with the highest risk (type 2 thoracoabdominal aneurysms) start just distal to the origin of the left subclavian artery and affect the whole of the descending thoracic aorta and the whole of the abdominal aorta. The major complications include blood loss, paraplegia, renal failure and mesenteric ischaemia. Those aneurysms associated with the lowest risk start at the level of the diaphragm and involve the origins of the mesenteric and renal vessels (type 4 thoracoabdominal aneurysms).[6] Any evidence of poor left ventricular function or chronic obstructive airways disease would mitigate against operative repair. Patients over the age of 80 are unlikely to survive the surgical onslaught.

## Popliteal aneurysms

These rarely rupture but more commonly cause limb ischaemia by thrombosis. This is usually severe, as the thrombosis propagates into the distal vessels. Popliteal pulses which are easily palpable should be deemed to be aneurysmal and the diameter ascertained by ultrasound examination. Vascular surgeons are divided into two camps as to the management of asymptomatic popliteal aneurysms. The first group considers surgery to be the best option, particularly if the aneurysm contains thrombus.[7] They are concerned that a popliteal aneurysm which thromboses often leads to the loss of the leg, frequently resulting in an above-knee amputation. The aneurysm is usually ligated proximally and distally and a bypass graft inserted. The second group suggests that many of these aneurysms do not thrombose, and even if they do, not all of them lead to a critically ischaemic limb.[8] They suggest that

aneurysms, particularly if they contain no thrombus, should be treated conservatively. If they thrombose they should be treated initially with thrombolytic therapy to restore patency to the distal vessels. Following this, definitive surgery can be performed. I believe that any popliteal aneurysm should be repaired if it measures more than 2 cm in diameter. Aneurysms which are between 1 and 2 cm should be treated conservatively unless they contain thrombus or are symptomatic. A further proviso is if the patient is likely to travel abroad where thrombolytic therapy and surgery may not be readily available; surgical repair then is advisable.

## Point 2

Abdominal aortic aneurysms are easily diagnosed on abdominal palpation. Aneurysms greater than 3 cm or those which cannot be easily palpated should have an ultrasound examination. Any aneurysm greater than 3 cm should be referred to a vascular surgeon. Easily palpable popliteal pulses should have an ultrasound examination. Those greater than 1 cm should be referred for a vascular surgical opinion.

# Stenosing disease of lower limb arteries

Stenosis or occlusion of arteries to the lower limb may cause distal ischaemia. Claudication is a pain which is worse with exercise and improves with rest. Disease of the femoral arteries provokes calf claudication, external iliac disease causes thigh claudication and aortic disease produces bilateral buttock claudication associated with impotence in men. Unilateral buttock claudication suggests common iliac occlusion. The more distal pulses are reduced or absent. A bruit may indicate that the artery is stenosed but patent, and may be suitable for balloon angioplasty. Critical ischaemia is associated with rest pain, ulceration or gangrene, and indicates multilevel disease.[9] Rest pain is a severe pain which keeps the patient awake at night and is due to ischaemia in the distal vascular beds. The pain is due to skin ischaemia and is sited usually in the hallux or the dorsum of the foot. This pain is improved by placing the foot in a dependent position. The patient will often go for a walk during the night, having been woken up by the pain, or may sleep with the foot out of bed. Some patients sleep in a chair. The most important measurement is the ankle systolic pressure. A torniquet is placed around the ankle, a Doppler probe is positioned over the dorsalis pedis and the pressure at which the signal disappears is noted. A pressure less than 50 mm Hg indicates critical ischaemia. Care should be taken in diabetic and renal failure patients as calcification in the arterial wall can lead to falsely elevated pressures being recorded. In these patients impalpable pedal pulses indicate arterial disease.

There are several diseases which cause pain in the lower limb which may mimic arterial insufficiency. The first is cardiac claudication.[10] These patients have very poor left ventricular function. During exercise the stroke volume decreases, resulting in reduced delivery of oxygenated blood to the periphery. It is the pump rather than the pipes which is to blame. Often these patients give a good history of claudication which affects both calves simultaneously. They develop chest pain or shortness of breath at the same time as the onset of calf pain. They usually have normal pedal pulses and Doppler pressures at rest. Such patients do not benefit from any intervention in their peripheral vascular disease, for any improvement in the peripheral arteries will not help the deterioration in left ventricular stroke volume produced by exercise. The most important treatment is to maximize their cardiac output by improving left ventricular function and to decrease peripheral resistance with vasodilating agents.

The second large group of patients have spinal claudication. These patients have a long history of back pain and frequently have suffered trauma to the spine. The pain is usually present at rest and radiates from the spine down the leg. It is often described as a burning sensation, and is not improved by putting the foot into a dependent position. The pain may be made better or worse with exercise and may be improved by changing the position of the spine, e.g. by sitting down. These patients often have spinal stenosis detected on magnetic resonance imaging, and should be referred to a rheumatologist, orthopaedic surgeon or neurologist with a special interest in this condition.

Venous claudication is described as a bursting pain which is relieved by elevating the limb. There is usually a history of deep venous thrombosis, and the patient has the typical features of the post-thrombotic limb, with ankle oedema, lipodermatosclerosis and ulceration of the medial aspect of the lower limb.

Any patient who has critical ischaemia should be referred for an urgent vascular surgical opinion. Intervention is always indicated. This is not the case with claudication. The results for any intervention must be weighed against alternative treatments and the complications of any procedure undertaken. Balloon dilatation of stenoses is associated with much better results than occlusions, and the length of the occlusion is another pertinent factor. Intervention in large-calibre arteries such as the aorta and iliacs is associated with better results than in smaller diameter vessels such as the superficial femoral or popliteal arteries.

Claudication is best treated conservatively by advising the patient to stop smoking, to exercise regularly by walking and to achieve their ideal body weight. The Oxford study showed that there was no difference at 2 years between patients treated with balloon dilatation and those encouraged to take regular exercise with no intervention.[11] The natural history of claudication is benign, with two-thirds of patients remaining either the same or improving. The only indications for intervention are firstly, if their occupation is at risk, or secondly, if they suffer from such short distance claudication that their quality of life is poor. It is well worth advising the patient that vascular intervention can go wrong, and that if complications do occur these could result in the loss of a limb. Such treatment should not be undertaken lightly. This is very different from pain on exercise related to myocardial ischaemia, which is always of a serious nature, and where failure to intervene may have severe repercussions on the viability of the myocardium.

## Investigations

The most basic test for peripheral vascular disease of the lower limb is to record the ankle systolic pressure. This is compared with the brachial systolic pressure to give the ankle/brachial systolic pressure index. Normal people have a ratio greater than 1. Patients who experience claudication usually have a ratio of 0.5–0.9, and patients with critical ischaemia have a ratio of 0.4 or less. An exercise test using a treadmill will show a fall in ankle pressure in patients with arterial disease and in those with cardiac claudication. There is a lot of interest in duplex scanning of peripheral arteries. Duplex scanning can differentiate arteries which are stenosed from those which are occluded. At Guy's we are fortunate to have the Doppler quickscan, which is a simple technique which records the frequency of a hand-held Doppler probe. This is matched to a grey scale image of the patient taken from an overhead wide-angle camera. The scan will detect stenoses and occlusions of peripheral vessels with acceptable accuracy. The development of non-invasive techniques to assess the arterial tree allows angiography to be used only as a prelude to treatment in the form of either angioplasty or surgery. Angiography should only be performed if intervention is contemplated, and there is no place for so-called 'baseline' angiograms.

Many patients presenting to cardiology clinics are hypertensive and may have renal artery stenosis. The only reliable method for detecting this is angiography, usually in the form of intra-arterial digital subtraction angiography. Intervention is indicated if there is proven renal artery stenosis causing uncontrollable hypertension, or if there is deteriorating renal function associated with loss of renal substance.

## Point 3

Claudication affecting the lower limb may be due to peripheral arterial disease. This does not have the same importance as angina and should be treated with conservative measures unless the patient's occupation is at risk, or unless it is severely affecting the quality of life. Poor left ventricular function can also cause cardiac claudication, and may exacerbate stenotic peripheral arterial disease. Treatment is aimed at improving left ventricular function. Patients with critical ischaemia always require intervention.

## Iatrogenic peripheral vascular disease

There is a significant (if small) percentage of problems caused by invasive arterial procedures which are involved in current medicine,

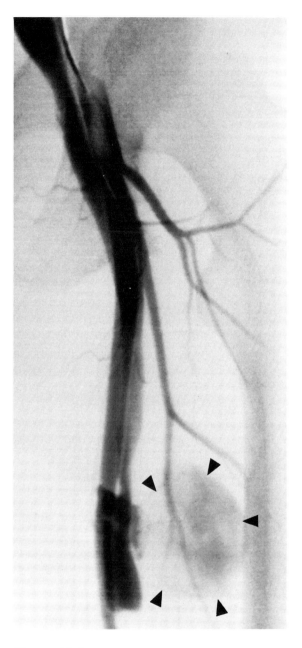

**Figure 12.3**
*A catheter positioned in the common femoral
artery. The arrows show a large false femoral
aneurysm and there is a connection at this level
between the superficial femoral artery and the
vein. The dye is well seen outlining the
superficial and common femoral vein.*

particularly in cardiological practice. These
include haematoma formation, false aneurysm
formation, occlusion of the vessel, and very
rarely the formation of an arteriovenous fistula
(Figure 12.3). Any complication caused by
invasive procedures should be referred to a
vascular surgeon for immediate repair.

Most haematomas will resolve by themselves,
unless they are false aneurysms. These can be
distinguished by the degree of expansile pulsation associated with the mass. A systolic bruit
would suggest turbulent flow within a false
aneurysm sac, and a machinery murmur
indicates an arteriovenous fistula. Both of these
conditions need surgical repair, although there
was a recent report suggesting that if the neck of
the false aneurysm was detected by duplex scan,
then pressure over the neck by the probe for
5–10 min such that no flow occurred into the sac
was often enough to thrombose the aneurysm
lumen. Occlusion of arteries following arterial
catheterization is always due to damage to the
intima, producing a dissection, and this must be
repaired surgically. Usually this can be treated
with a vein patch, but sometimes there is so
much damage to the artery that a bypass graft is
required. Those patients who are referred late
have often thrombosed proximally and distally
for a much longer segment and require longer
arterial bypass procedures. Neglect of this condition can result in joint flexion contractures,
Volkmann's ischaemic contracture, rest pain or
ischaemic pain on exercise. For this reason,
puncture of large arteries reduces the risk of
iatrogenic damage, and increases the chances of
success in any subsequent surgical repair. The
brachial artery is of small diameter and occlusion
is often followed by serious consequences for the
distal limb. If both femoral arteries are for some
reason unusable the brachial artery of the non-
dominant hand should be used. It makes no
sense to use the artery of the dominant hand
when the results of occlusion can be so dire.

Most of the problems encountered in the femoral region seem to occur when the catheter is placed in either the profunda or superficial femoral artery rather than the common femoral artery. This artery lies at its most superficial in the groin skin crease in the majority of patients, although there is considerable variation in anatomy. Catheterization high above the groin crease usually punctures the external iliac artery, and problems can be encountered in obtaining adequate pressure for haemostasis following removal of the catheter. A final word of caution: beware of patients who are taking non-steroidal anti-inflammatory drugs, as these can lead to a decreased effectiveness of platelets, and therefore haemostasis and pressure may have to be applied for longer than usual.

## Point 4

Iatrogenic injuries associated with arterial catheterization should be immediately repaired.

# If I had ...

1 A tight symptomatic carotid artery stenosis—I would find a vascular surgeon who did more than 30 endarterectomies a year with a morbidity and mortality of less than 3 per cent and undergo surgery.

2 Unstable angina and a tight symptomatic carotid artery stenosis—I would elect for a combined carotid endarterectomy and coronary artery bypass operation.

3 An aortic aneurysm—I would seek the advice of an experienced vascular surgeon with a low morbidity and mortality who would refer me for a cardiological opinion before surgery.

4 A popliteal aneurysm—I would have it repaired if it was greater than 2 cm or if it was larger than 1 cm and contained clot.

5 Claudication—I would firstly give up smoking, secondly make sure I took lots of exercise in the form of walking, thirdly take one aspirin a day and finally take measures to achieve my ideal body weight. If there was shortness of breath or chest pain associated with the leg pain I would seek the advice of a cardiologist.

6 Rest pain—I would find a vascular surgeon trained in the techniques of distal bypass, and subject myself to the knife.

# References

1 Hertzer NR et al, Coronary artery disease in peripheral vascular patients. A classification of 1000 coronary angiograms and results of surgical management, *Ann Surg* (1984) **199**:223–33.

2 Browse NL, Current status of carotid endarterectomy, *Br J Surg* (1991) **78**:1153–5.

3 Merritt CRB, ed. *Doppler color imaging* (Churchill Livingstone: London 1992).

4 Nicolaides AN, Hertzer NR, The arteriosclerotic patient. In: Eastcott HHG, ed. *Arterial surgery*, 3rd edn (Churchill Livingstone: Edinburgh 1992) 615–44.

5 Taylor PR, Wolfe JHN, Treating aortic aneurysm, *Br Med J* (1991) **303**:1127–9.

6 Crawford ES et al, Thoracoabdominal aortic aneurysms: peroperative and intraoperative factors determining immediate and long term results of operations in 605 patients, *J Vasc Surg* (1986) **3**:389–404.

7 Halliday AW et al, The management of popliteal aneurysms; the importance of early surgical repair, *Ann R Coll Surg Engl* (1991) **73**:253–7.

8 Bowyer RC et al, Conservative management of asymptomatic popliteal aneurysm, *Br J Surg* (1990) **77**:1132–5.

9 Dormandy J, *European consensus document on critical limb ischaemia* (Springer-Verlag: Berlin 1989).

10 Salmasi A-M et al, Intermittent claudication as a manifestation of silent myocardial ischaemia: a pilot study, *J Vasc Surg* (1991) **14**:78–85.

11 Creasy TS et al, Is percutaneous transluminal angioplasty better than exercise for claudication?—preliminary results from a prospective randomised trial, *Eur J Vasc Surg* (1990) **4**:135–40.

# 13

# Primary pulmonary hypertension
## A Yazdani Butt and Tim W Higenbottam

Primary pulmonary hypertension (PPH) is a serious disease with a fatal outcome in the majority of patients. In a retrospective series of 120 patients, only 24 patients (21 per cent) were alive after 5 years.[1] Although it is an uncommon disease, its importance cannot be overemphasized as it generally affects young people, mostly in their third or fourth decades. Females are affected more than males, with a female to male ratio of 1.7 : 1; occasionally children and the elderly also suffer from this disease.[2] In a small proportion of patients, especially those with a maintained cardiac output, disease regresses, leading to 'spontaneous' recovery. Most patients, however, face a bleak outlook with a downhill course resulting in terminal right heart failure,[1,3,4] which is the main cause of death (Figure 13.1).

Investigations are directed towards finding an underlying cause of pulmonary hypertension, such as intracardiac left-to-right shunt,

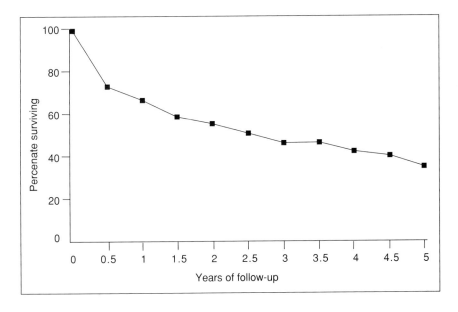

**Figure 13.1**
Estimated percentage of patients surviving over time from the baseline catheterization. Number of patients at risk are shown for 0 through 5 years. Median survival is estimated at 2.8 years. Estimated percentage of patients surviving at 1, 3 and 5 years are 68, 48 and 34 per cent respectively. (From D'Alonzo GE et al, Survival in patients with primary pulmonary hypertension, Ann Intern Med (1991) **115**:344.)

*Causes of pulmonary hypertension.*

- **Secondary pulmonary hypertension**
  Congenital heart disease with left-to-right shunt
  Mitral valve disease
  Primary or secondary myocardial disease
  Pulmonary embolism
  Intravenous drug abuse
  Chronic obstructive lung disease
  Interstitial lung disease
  Neuromuscular diseases causing hypoventilation
  Pickwickian syndrome
  Ankylosing spondylitis
  Connective tissue disease, e.g. systemic sclerosis
  Pulmonary venous obstruction
  Chronic liver disease
  HIV infection

- **Primary pulmonary hypertension**
  Plexogenic arteriopathy
  Thrombotic arterial disease
  Veno-occlusive disease
  Pulmonary capillary haemangiomatosis

*Adapted from* Rich S, Primary pulmonary hypertension, *Prog Cardiovasc Dis* (1988) **XXXI**:212.

chronic hypoxic lung disease, pulmonary embolism, left ventricular failure, HIV infection or mitral valve disease. Patients are also screened for connective tissue diseases and systemic arteritides. Once such a cause cannot be identified, a diagnosis of unexplained or primary pulmonary hypertension is made. Physiological measurement of pulmonary artery pressure and cardiac output are essential in order to diagnose pulmonary hypertension. At sea level a normal systolic pulmonary artery pressure is approximately 20 mm Hg and the diastolic pressure is 12 mm Hg for a cardiac output of 5 l/min. However, for practical purposes a mean pulmonary artery pressure in

excess of 25 mm Hg at rest and 30 mm Hg on exercise is considered abnormal.[5]

## Historical background

It was described for the first time by Romberg in 1891 after an autopsy when he found sclerosis of the pulmonary arteries in the absence of any cardiopulmonary disease.[6] The first description of PPH giving the clinical and histological findings was made by Monckeberg in 1907.[7] This was a single case report, but in 1935 Brenner published the first series of patients with primary pulmonary vascular disease, outlining the clinical and histological criteria.[8] However, a lot of confusion prevailed in these decades regarding diagnosing the disease before death, and it was not until 1951 that Dresdale published the first series of PPH[9] based on cardiac catheterization which provided direct evidence of raised pulmonary artery pressure in these patients. The possibility of vasoconstrictive factors playing a role in PPH was raised by Wood[10] in 1958. This idea supported the use of vasodilator treatments of PPH. In 1967 there was an epidemic of PPH in Europe which has been related to the use of slimming agent aminorex fumarate.[11] This led to an international symposium organized by the World Health Organization in order to gain further insight into this disease.[12] A classification of PPH emerged which was based on histopathological findings. It provides a generally accepted scheme with the following categories: plexogenic pulmonary arteriopathy, thrombotic arterial disease and veno-occlusive disease. Much depended upon the work of Wagenvoort, who, in 1970, had published a pathological study of lung vessels in 156 clinically diagnosed cases of PPH.[13] A patient registry of primary pulmonary hypertension was set up in the USA in 1987 where data were supplied by 32 cardiothoracic centres. Impetus was provided by the introduction of successful lung transplantation as a treatment. The registry has provided clinical and haemodynamic data which are valuable for determining the prognosis of the disease.[2,4] An international primary pulmonary hypertension study (IPPHS) is underway, involving five European countries and Canada, to examine the incidence and risk factors for this disease.

## Pathophysiology of primary pulmonary hypertension

As its name suggests, the cause of this condition is not known but there are various factors which could contribute to the disease. The low-pressure and low-resistance pulmonary vasculature can react differently to various stimuli such as hypoxia, increased bloodflow or various pharmacological agents. It is possible that susceptible patients hyperreact to such stimuli with an augmented vasocontrictor response. This could lead to the development of pulmonary hypertension. As intimal thickening is a prominent feature of PPH, endothelial dysfunction of pulmonary vasculature has been suggested to contribute in the genesis of pulmonary hypertension.[14] A number of powerful vasodilator substances, such as prostacyclin ($PGI_2$) and endothelium-derived nitric oxide (EDNO),[15,16] are released from the endothelium together with vasoconstrictor peptides such as endothelin-1 (ET-1).[17] The release of vasodilators may be impaired as a result of endothelial injury. Such a mechanism could lead to pulmonary vasoconstriction. $PGI_2$ and EDNO also prevent platelet aggregation[15,18] and clot formation and one can speculate that local deficiency of $PGI_2$ and EDNO may contribute to the formation of microthrombi, which is a common terminal finding in PPH. The potent vasoconstrictor peptide called endothelin-1 could be released in increased quantities, which could lead to pulmonary vasoconstriction. The structural changes of pulmonary vasculature such as intimal thickening could result from an imbalance of proliferative and antiproliferative factors released by the endothelium.

Various autoimmune diseases such as systemic lupus erythematosis (SLE) are associated with PPH.[19,20] A proportion of patients with lupus may develop pulmonary hypertension in the absence of any parenchymal lung involvement. Circulating lupus anticoagulant which may be present in some patients with SLE is a possible contributing factor. Lupus anticoagulant is an IgG or IgM[21] which may also interfere with the formation of prostacy-clin.[22–24]

Antithrombin III deficiency has been recognized to be associated particularly with familial-type PPH.[25] In the NIH registry 7 per cent of patients had familial disease.

# Histopathology of PPH

PPH has been classified into three main pathological entities: plexogenic pulmonary arteriopathy (PPA), thrombotic pulmonary arteriopathy (TPA) and veno-occlusive disease.[12,13] Plexogenic pulmonary arteriopathy may suggest an underlying pulmonary vasoconstrictor phenomenon which could trigger the disease process and may also involve migration of the myofibroblasts[26] towards intimal layers. PPA is characterized by medial hypertrophy, intimal thickening leading to concentric intimal fibrosis and dilatations in small pulmonary arteries. At times, intimal thickening can be severe enough to cause arterial occlusion, giving the appearance of so-called 'onion skinning'.[27] In advanced pulmonary hypertension, typical plexiform lesions[28] develop due to multichannelled outpouching of the pulmonary arterioles. Pulmonary thrombotic arteriopathy (PTA) is mainly featured as eccentric intimal thickening and recanalized thrombi.[28] In veno-occlusive disease, the pulmonary venous system is mainly involved due to intimal proliferation and fibrosis, often resulting in complete obliteration of the venous channels.[29] Pulmonary capillary haemangiomatosis is a rare histological entity which may lead to pulmonary hypertension. It is a form of microangiopathy in which marked proliferation of small blood vessels occurs in alveolar septa.

# Diagnosis

## Clinical features

It is important that physicians should have a high index of suspicion. Many patients are treated for asthma or psychological illness. There is usually a delay of up to 2 years from the onset of symptoms to the diagnosis of PPH.[2] The main symptoms are dyspnoea, chest pain and syncope.[2,30,31] Dyspnoea is the most common symptom and reflects increased ventilation as a result of hypoxia. These patients are hypoxic as a result of a low cardiac output which cannot increase sufficiently during exercise, leading to increased tissue extraction and falling pulmonary artery oxygen content. This leads to increasing arterial hypoxia on exercise. Initially dyspnoea is mild and may only be noticed on exertion but as the disease progresses it may occur on rest. Chest pains which have characteristics of angina are common. Angiographic appearance of the coronary arteries is normal. Syncope occurs on exercise and represents impending terminal right ventricular failure. Syncope on rest may be triggered by an arrhythmia. Lethargy is another common symptom and represents poor oxygen tissue delivery. Peripheral oedema occurs late, probably because of a raised circulatory concentration of atrial natriuretic peptide (ANP) levels in patients with PPH.[32] There may be associated Raynaud's phenomenon, which is associated with a poor prognosis.[4]

The onset of symptoms is usually insidious and may be triggered by pregnancy,[33] travel to high altitude or certain drugs such as aminorex,[11] fenfluramine[34] or oral contraceptives.[35,36] The course of the disease is usually progressive and the patient is often greatly disabled at the time of presentation. On physical examination the patient usually has a low pulse volume. Both peripheral and central cyanosis are often present. Jugular venous pressure may be raised along with prominent 'a' waves.[37] There may be audible right-sided third and fourth heart sound and loud pulmonary component of the second heart sound along with flow and regurgitant murmurs across the pulmonary valve. Murmur due to tricuspid regurgitation is a common finding and is associated with prominent 'v' wave. Palpable second heart sound and left parasternal heave are often present.

## Investigations

Electrocardiogram and chest X-ray are abnormal in approximately 90 per cent of cases showing respectively signs of right ventricular hypertrophy along with right axis deviation (Figure 13.2) and enlargement of proximal pulmonary arteries with peripheral pruning (Figure 13.3). Presence of right ventricular strain on ECG indicates severe pulmonary hypertension. Immunological assays may demonstrate raised antinuclear factor (ANF) in

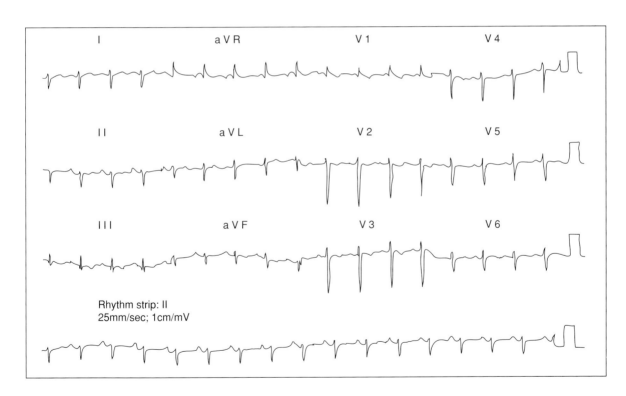

**Figure 13.2**
*Electrocardiogram of a patient with pulmonary hypertension showing evidence of right ventricular hypertrophy with some strain.*

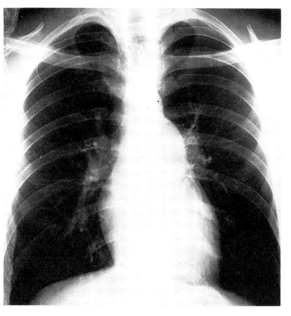

*a*

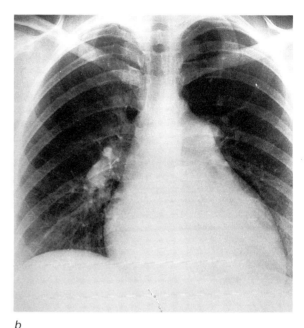

*b*

**Figure 13.3**
*Chest radiographs from patients with primary pulmonary hypertension showing: (a) enlargement of the central pulmonary arteries and some peripheral pruning; (b) dilated proximal pulmonary arteries as well as marked enlargement of the cardiac silhouette.*

29 per cent of patients.[1,38] Transthoracic echocardiography shows dilated right-sided chambers, distortion of interventricular septum and right ventricular hypertrophy.[39–41] An estimate of pulmonary artery pressure using Doppler may be possible in the presence of tricuspid regurgitation (Figure 13.4). Enlargement of the pulmonary trunk along with some pulmonary regurgitation may also be detected. Patent foramen ovale may be present and there is some evidence that it may be associated with longer survival.[42] Echocardiography is used to exclude a cardiac cause, such as septal defects, mitral valve disease or left ventricular failure. Ventilation and perfusion lung scintigraphy (V/Q lung scan) is of value.[43,44] In pulmonary embolism the scan shows segmental or subsegmental perfusion defects which are normally ventilated (Figure 13.5). Pulmonary angiography should be then performed in order to detect any clot in the proximal arteries. Such proximal occlusions are amenable to thromboendarterectomy[45] (Figure 13.6). In PPH, V/Q scan usually is either normal or shows patchy perfusion defects (Figure 13.5) and does not distinguish

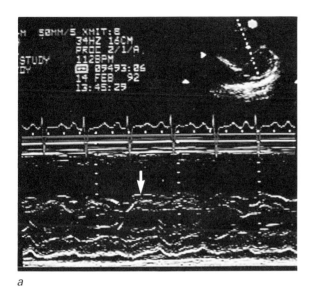

a

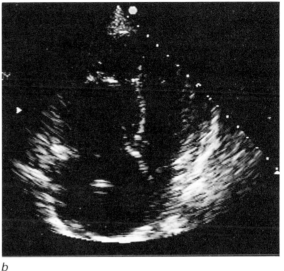

b

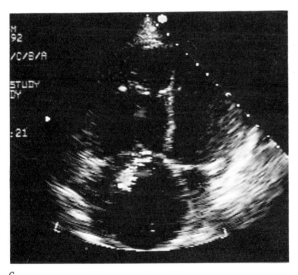

c

**Figure 13.4**
*Echocardiographic pictures from a patient with severe pulmonary hypertension. (a) M-mode; (b) four-chamber view of cross-sectional echocardiogram showing dilated right-sided chambers and septal hypertrophy (arrow); (c) colourflow imaging demonstrates a jet due to tricuspid regurgitation.*

between predominantly plexogenic and thrombotic pulmonary arteriopathy.[46] High-resolution computerized tomography is now being used as a non-invasive technique to define the proximal clot in pulmonary arteries of patients with pulmonary embolism (Figure 13.7). It also provides evidence of any interstitial lung disease.

Pulmonary function tests are either normal or may show slightly a restrictive pattern in the lung volume studies along with impairment of gas transfer.[2] Arterial blood gas analysis shows

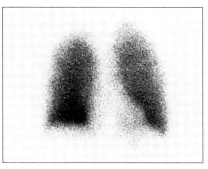

a    ventilation

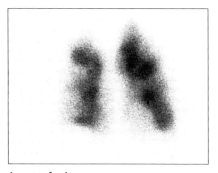

b    perfusion

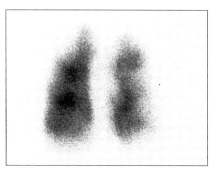

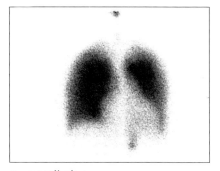

c    ventilation

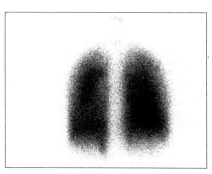

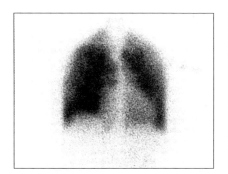

d    perfusion

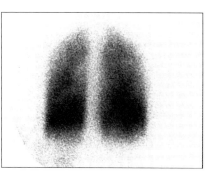

**Figure 13.5**
*(a) Ventilation and (b) perfusion scans showing multiple areas of segmental V/Q mismatches suggestive of pulmonary embolism. Scans from a patient with PPH, (c) ventilation and (d) perfusion, shows no significant V/Q mismatches; however, there is some patchy reduction in peripheral perfusion of the upper holes.*

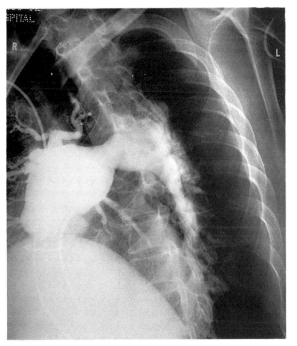

*a*

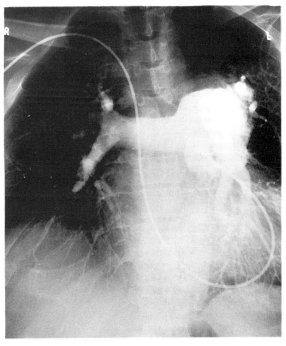

*b*

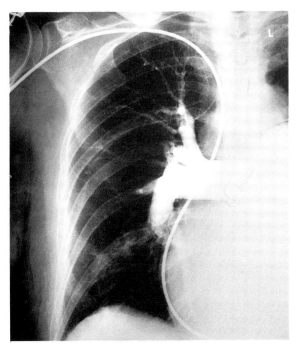

*c*

**Figure 13.6**
*(a) Pulmonary angiogram showing funnel-shaped
appearance of left main pulmonary artery
suggestive of an organized thrombus. (b) Right
pulmonary arterial tree from the same patient
shows occlusions of the right upper lobe and
basal pulmonary arteries due to organized
thrombi but the main pulmonary artery is clear
of any clots. (By courtesy of JW Wallwork and
CDR Flower.) (c) Pulmonary angiogram from
another patient with severe pulmonary
hypertension showing occlusion of right middle
lobe and basal pulmonary arteries suggestive of
pulmonary embolism. (By courtesy of Dr PM
Schofield.)*

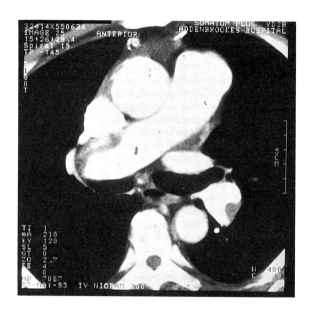

**Figure 13.7**
*CT scan of a patient with severe pulmonary hypertension taken after intravenous contrast enhancement; a slice with spiral acquisition showing a large thrombus in the right main pulmonary artery (arrow). A smaller thrombus is also seen in a basal branch of the left pulmonary artery. Note area of calcification in the right pulmonary artery thrombus. By courtesy of Dr Richard Coulden.*

hypoxia and hypocapnia. Multiple-gated acquisition (MUGA) scan may not only show dilated right ventricle but also indicate impaired left ventricular function. The diagnosis of pulmonary hypertension depends on direct measurement of elevation of pulmonary vascular resistance.

### Right heart catheterization

Right heart catheterization (RHC) not only establishes the diagnosis of pulmonary hypertension but also provides the necessary data to determine the patient's prognosis and so the best treatment regime.[1,2,5] After an overnight fast and avoidance of any vasodilators for up to 24 h, right heart catheterization is performed by inserting the triple-lumen flow-directed balloon-tipped catheter[47] through the right internal jugular vein. It is positioned using fluoroscopic screening in a branch of a descending pulmonary artery. Mean right atrial pressure (RAP) and mean pulmonary artery pressure (PAP) are measured and mean systemic arterial pressure (SAP) is monitored through an indwelling radial arterial cannula. Cardiac output is measured using the thermodilution method and pulmonary wedge pressure is also measured. Pulmonary and systemic arterial blood samples are taken for arterial ($SaO_2$) and mixed venous oxygen saturation ($SvO_2$) measurements. Mixed venous oxygen saturation of less than 63 per cent indicates advanced disease and is

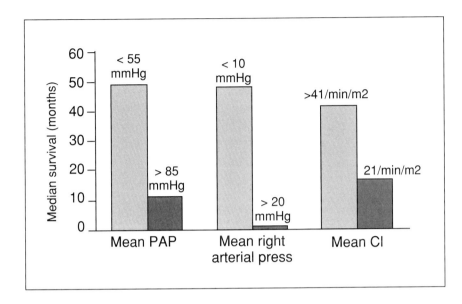

**Figure 13.8**
*Median survival in months from patients with primary pulmonary hypertension compared with three haemodynamic variables. (From D'Alonzo GE et al, Survival in patients with primary pulmonary hypertension, Ann Intern Med (1991) **115**:346.)*

associated with 3-year survival of only 17 per cent, while $SvO_2$ of greater than 63 per cent is associated with a 55 per cent chance of survival in 3 years.[1] Haemodynamic measurements also carry prognostic significance. Data obtained from the National Registry on 194 patients with PPH were published in 1991,[4] analysing factors affecting survival. In this study, an increase in the PAP from less than 55 mm Hg to 85 mm Hg or more reduced the median survival time from 48 months to 12 months. More importantly, a raised RAP and low cardiac output were particularly associated with poor prognosis. An increase in RAP from less than 10 mm Hg to 20 mm Hg or more was associated with a drop in median survival time from 46 months to only 1

month, and an increase in cardiac index from less than 2.0 l/min per m² body surface area to at least 4.0 l/min per m² was associated with the improvement in survival time from 17 months to 43 months (Figure 13.8). Similarly, variables derived from these haemodynamic measurements, e.g. higher pulmonary vascular resistance index, higher systemic vascular resistance index and a low stroke volume index, were also significantly related to mortality.[4]

Although not in common use, a new system for ambulatory PA pressure monitoring has been developed comprising a micromanometer-tipped catheter attached to a small battery-powered recorder.[48] This development looks promising for the future.

| Patient | Max. dose of epoprostenol | SAP (mm Hg) | PAP (mm Hg) | CI (l/min per m²) | PVR (dyn/s per cm⁻⁵) | SVR (dyn/s per cm⁻⁵) | HR (beats/min) | PaO₂ saturation | O₂ delivery (ml/kg per min) |
|---|---|---|---|---|---|---|---|---|---|
| 1 | Baseline | 78 | 100 | 1.7 | 2133 | 1600 | 104 | 45 | 5.8 |
|   | 4 ng/kg per min | 77 | 81 | 2.3 | 1190 | 1200 | 120 | 50 | 8.2 |
| 2 | Baseline | 82 | 71 | 1.5 | 1899 | 1992 | 70 | 38 | – |
|   | 6 ng/kg per min | 66 | 68 | 1.9 | 1365 | 1223 | 82 | 45 | – |
| 3 | Baseline | 80 | 55 | 1.7 | 1376 | 1952 | 98 | 52 | 10.9 |
|   | 5 ng/kg per min | 65 | 65 | 1.8 | 1629 | 1425 | 104 | 53 | 11.9 |
| 4 | Baseline | 83 | 80 | 2.1 | 1558 | 1684 | 87 | 60 | 9.5 |
|   | 4 ng/kg per min | 75 | 80 | 2.6 | 1242 | 1174 | 90 | 70 | 11.6 |
| 5 | Baseline | 73 | 62 | 3.0 | 784 | 1094 | 90 | 51 | 15.2 |
|   | 4 ng/kg per min | 72 | 48 | 3.1 | 580 | 1020 | 90 | 61 | 16.8 |
| 6 | Baseline | 93 | 60 | 1.5 | 1583 | 2187 | 77 | 42 | 8.5 |
|   | 6 ng/kg per min | 80 | 60 | 1.8 | 1358 | 1457 | 84 | 56 | 9.5 |
| 7 | Baseline | 100 | 80 | 1.8 | 1800 | 2275 | 78 | 51 | 12.4 |
|   | 6 ng/kg per min | 80 | 80 | 2.1 | 1516 | 1579 | 82 | 57 | 14.3 |
| 8 | Baseline | 70 | 50 | 2.2 | 869 | 1440 | 63 | 60 | 11.8 |
|   | 6 ng/kg per min | 61 | 48 | 2.8 | 675 | 1031 | 68 | 68 | 15.1 |
| 9 | Baseline | 95 | 105 | 1.5 | 2744 | 2425 | 84 | 43 | 8.3 |
|   | 8 ng/kg per min | 70 | 105 | 2.0 | 2054 | 1340 | 96 | 57 | 10.9 |
| 10 | Baseline | 76 | 93 | 1.3 | 2523 | 1723 | 82 | 42 | 7.3 |
|   | 6 ng/kg per min | 62 | 98 | 1.45 | 2400 | 1048 | 82 | 51 | 8.1 |
| Mean | Baseline | 83 (3) | 76 (6) | 1.83 (0.2) | 1727 (202) | 1837 (129) | 83 (4) | 48 (2) | 10.0 (1) |
| (SEM) | 5.5 ng/kg per min | 71 (2) | 73 (6) | 2.19 (0.2) | 1401 (175) | 1250 (61) | 90 (4) | 57 (2) | 11.8 (1) |
| p value | | <0.001 | >0.4 | <0.005 | <0.02 | <0.001 | <0.005 | <0.001 | <0.001 |

*Source*: Jones et al, Treatment of primary pulmonary hypertension with intravenous epoprostenol, *Br Heart J* (1987) **57**:273.

SAP = systemic arterial pressure
CI = cardiac index
SVR = systemic vascular resistance
PaO₂ = pulmonary arterial oxygen saturation

PAP = pulmonary artery pressure
PVR = pulmonary vascular resistance
HR = heart rate
O₂ delivery = peripheral oxygen delivery

**Table 13.1**
*Values for haemodynamic data at baseline and during maximal dose infusion during short-term epoprostenol trial on 10 patients with primary pulmonary hypertensicn*

*Acute vasodilator trial with PGI$_2$*

The vasodilatory capacity of the pulmonary vasculature is tested acutely at RHC with prostacyclin (PGI$_2$). Prostacyclin is a product of arachidonic acid metabolism involving the cyclo-oxygenase pathway. It is a potent vasodilator but it is labile, with a short half-life in the circulation of approximately 5 min. As it has a rapid onset of action it is possible to titrate the continuously infused intra-venously administered dose of PGI$_2$ to obtain an optimum fall in PVR by gradual increase in PGI$_2$ infusion without a risk of sustained systemic hypotension.[49] PGI$_2$ was used for the first time in 1980 as an acute pulmonary vasodilator in a child.[50] Since then, interest in its use has grown and many centres now use PGI$_2$ routinely to assess the vasodilatory capacity of the pulmonary vasculature.[51,52] After taking baseline measurements during RHC, prostacyclin infusion is commenced at approximately 2 ng/kg per min. Haemodynamic measurements and arterial and mixed venous blood samples are taken at intervals of 5–15 min before the dose is increased by 1–2 ng/kg per min. Prostacyclin infusion is continued with stepwise incremental doses until a significant 20 per cent drop in pulmonary vascular resistance (PVR) or a 20 per cent fall in systemic vascular resistance (SVR) is achieved or until the patient suffers significant side-effects. These can include headaches or flushing and occasionally syncope. The capacity to vasodilate has been suggested to be of value in deciding which patients should receive vasodilator therapy[53–55] (Table 13.1). Whilst this may be true in the earlier stages of the disease in the severely affected patients, we have noticed improvement in exercise tolerance of patients treated with PGI$_2$ who showed little acute vasodilatory response during right heart catheterization.[56] Similarly, enhanced survival on PGI$_2$ is seen to be greatest in those patients without much capacity to vasodilate.

# Treatment

As the cause of PPH is not known, treatment is mainly directed towards alleviating the effects of low cardiac output and pulmonary vasoconstriction.[53,57]

## Anticoagulants

Anticoagulants are recommended as they improve survival in PPH.[1] The mechanism of this effect is not clear; however, anticoagulants are likely to prevent the thrombosis in the pulmonary vasculature which is a risk in PPH due to low cardiac output state.

## Vasodilators

Various parenteral vasodilators have been used with conflicting results[58] and they include acetylcholine, tolazoline, phentolamine and isoprenaline. Oral vasodilators such as capto-pril[59] and hydralazine[60] have also been used with some early success but their long-term use has been disappointing. Calcium channel blockers[61] are currently favoured, particularly for patients with a maintained cardiac output and a mixed venous oxygen saturation of more than 63 per cent. Diltiazem is preferred to nifedipine in view of fewer side-effects and smaller effect on systemic circulation. Usually we commence with 180 mg of diltiazem daily in divided doses which may be increased in a stepwise fashion to 720 mg if necessary, depending upon the patient's response. Rich et al have demonstrated sustained haemodynamic as well as symptomatic and electrocardio-graphic improvement with high-dose calcium channel blocker therapy with nifedipine (240

| Patient no. | Maintenance (mg/day) | FC | Follow-up (months) | QRS axis (degrees) | RV$_1$ (mm) | RVID (mm) |
|---|---|---|---|---|---|---|
| 1 | 720 dil | I | 20 | 95→66 | 2→1 | 31→21 |
| 2 | 240 dil[a] | II | 19 | 115→110 | 4→2 | 32→36 |
| 3 | 120 nif | I | 17 | 98→76 | 4→1 | 28→16 |
| 4 | 120 nif | I | 16 | 110→78 | 7→1 | 40→28 |
| 5 | 120 nif | I | 13 | 125→105 | 5→3 | 34→26 |
| 6 | 180 nif | I | 6 | | | |
| 7 | 160 nif | (died) | 6 | | | |
| 8 | 240 nif | I | 4 | | | |

*Source:* Rich and Brundage, High-dose calcium blocking therapy for primary pulmonary hypertension, *Circulation* (1987) **76**:138.
Maintenance = daily dose of drug taken after outpatient readjustments
FC = NYHA functional class at follow-up
Follow-up = current length of follow-up period
QRS axis = initial QRS axis from electrocardiogram and changes after 1 year
RV$_1$ = height of R-wave from lead V$_1$ initially and after 1 year
RVID = right ventricular internal dimension by M-mode echocardiogram initially and after 1 year
dil = diltiazem
nif = nifedipine
[a]Patient who reduced her dose.

**Table 13.2**
*Results of long-term treatment with high-dose calcium channel blockers.*

mg/day) and diltiazem[62] (720 mg/day) (Table 13.2). More recently they have also shown improved survival with high-dose calcium channel blockers in the group of patients who responded with more than a 20 per cent drop in pulmonary artery (PA) pressure and PVR when challenged with a calcium channel blocker. Of the 17 patients, 16 (94 per cent) were alive after a 5-year period, which was significantly better than the patients enrolled in the NIH registry. However, those patients who did not drop their PA pressure and PVR significantly to acute challenge did less well and the survival rate in this group was similar to that of the NIH registry patients.[63]

We recommend calcium channel blockers along with anticoagulant therapy in patients who show significant acute pulmonary vasodilation to PGI$_2$ during RHC. They must not, however, be in right heart failure. An elevated right atrial pressure of greater than 10 mm Hg, or cardiac index of less than 1.95 l/min per m², excludes the use of this treatment. Patients who show no acute vasodilatory responses to PGI$_2$ are treated with anticoagulants only. These patients have NYHA grade I to II and have got a relatively good prognosis. They comprise 25–30 per cent of the patients with PPH.

## *Long-term treatment with prostacyclin in PPH*

Prostacyclin is a potent vasodilator. It can be used in the long-term treatment of PPH but only by continuous intravenous infusion. As it is quickly inactivated due to its short half-life, an optimum dose to achieve adequate pulmonary vasorelaxation can be titrated during right heart catheterization,[49] but because it is expensive and can only be administered parenterally it has to be reserved for selected patients with a poor prognosis.

The first case report using long-term prostacyclin came from our centre, showing improvement of a young woman bed-bound with severe pulmonary hypertension.[54] This was followed by a study of 10 patients treated with long-term intravenous $PGI_2$. The majority of these patients showed significant improvement in exercise tolerance and general well-being.[64] A decrease in PVR by $PGI_2$ leads to increase in cardiac output and oxygen tissue delivery which is translated into clinical improvement. However, there is no evidence that prostacyclin actually reverses the underlying disease process. Rubin et al have reported sustained haemodynamic and symptomatic improvement with prostacyclin in PPH.[65] In a randomized trial they demonstrated a significant drop in PVR (by 7.9 units from 21.6 units) in the group treated with prostacyclin for 8 weeks while there was no significant change in PVR (from 20.6 to 20.4 units) in a conventional therapy group in the same period. At our centre, long-term $PGI_2$ infusion is used in patients with a relatively poor prognosis, i.e. those who have evidence of right ventricular dysfunction as demonstrated during the right heart catheter study and have pulmonary artery oxygen saturation of less than 63 per cent. These patients are usually considered for heart–lung transplantation[66] but prostacyclin is used to stabilize their condition before a suitable donor is available. Generally, right heart catheterization with acute vasodilator trial is a prerequisite for initiating this treatment; however, in moribund cases where earlier investigations at the referring hospital had confirmed pulmonary hypertension, we have commenced prostacyclin before a formal right heart catheterization in order to achieve clinical improvement. Once the condition stabilizes, we undertake a so-called 'reverse' catheter study in order to establish objective evidence of haemodynamic change which may be obtained on withdrawing prostacyclin. In such a study we first take measurements during $PGI_2$ infusion and then a second set of readings up to 15 min after stopping the infusion. Patients who have had a vasodilator response to $PGI_2$ would show significant worsening of the right ventricular haemodynamics and pulmonary oxygen saturation on withdrawing $PGI_2$, thus underlining the need to continue with this form of therapy.

Long-term administration of prostacyclin poses a number of practical problems. Patients need up to 2 weeks to be adequately trained in self-administration of this drug, which includes aseptic preparation of the solution and its storage, running of the Graseby pump and looking after the central line and its connections (Figure 13.9). A long intravenous cannula has to be inserted through a subcutaneous tunnel in order to minimize the risk of systemic infection (Figure 13.10). The solution of prostacyclin is prepared by dissolving sodium salt of epoprostenol in the sterile glycine buffer. The solution is drawn into a 20-ml plastic syringe and is mounted on the electrically driven pump, also called a Graseby pump (MS16A,

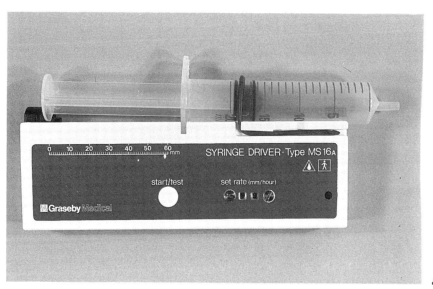

a

**Figure 13.9**
*Electrically driven Graseby pump with a mounted syringe (a) and apparatus used to prepare prostacyclin infusion (b).*

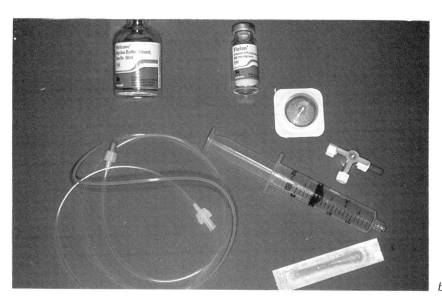

b

Graseby Dynamics, Bushey, Hertfordshire). The pump has an automatic auditory alarm in order to indicate any pump failure. The $PGI_2$ solution is quite unstable, should be protected from light and should not be used more than 12 h after its preparation as it tends to lose its efficacy. An optimum dose of prostacyclin is determined during a therapeutic trial lasting for a week to 10 days, while the patient's progress is monitored. Usually the commencing dose is 1–2 ng/kg per min, which is increased in a stepwise fashion by 1–2 ng/kg per min after every 12–24 h. Serial 12-min measured walks are carried out

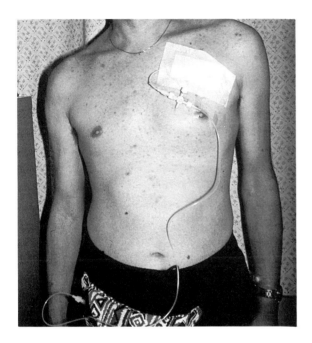

**Figure 13.10**
*Tunnelled central line with PGI₂ infusion set-up shown in a patient with primary pulmonary hypertension.*

during this period in order to measure clinical response and satisfy the need for long-term therapy. Long-term treatment with prostacyclin is at present indeed expensive and somewhat complicated, but it works well for many patient with severe pulmonary hypertension who are critically ill.

### Complications of PGI₂ therapy

Problems associated with prostacyclin therapy can be related to either the delivery system or the drug itself. Generally the drug is tolerated well provided the necessary precautions are taken. Common side-effects of prostacyclin include loose stools, jaw pain and photosensitivity and have been reported in 100, 57 and 36 per cent of cases respectively.[65] Other common side-effects are headache, abdominal pain and cutaneous flushing, which are observed either on commencing therapy or increasing the dose, but often settle within 24 h.[49] Vasovagal episodes may occur, especially during acute vasodilator trial, but fortunately are uncommon. Pulmonary oedema and ascites are occasionally seen with prostacyclin[65] therapy. The exact mechanism is not known and could be related to the underlying disease process. It may be due to increased vascular permeability in the lungs and peritoneum respectively. In our report 3 out of 10 patients developed ascites.[64] The exudative nature of the ascitic fluid indicated leakage from the peritoneal vasculature rather than right heart failure. One patient had developed chylous ascites before death.

The complications related to the delivery system could either occur at the time of central line insertion, e.g. pneumothorax or malpositioning of the line, or might happen subsequently. Line sepsis is not uncommon and accounts for one of the main problems necessitating line replacement. Displacement of the line either within the vein or into subcutaneous tissue and broken or kinked line barrel occasionally pose problems. One-third of the patients may become more symptomatic during heparin flushing of the cannula; this may persist for up to 30 min after recommencing prostacyclin and can be prevented by removing the dead space created by heparin flush.[65] Mechanical faults may occur in the electric

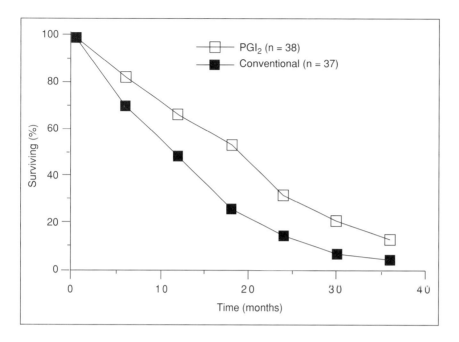

**Figure 13.11**
*Improvement of survival in primary pulmonary hypertension with continuous prostacyclin infusion as compared to conventional therapy; experience from Papworth Hospital.*

pump, causing underdosing or interruption of the infusion. We usually supply an extra Graseby pump to ensure uninterrupted infusion in the event of any pump malfunction. A few patients have noticed a return of symptoms like presyncope on changing brand of the syringe, suggesting underdosing of prostacyclin.[65]

In spite of the problems encountered occasionally with prostacyclin therapy, we have found it useful in many patients with severe disease. It has improved not only quality of life, but in some cases survival as well (Figure 13.11). We have witnessed an improved survival in the first year with prostacyclin for patients with severe PPH awaiting transplantation.[67] It may be pointed out that improved survival of patients treated with prostacyclin was not related to the degree of acute vasodilator response achieved during right heart catheterization, suggesting an additional mechanism of action by prostacyclin besides vasodilatation. This is an interesting observation and needs to be evaluated by further studies.

We have observed a significant clinical response to relatively small doses of $PGI_2$ during the early stages, but with the passage of time many patients require a gradual increase in dosage. This is not necessarily always due to progression of the disease, as clinical stability can be obtained with a small increase in $PGI_2$. Furthermore, many of those patients who may be quite sensitive to a small dose of $PGI_2$ may tolerate a much higher dose subsequently, suggesting an element of tachyphylaxis with long-term administration of prostacyclin.

|  | Inclusion | PGI$_2$ | Iloprost |
|---|---|---|---|
| Distance (m) | 463 ± 43 | 640 ± 25** | 653 ± 38** |
| Rest time (s) | 197 ± 127 | 0** | 50 ± 41* |
| ΔSaO$_2$ (%) | 16 ± 9 | 5 ± 3* | 3 ± 1** |
| ΔHR (min$^{-1}$) | 45 ± 6 | 39 ± 3 NS | 31 ± 4 NS |

*Source:* Dinh-Xuan et al, Effects of long-term treatment with iloprost, a prostacyclin analogue, on exercise tolerance in patients with primary pulmonary hypertension, *Am Rev Resp Dis* (1990) **141**:A889.
*P < 0.05; **P < 0.01
ΔSaO$_2$ (%) = arterial oxygen desaturation
ΔHR (min$^{-1}$) = increase in heart rate

**Table 13.3**
*Data from 12-min walk showing comparable improvement with PGI$_2$ and iloprost*

## Iloprost

Prostacyclin (PGI$_2$), although a useful investigational as well as a therapeutic agent in PPH, has got some drawbacks. It is fairly unstable at room temperature, photosensitive, orally inactive and quite expensive. So there has been a need for a synthetic analogue which is more stable and possibly cheaper. Iloprost, a synthetic prostacyclin analogue produced by Schering, fulfils that role to a certain extent. Its molecule is similar to prostacyclin and its vasorelaxant effect seems to be mediated through prostacyclin receptors.[68] Iloprost is supplied in an ethanol-Tris-HCl buffered solution[69] and can be diluted in isotonic solution. It is more stable, can be stored at room temperature and does not have to be protected from light. It has got a somewhat longer half-life of 13 min after intravenous administration[70] and also has an oral bioavailability of 13 per cent,[71] suggesting that an oral preparation may become available in the future. Apart from its pulmonary vasodilatory action, studies have demonstrated its antiplatelet[72] and anti-arrhythmic[73] activities as well as its favourable effect on glomerular filtration[74] and coronary bloodflow.[75]

We have shown that iloprost is equally effective as prostacyclin in decreasing pulmonary vascular resistance in severe PPH; however, a lower dose was required to obtain similar haemodynamic effects.[69] Long-term use of iloprost also produced comparable benefits in terms of improved exercise tolerance for patients with severe pulmonary hypertension[76] (Table 13.3). Iloprost may not only be useful in the acute assessment but also might replace prostacyclin in the long-term treatment of PPH.

## New possible therapies

In those patients where proximal pulmonary arteries are occluded by emboli, surgical endarterectomy[45] is now offered, which can restore normal haemodynamics and improve quality of life dramatically. These patients are usually older and more frequently male. Surgical endarterectomy is carried out when risk of further emboli has decreased.

There is a proportion of patients with severe PPH who do not demonstrate an acute vasodilatory response to $PGI_2$ during right heart catheterization or show any improvement in exercise tolerance with prostacyclin therapy. They are likely to do less well and could develop right heart failure quite quickly. Additional use of a nitrovasodilator along with prostacyclin may be an option that clinicians may like to choose to achieve effective pulmonary vasodilatation for these selected patients. We have seen this approach succeed in one patient who was unresponsive to high doses of prostacyclin but showed a dramatic fall in pulmonary vascular resistance after nitroprusside[77] was added to the regime. A nitrovasodilator acts like an exogenous source of nitric oxide (NO) for the vascular smooth muscle cells. NO stimulates guanylate cyclase enzyme, leading to increased formation of cyclic 3,5-guanosine monophosphate (cGMP),[78] which promotes vascular relaxation by causing a fall in intracellular calcium levels. Prostacyclin works on the parallel pathway by causing a rise in another cyclic nucleotide, i.e. cyclic 3,5-adenosine monophosphate (cAMP),[79] which also leads to vascular relaxation. Therefore it seems rational to use combined therapy for difficult cases of PPH; however, properly randomized studies would be required to establish such a strategy.

Enoximone is a type III phosphodiesterase inhibitor[80] which is currently available in injectable form. It has been used in cardiac failure[81–83] because of its positive inotropic and systemic vasorelaxant activities. It causes a rise in cAMP in myocardial cells and a rise in cGMP in vascular smooth muscle cells by preventing breakdown of these cyclic nucleotides.[84,85] In an experimental study on vascular rings we have demonstrated that enoximone is also a potent pulmonary vasodilator.[86] Its pulmonary vasorelaxant effect is not influenced by the presence of endothelium or its relaxing factors, and is mediated by a rise in cGMP in pulmonary vascular smooth muscle cells. This endothelium-independent vasodilatory effect of enoximone makes it a potentially useful drug in the management of pulmonary hypertension, especially where endothelial function is impaired. We have used enoximone infusion in one patient with severe PPH who started to deteriorate while on $PGI_2$ but showed significant improvement with enoximone and was successfully bridged to have a heart–lung transplantation. We believe there is an opportunity to explore new pharmacological applications in the management of PPH as our understanding of molecular mechanisms of prostacyclin, nitrovasodilators and phosphodiesterase inhibitors improves.

There is a scope for inhaled NO to be used in pulmonary hypertension, provided a safe and effective delivery apparatus for this gas is available. Properly randomized studies are required to explore this possibility. EDNO[87–89] is a highly labile gas with a half-life of only a few seconds. It is quickly inactivated by haemoglobin, and therefore any vasorelaxant effect downstream in pulmonary arteries would be negligible. After its release from the endothelial cells it quickly diffuses into the underlying vascular smooth muscle cells, where it promotes relaxation. Inhaled NO provides an alternative route, as it reaches the vascular smooth muscle cells abluminally and thus avoids the risk of being neutralized by blood. Frostell et al have demonstrated substantial reversal of hypoxic pulmonary vasoconstriction by inhaled NO (80 ppm in air) in sheep.[90] At our centre we have shown a pulmonary vasodilatory response to inhaled NO (40 ppm

|  | Baseline | PGE$_1$ | *p* |
|---|---|---|---|
| CI (l/min per m²) | 3.9 ± 0.3 | 4.5 ± 0.3 | <0.001 |
| HR (beats/min) | 110 ± 7 | 116 ± 7 | <0.01 |
| RAM (mm Hg) | 6 ± 3 | 5 ± 1 | NS |
| MAP (mm Hg) | 88 ± 6 | 82 ± 7 | <0.05 |
| SVR (dyne/s per cm$^{-5}$) | 1082 ± 107 | 814 ± 131 | <0.001 |
| PAM (mm Hg) | 48 ± 5 | 38 ± 4 | <0.001 |
| PVR (dyne/s per cm$^{-5}$) | 532 ± 65 | 368 ± 51 | <0.001 |
| PaO$_2$ (mm Hg) | 38 ± 3 | 37 ± 2 | NS |
| PvO$_2$ (mm Hg) | 26 ± 3 | 27 ± 2 | NS |
| C(a-v)O$_2$ (ml/dl) | 4.6 ± 0.3 | 3.9 ± 0.3 | <0.01 |
| TO$_2$ (ml/min per m²) | 586 ± 61 | 657 ± 56 | <0.001 |

*Source:* Naeije et al, Reduction in pulmonary hypertension by prostaglandin $E_1$ in decompensated chronic obstructive pulmonary disease, *Am Rev Resp Dis* (1982) **125**:2.
CI = cardiac index
HR = heart rate
RAM = right atrial mean pressure
MAP = mean systemic arterial pressure
SVR = systemic vascular resistance
PAM = pulmonary artery mean pressure
PVR = pulmonary vascular resistance
PaO$_2$ = arterial PO$_2$
PvO$_2$ = mixed venous PO$_2$
C(a-v)O$_2$ = arteriovenous O$_2$ content difference
TO$_2$ = O$_2$ delivery

**Table 13.4**
*Mean ± SEM gasometric and haemodynamic measurements before and at 13 min of PGE$_1$ infusion 0.02 μg/kg per min in 10 patients with secondary pulmonary hypertension due to chronic obstructive pulmonary disease*

in air) which was comparable to that to prostacyclin in patients with PPH.[91] We have also demonstrated a decrease in pulmonary vascular resistance with inhaled NO in cardiac patients with normal PVR. This suggests that inhaled NO can act as a selective pulmonary vasodilator and may have a role in the management of pulmonary hypertension.

## Role of prostaglandins and NO in secondary pulmonary hypertension

As opposed to PPH, secondary pulmonary hypertension is relatively common. End-stage chronic lung disease, left heart disease and pulmonary embolism are major causes. Development of pulmonary hypertension indicates a poor outlook for these patients. In secondary pulmonary hypertension due to chronic hypoxic lung disease, the only agent to have improved the mortality is domiciliary oxygen.[92] We have shown a decrease in pulmonary vascular resistance with prostacyclin in chronic obstructive lung disease and pulmonary fibrosis due to sarcoidosis.[53] Naeije et al have also demonstrated improvement in haemodynamics and pulmonary gas exchange using PGE$_1$ in pulmonary hypertension due to decompensated chronic obstructive pulmonary disease (Table 13.4).[93] In some patients with chronic lung disease a pulmonary vasodilator, by overcoming hypoxic vasoconstriction, might aggravate ventilation/perfusion imbalance, leading to increased arterial desaturation. However, it has been argued that tissue oxygen delivery is more important than $PaO_2$.[94] Although tissue oxygen delivery is likely to improve in many such patients as a direct effect of increased cardiac output, it would be advisable to demonstrate beneficial effects on haemodynamic and pulmonary gas exchange in each patient before resorting to long-term vasodilator therapy.

Inhaled NO may also have a role in secondary pulmonary hypertension, as there is evidence of impaired EDRF release from the pulmonary arteries of patients with chronic hypoxic lung disease.[95] Inhaled NO is likely to improve haemodynamics and pulmonary gas exchange by supplementing that deficiency.

A pulmonary vasodilator may also play a useful role during the early postoperative period of heart transplantation. Most patients with severe cardiac failure requiring heart transplantation have secondary pulmonary vascular disease. The right ventricle of the donor heart is under considerable stress in the postoperative period and impairment of its function plays an important role in early postoperative mortality. Intravenous $PGI_2$ or inhaled NO acting as potent pulmonary vasodilators may alleviate right ventricular stress during this crucial period and may have a beneficial effect on morbidity and mortality of these patients.

## Heart–Lung transplantation in PPH

In selected patients where medical therapy does not halt the progress of disease, heart and lung transplantation (HLT) remains an option[66] from which some patients can benefit more than others (Figure 13.12). Younger patients who have no other systemic disease are likely to do better. Effective immunosuppressive regime and periodic use of transbronchial pulmonary biopsies[96] (TBB) to detect any acute rejection have improved the survival to 65 per cent in 3 years, as the incidence of obliterative bronchiolitis is now reduced in HLT.[97] in HLT recipients transbronchial biopsy is also essential to diagnose any pulmonary infection,[98–101] which otherwise is often difficult to distinguish from rejection,[102,103] and if not treated early may prove fatal.[104] Use of prostacyclin in perfusing the heart and lung grafts and improved techniques in preservation of the donor organs to allow distant procurements have also contributed to improved survival after surgery.[105,106]

At our centre, patients with severe pulmonary hypertension, i.e. having evidence of right ventricular dysfunction and pulmonary artery oxygen saturation ($SvO_2$) of less than 63 per cent, are considered for heart and lung transplantation. Age (generally less than 50 years), psychosocial stability and absence of non-reversible organ dysfunction and systemic disease are also taken into account. In the interim period continuous prostacyclin infusion is offered.

Long-term survival data are lacking at this stage; however, some early evidence from Pasque et al cautiously supports the option of single lung transplantation in pulmonary hypertension.[107] Doig et al have also demonstrated considerable haemodynamic improvement after single lung transplantation for moderately severe pulmonary hypertension.[108] Once the role of single lung transplantation is established, it will solve many problems.[109] Apart from the simpler surgical technique and shorter operating time, all to the benefit of postoperative recovery, single lung transplantation would also ease the stress on the

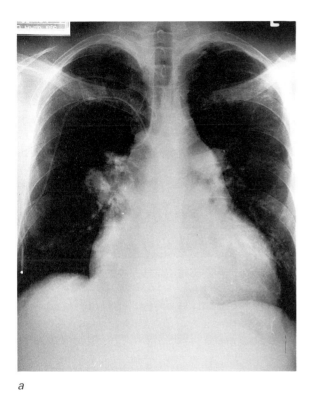

a

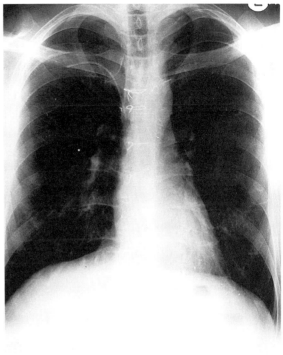

b

**Figure 13.12**
*Chest X-ray of a patient with severe pulmonary hypertension before (a) and after (b) heart–lung transplantation. Central line used for PGI$_2$ infusion can also be seen in (a).*

scarce resource of donor organs, as only one healthy lung would be required per patient. Moreover, patients would not run the risk of graft-related coronary occlusive disease, which is a major cause of late mortality associated with heart transplantation.[110,111] At present, the need for a suitable heart and two healthy lungs makes many organ blocks not fit for transplantation, which prolongs a long waiting period further for these patients. While we await convincing evidence of long-term benefit with single lung transplantation in pulmonary hypertension, HLT remains the main surgical option for these patients.

## Summary

PPH is a serious disease with a fearful prognosis. Its aetiology and exact pathogenesis are not known. Clinicians should have a high index of suspicion for this disease to avoid undue delay in its diagnosis. Right heart catheterization is the cornerstone investigation which confirms the diagnosis and provides prognostic information. Patients with adequate cardiac output and $SvO_2$ of more than 63 per cent should be treated with anticoagulants and calcium channel blockers. Those with $SvO_2$ of less than 63 per cent and evidence of right ventricular dysfunction carry a poor prognosis and should be considered for HLT[112] or single lung transplantation, once its role has been established. Before suitable donor organs are available, these patients may be treated with continuous prostacyclin infusion, which improves quality of life and may improve long-term survival. As we have seen clinical improvement with $PGI_2$ even in patients who do not show an acute pulmonary vasodilatory response to prostacyclin, there may be an additional mechanism for this agent which needs to be explored. Further developments in understanding the pathogenesis of PPH may open the possibility of new pharmacological approaches to deal with this disease, which so far has carried a bleak outlook.

## *If I had …*

I would like it to be diagnosed sooner rather than later and would prefer to be sent to a hospital which has a physician with a special interest in PPH and also has the transplantation facility. I would like to have a complete work-up to ensure that there is no underlying cause of pulmonary hypertension, particularly any clot in the proximal pulmonary artery which could be removed by thromboendarterectomy, but I would not favour having a lung biopsy. I would prefer to have a right

heart catheter study done by an experienced operator and would like to know how I responded to a vasodilator challenge, but I may not be interested in knowing the survival chance. If I have mild to moderate disease, and there is no right ventricular dysfunction, I would like it to be treated with anticoagulants with or without a calcium channel blocker, depending upon the degree of my vasodilatory response during RHC study. If the acute vasodilatory response was significant, then the calcium channel blocker could be increased to a high dose range.

If I had severe disease I would like to be considered for heart–lung transplantation, but I would enquire about the feasibility of single lung transplantation on the basis of the current state of knowledge and whether my surgeon was comfortable with this option. In either case I would like my explanted tissue used for further research. In the interim period I would agree to be treated with continuous prostacyclin infusion before suitable donor organs become available; however, if I had a good response to $PGI_2$ I would not mind waiting for transplantation for as long as was necessary. At the time of central tunnel line insertion I would expect my operator to be skilled, and to take all necessary measures to minimize the risk of complications. If my physician offered an alternative therapy with inhaled NO, I would like to confirm that the delivery apparatus for this gas is effective and absolutely safe.

Lastly, although I would not want my family members to be screened for PPH if they were asymptomatic, I would expect my doctor to rule out this possibility if they presented even with very mild dyspnoea, chest pain or syncope.

# References

1   Fuster V et al, Primary pulmonary hypertension: natural history and the importance of thrombosis, *Circulation* (1984) **70**:580–7.

2   Rich S et al, Primary pulmonary hypertension. A national prospective study, *Ann Intern Med* (1987) **107**:216–23.

3   Voelkel NF, Reeves JT, Primary pulmonary hypertension. In: Mosesr KM, ed, *Pulmonary vascular diseases* (Marcel Dekker: New York 1979) 573–628.

4   D'Alonzo GE et al, Survival in patients with primary pulmonary hypertension, *Ann Intern Med* (1991) **115**:343–9.

5   Weir EK, Diagnosis and management of primary pulmonary hypertension. In: Weir EK, Reeves JT, eds. *Pulmonary hypertension* (Futura Publishing Company: New York 1984) 115–68.

6   Romberg E, Uver sklerose der lungenarterien, *Dtsch Arch Klin Med* (1891) **48**:197.

7   Monckeberg JG, Ube die genuine arteriosklerose der lungenarterie, *Dtsch Med Wochenschr* (1907) **33**:1243.

8   Brenner O, Pathology of the vessels of the pulmonary circulation, *Arch Intern Med* (1935) **56**:211–19.

9   Dresdale DT, Schultz M, Michtom RJ, Primary pulmonary hypertension 1. Clinical and hemodynamic study, *Am J Med* (1951) **11**:686–705.

10  Wood P, Pulmonary hypertension with special reference to the vaso constrictive factor, *Br Heart J* (1958) **20**:557–70.

11  Gurtner HP, Aminorex and pulmonary hypertension, *Cor Vasa* (1985) **27**:160–71.

12  Hatano S, Strasser T, eds. *Primary pulmonary hypertension* (World Health Organisation: Geneva 1975) 7–45.

13  Wagenvoort CA, Wagenvoort N, Primary pulmonary hypertension: a pathologic study on the lung vessels in 156 clinically diagnosed cases, *Circulation* (1970) **42**:1163–84.

14  Reid LM, Structure and function in pulmonary hypertension: new perceptions, *Chest* (1986) **89**:279–88.

15  Moncada S et al, An enzyme isolated from arteries transforms prostaglandin endoperoxides to an unstable substance that inhibits platelet aggregation, *Nature* (1976) **263**:663–5.

16  Palmer RMJ, Ferrige AG, Moncada S, Nitric oxide release accounts for the biological activity of endothelium-derived relaxing factor, *Nature* (1987) **327**:524–6.

17  Yanagisawa M et al, A novel potent vasoconstrictor peptide produced by vascular endothelial cells, *Nature* (1988) **332**:411–15.

18  Radomski MW, Palmer RMJ, Moncada S, Endogenous nitric oxide inhibits human platelet adhesion to vascular endothelium, *Lancet* (1987) **ii**:1057–8.

19  Asherson RA et al, Pulmonary hypertension in systemic lupus erythematosis, *Br Med J* (1983) **287**:1024–5.

20  Anderson NE, Ali MR, The lupus anticoagulant, pulmonary thromboembolus and fatal pulmonary hypertension, *Ann Rheum Dis* (1984) **43**:760–3.

21  Harris EN, Gharavi AE, Boey RG, Antiplatelet antibodies: detection by radioimmunoassay and association with thrombosis in lupus erythematosis, *Lancet* (1983) **ii**:1211–14.

22  Cerreras LO, Defreyn G, Machin SJ, Arterial thrombosis, intra-uterine death and 'lupus' anticoagulant: detection of immuno-globulin interfering with prostacyclin formation, *Lancet* (1981) **i**:244–6.

23  McVerry BA et al, Reduced prostacyclin activity in systemic lupus erythematosis, *Ann Rheum Dis* (1980) **39**:524–5.

24  Lanham JG et al, Prostacyclin deficiency in a young woman with recurrent thrombosis, *Br Med J* (1986) **292**:435–6.

25  Eigeberg O, Inherited antithrombin deficiency causing thrombophilia, *Thromb Diath Haem* (1965) **13**:516–30.

26  Heath D, Smith P, Gosney J, The pathology of the early and late stages of primary pulmonary hypertension, *Br Heart J* (1987) **58**:204–13.

27 Wagenvoort CA, Hypertensive pulmonary vascular disease. The point of no return, *Minn Med* (1985) **73**:45–8.

28 Giuseppe G et al, Histopathology of primary pulmonary hypertension, *Circulation* (1989) **80**:1198–206.

29 Dail DH et al, A study of 43 cases of pulmonary veno-occlusive disease, *Lab Invest* (1978) **38**:340–50.

30 Wallcott G, Burchell HB, Brown AL, Primary pulmonary hypertension, *Am J Med* (1970) **49**:70–9.

31 Hughes JD, Rubin LJ, Primary pulmonary hypertension. An analysis of 28 cases and a review of the literature, *Medicine* (1986) **65**:65–72.

32 Morice AH et al, Atrial natriuretic peptide in primary pulmonary hypertension, *Eur Respir J* (1990) **3**:910–13.

33 McCaffrey RM, Dunn LJ, Primary pulmonary hypertension in pregnancy, *Obstet Gynecol Surv* (1964) **19**:567–91.

34 Douglas JG et al, Pulmonary hypertension and fenfluramine, *Br Med J* (1981) **283**:881–3.

35 Oakley C, Somerville J, Oral contraceptives and progressive pulmonary vascular disease, *Lancet* (1968) **1**:890–3.

36 Kleiger RE et al, Pulmonary hypertension in patients using oral contraceptives. A report of six cases, *Chest* (1976) **69**:143–7.

37 Stojnic B et al, Jugular venous 'a' wave in pulmonary hypertension: new insights from a Doppler echocardiographic study. *Br Heart J* (1992) **68**:187–91.

38 Rawson AJ, Woske HM, A study of etiologic factors in so-called primary pulmonary hypertension, *Arch Intern Med* (1960) **105**:233–43.

39 Goodman J, Harrison DC, Popp RL, Echocardiographic features of primary pulmonary hypertension, *Am J Cardiol* (1974) **33**:438–43.

40 Visner MS et al, The effects of pressure-induced right ventricular hypertrophy on left ventricular diastolic properties and dynamic geometry in the conscious dog, *Circulation* (1986) **74**:410–19.

41 King ME et al, Interventricular septal configuration as a predictor of right ventricular systolic hypertension in children: a cross-sectional echocardiographic study, *Circulation* (1983) **68**:68–75.

42 Rozkovec A, Montanes P, Oakley C, Factors that influence the outcome of primary pulmonary hypertension, *Br Heart J* (1986) **55**:449–58.

43 D'Alonzo G, Bower J, Dantzker D, Differentiation of patients with primary and thromboembolic pulmonary hypertension, *Chest* (1984) **85**:457–61.

44 Hull RD, Raskob GE, Heish J, The diagnosis of clinically suspected pulmonary embolism. Practical approaches, *Chest* (1986) **89** (suppl):417–25.

45 Moser KM et al, Chronic thrombotic obstruction of major pulmonary arteries. Results of thromboendarterectomy in 15 patients, *Ann Intern Med* (1983) **99**:299–305.

46 Wilson AG, Harris CN, Lavender JP, Perfusion lung scanning in obliterative pulmonary hypertension, *Br Heart J* (1973) **35**:917–30.

47 Swan HJC et al, Catheterisation of the heart in man with use of a flow-directed balloon-tipped catheter, *N Engl J Med* (1970) **283**:447–51.

48 Gibbs S, MacLachlan D, Fox K, A new system for ambulatory pulmonary artery pressure recording, *Br Heart J* (1992) **68**:230–5.

49 Higenbottam T, The place of prostacyclin in the clinical management of primary pulmonary hypertension, *Am Rev Respir Dis* (1987) **136**:782–5.

50 Watkins WD et al, Prostacyclin and prostaglandin E$_1$ for severe idiopathic pulmonary artery hypertension (letter to the editor), *Lancet* (1980) **i**:1083.

51 Guadagni DN, Ikram H, Maslowski AH, Haemodynamic effects of prostacyclin (PGI$_2$) in pulmonary hypertension, *Br Heart J* (1981) **45**:385–8.

52 Jones DK, Higenbottam TW, Wallwork J, Pulmonary vasodilation with prostacyclin in primary and secondary pulmonary hypertension, *Chest* (1989) **96**:784–9.

53 Reeves JT, Groves BM, Turkevich D, The case for treatment of selected patients with primary pulmonary hypertension, *Am Rev Respir Dis* (1986) **134**:342–6.

54  Higenbottam TW et al, Long-term treatment of primary pulmonary hypertension with continuous intravenous epoprostenol (prostacyclin), *Lancet* (1984) i:1046–7.

55  Roskovec A et al, Prediction of favourable response to long term vasodilation of pulmonary hypertension by short term administration of epoprostenol (Prostacyclin) or nifedipine, *Br Heart J* (1988) 59:696–705.

56  Butt AY et al, Lack of acute pulmonary vasodilatation does not preclude successful clinical response to prostacyclin (PgI₂) in severe pulmonary hypertension (SPH), *Br Heart J* (1993) 69(5)[suppl]:77 (abstr.).

57  Oakley CM, Management of primary pulmonary hypertension, *Br Heart J* (1985) 53:1–4.

58  Rich S, Brundage BH, The pharmacologic treatment of primary pulmonary hypertension. In: Bergofsky EH ed. *Abnormal pulmonary circulation* (Churchill Livingstone: New York 1986) 283–311.

59  Rich S et al, Captopril as treatment for patients with pulmonary hypertension: problem of variability in assessing chronic drug treatment, *Br Heart J* (1982) 48:272–7.

60  Hermiller JB et al, Vasodilators and prostaglandin inhibitors in primary pulmonary hypertension, *Ann Intern Med* (1982) 97:470–89.

61  Camerini F et al, Primary pulmonary hypertension: effects of nifedipine, *Br Heart J* (1980) 44:352–6.

62  Rich S, Brundage BH, High-dose calcium channel-blocking therapy for primary pulmonary hypertension: evidence for long-term reduction in pulmonary arterial pressure and regression of right ventricular hypertrophy, *Circulation* (1987) 76:135–41.

63  Rich S, Kaufmann E, Levy P, The effect of high doses of calcium-channel blockers on survival in primary pulmonary hypertension, *N Engl J Med* (1992) 327:76–81.

64  Jones DK, Higenbottam TW, Wallwork J, Treatment of primary pulmonary hypertension with intravenous epoprostenol (prostacyclin), *Br Heart J* (1987) 57:270–8.

65  Rubin LJ et al, Treatment of primary pulmonary hypertension with continuous intravenous prostacyclin (epoprostenol), *Ann Intern Med* (1990) 112:485–91.

66  Reitz BA et al, Heart–lung transplantation: successful therapy for patients with pulmonary vascular disease, *N Engl J Med* (1982) 306:557–64.

67  Cremona G, Higenbottam TW, Scott JP, Continuous intravenous infusion of prostacyclin (PGI₂) improves survival in primary pulmonary hypertension, *Am Rev Respir Dis* (1991) 143:A180 (abstr.).

68  Schror et al, The anti-platelet and cardiovascular actions of a new carbacyclin derivative (ZK36374)—equipotent to PG12 *in vitro*, *Arch Pharmacol* (1981) 316:252–5.

69  Scott JP, Higenbottam TW, Wallwork J, The acute effect of the synthetic prostacyclin analogue iloprost in primary pulmonary hypertension, *Br J Clin Pharmacol* (1990) 6:231–4.

70  Kaukinen S et al, Hemodynamic effects of iloprost, a prostacyclin analog, *Clin Pharmacol Ther* (1984) 36:464–9.

71  Krause W, Humpel M, Hoyer GA, Biotransformation of the stable prostacyclin analogue, iloprost, in the rat, *Drug Metab Dispos* (1984) 12:645–51.

72  Bugiardini R et al, Effects of iloprost, a stable prostacyclin analog, on exercise capacity and platelet aggregation in stable angina pectoris, *Am J Cardiol* (1986) 58:453–9.

73  Coker SK, Parrat JR, Prostacyclin—antiarrhythmic or arrhythmogenic? Comparison of the effects of intravenous and intracoronary prostacyclin and ZK 36374 during coronary arterial occlusion and reperfusion in anaesthetised greyhouds, *J Cardiovasc Pharmacol* (1983) 5(5):557–67.

74  Yitalo P et al, Effects of a prostacyclin analog iloprost on kidney function, renin–angiotensin and kallikrein–kinin systems, prostanoids and catecholamines in man, *Prostaglandins* (1985) 29:1063–71.

75  Uchida Y, Murao S, Effects of prostaglandin 12 analogue, ZK 36374, on recurring reduction of coronary blood flow, *Jap Heart J* (1983) 24(4):641–7.

76  Dinh Xuan AT et al, Effects of long-term treatment with iloprost, a prostacyclin analogue, on exercise tolerance in patients with primary pulmonary hypertension, *Am Rev Respir Dis* (1990) 141:A889.

77  Fuleihan DS et al, Sodium nitroprusside: a new role as a pulmonary vasodilator. *Am J Cardiol* (1979) **43**:405 (abstr.).

78  Dinh-Xuan AT, Higenbottam TW, Non-prostanoid endothelium-derived vasoactive factors, *J Int Med Res* (1989) **17**:305–15.

79  Moncada S, Palmer RMJ, Higgs EA, Prostacyclin and endothelium-derived relaxing factor: biological inter-actions and significance. In: Verstraete M, Vermylen J, Lijnen HR, Arnout J, eds. *Thrombosis and haemostasis* (Leuven University Press: Leuven 1987) 597–618.

80  Dage RC et al, Pharmacology of enoximone, *Am J Cardiol* (1987) **60**:10C–14C.

81  Vincent JL et al, Administration of Enoximone in cardiogenic shock, *Am J Cardiol* (1988) **62**:419–23.

82  Weber KT, Janicki JS, Jain MC, Enoximone (MDL 17,043) for stable, chronic heart failure secondary to ischemic or idiopathic cardiomyopathy, *Am J Cardiol* (1986) **58**:589–95.

83  Treese N et al, Long-term treatment with oral Enoximone for chronic congestive heart failure. The European experience, *Am J Cardiol* (1987) **60**:85C–90C.

84  Kauffman RF et al, In vitro vascular relaxation by new inotropic agents: relationship to phosphodiesterase and cyclic nucleotides, *J Pharmacol Exp Ther* (1987) **242**:864–72.

85  Kariya T, Dage RC, Tissue distribution and selective inhibition of subtypes of high affinity cAMP phosphodiesterase, *Biochem Pharmacol* (1988) **37**:3267–70.

86  Butt AY et al, In vitro pulmonary vasorelaxant effect of the phosphodiesterase inhibitor Enoximone, *Angiology* (1992) **44**(4):289–94.

87  Furchgott RF, Zawadzki JV, The obligatory role of endothelial cells in the relaxation of arterial smooth muscle by acetylcholine, *Nature* (1980) **288**:373–6.

88  Palmer RM, Ferrige AG, Moncada S, Nitric oxide release accounts for the biological activity of endothelium-derived relaxing factor, *Nature* (1987) **327**:524–6.

89  Ignarro LJ, Biological actions and properties of endothelium-derived nitric oxide formed and released from artery and vein, *Circ Res* (1989) **65**:1–21.

90  Frostell C et al, Inhaled nitric oxide, a selective pulmonary vasodilator reversing hypoxic pulmonary vasoconstriction, *Circulation* (1991) **83**:2038–47.

91  Pepke-Zaba J et al, Inhaled nitric oxide as a cause of selective pulmonary vasodilatation in pulmonary hypertension, *Lancet* (1991) **338**:1173–4.

92  Report of the MRC Working Party, Long-term domiciliary oxygen therapy in chronic hypoxic cor pulmonale complicating chronic bronchitis and emphysema, *Lancet* (1981) i:681–6.

93  Naeije R et al, Reduction in pulmonary hypertension by prostaglandin $E_1$ in decompensated chronic obstructive pulmonary disease, *Am Rev Respir Dis* (1982) **125**:1–5.

94  Bergofsky EH, Tissue oxygen delivery and corpulmonale in chronic obstructive pulmonary disease, *N Engl J Med* (1983) **308**:1092–4.

95  Dinh-Xuan AT et al, Impairment of endothelium-dependent pulmonary artery relaxation in chronic obstructive lung disease, *N Engl J Med* (1991) **324**:1539–47.

96  Higenbottam TW et al, Transbronchial lung biopsy for the diagnosis of rejection in heart–lung transplant patients, *Transplantation* (1988) **46**:532–9.

97  McCarthy PM et al, Improved survival after heart–lung transplantation, *J Thorac Cardiovasc Surg* (1990) **99**:54–9.

98  Hutter JA et al, The importance of cytomegalovirus in heart–lung transplant recipients, *Chest* (1989) **95**:627–31.

99  Smyth RL et al, Experience of cytomegalovirus infection in heart–lung transplant recipients, *Transplant Proc* (1990) **22**:1822–3.

100  Smyth RL et al, Herpes simplex virus infection in heart–lung transplant recipients, *Transplantation* (1990) **49**:735–9.

101  Smyth RL et al, Successful use of repeated transbronchial lung biopsies in a patient with multiple opportunistic infections, *Respir Med* (1989) **83**:505–7.

102  Penketh ARL et al, Clinical experience in the management of pulmonary opportunist infection and rejection in recipients of heart–lung transplants, *Thorax* (1988) **43**:762–9.

103  Millet B et al, The radiographic appearances of infection and acute rejection of the lung after heart–lung transplantation, *Am Rev Respir Dis* (1989) **140:**62–7.

104  Brooks RG et al, Infectious complications in heart–lung transplant recipients, *Am J Med* (1985) **79:**412–22.

105  Hakim M et al, Selection and procurement of combined heart and lung grafts for transplantation, *J Thorac Cardiovasc Surg* (1988) **98:**474–9.

106  Wallwork J et al, Distant procurement of organs for clinical heart–lung transplantation using a single flush technique, *Transplantation* (1987) **44:**654–8.

107  Pasque M et al, Single-lung transplantation for pulmonary hypertension. Three-month hemodynamic follow-up, *Circulation* (1991) **84:**2275–9.

108  Doig JC et al, Effect of single lung transplantation on pulmonary hypertension in patients with end stage fibrosing lung disease, *Br Heart J* (1991) **66:**431–4.

109  Higenbottam T, Single lung transplantation and pulmonary hypertension, *Br Heart J* (1992) **67:**121.

110  Bodek A, Need donor hearts be entirely free from disease? *N Engl J Med* (1989) **320:**1628.

111  Mullins PA et al, Coronary occlusive disease and late graft failure after cardiac transplantation, *Br Heart J* (1992) **68:**260–5.

112  Uren NG, Oakley CM, The treatment of primary pulmonary hypertension, *Br Heart J* (1991) **66:**119–21.

# 14

# Managing resistant hypertension

*Alasdair Breckenridge and Thomas Walley*

## Definition of resistant hypertension

If the definition of hypertension itself is difficult, what is precisely meant by resistant hypertension poses even greater problems. A recent review[1] suggested the following criteria:

1 Blood pressure remaining above 140/90 mm Hg (160/90 for patients over 60 years).
2 Routine evaluation does not suggest a secondary cause for the raised blood pressure.
3 Treatment with maximal doses of at least two appropriate antihypertensive agents has been initiated.
4 The antihypertensive regime has been given adequate time to be effective.

Other reviewers[2] have settled for simpler definitions such as 'the failure of arterial pressure to be reduced and controlled despite the use of acceptable therapy'. Clearly, this begs the questions of what is precisely meant by 'failure' and what is deemed to be 'acceptable therapy'. Should a figure of 140/90 or 160/100 mm Hg or some other arbitrary value be chosen; or should the level remain undefined? Is 'acceptable' therapy a two- or three-drug regime, and, if so, which drugs and in what doses? There are no absolute answers to these questions and so for the purpose of this chapter we propose to adopt the first set of criteria outlined above.[1] What is clear,

however, is that resistant hypertension cannot be defined by the height or the severity of blood pressure prior to therapy; even the most severe hypertension (in terms of blood pressure and target organ involvement) may be easily controlled by antihypertensive therapy. Similarly, resistant hypertension must be separated from hypertensive emergencies (such as malignant hypertension, hypertensive encephalopathy or the like) when adequate therapy may lower the blood pressure very satisfactorily. This chapter will not specifically address the issue of resistant isolated systolic hypertension, an area which is still the subject of considerable discussion.

## Classification of resistant hypertension

Frohlich[2] divides resistant hypertension into three categories—physician-resistant hypertension, patient-resistant hypertension and resistant hypertensive disease—and this has many attractions. It is important to discuss these categories in some detail, since the management will obviously depend on this and a 'checklist' approach to individual cases has much to commend it. One of the possible causes of resistance is failure to recognize secondary hypertension; while our working definition presupposes that routine evaluation does not suggest a secondary cause (see above),

- **Physician-resistant hypertension**
  Inadequate patient education
  Inaccurate assessment of dietary sodium
  Failure to recognize drug interactions
  Inadequate therapeutic regime

- **Patient-resistant hypertension**
  Inadequate adherence to a therapeutic regime
  1  Dietary:        (a) excessive sodium intake
                     (b) excessive alcohol consumption
                     (c) failure to lose weight adequately
  2  Pharmacological: (a) did not take prescribed drugs
                     (b) did not follow prescribed dosing schedule
  Discontinued medication
  Did not return for follow-up

- **Resistant hypertensive disease**
  White coat hypertension
  Failure to recognize secondary hypertension

*Source:* Frohlich.[2]

Classification of resistant hypertension.

we shall discuss secondary causes briefly because 'routine evaluation' may not bring to light the more obscure yet relevant aetiology.

## Physician-resistant hypertension

Inadequate patient education is an important issue. If the patient is not aware that hypertension is a condition requiring continuous and long-term therapy, any therapeutic stratagem is doomed to failure and resistance may appear. Any programme of treatment should be discussed on a contractual basis between patient and doctor, with both parties aware of its requirements. The rationale of the programme, and its goals, should be made clear.

Other causes of physician-resistant hypertension may appear self-evident, but may be of the highest relevance in the management of the patient whose blood pressure is difficult to control. Excessive sodium intake will reduce the effectiveness of most antihypertensive drugs, and while a simple dietary history may be sufficient to establish an excessive sodium intake in other instances, measurement of 24-h sodium excretion may be needed to confirm this. Documentation abounds on the drugs which may antagonize the therapeutic effects of antihypertensive agents, or which may raise the blood pressure in their own right. These can be classified according to whether they are usually prescribed, or whether the patient obtains them from other sources. As part of

- **Prescribed drugs which may antagonize antihypertensive medication**

  | *Drug* | *Medication antagonized* |
  | --- | --- |
  | Non-steroidal and anti-inflammatory drugs | Most antihypertensive drugs |
  | Oral contraceptive steroids | Most antihypertensive drugs |
  | Sympathomimetic amines | Most antihypertensive drugs |

- **Prescribed drugs which may cause a rise in blood pressure**
  Corticosteroids
  Cyclosporin
  Erythropoietin
  Monoamine oxidase inhibitors

- **Exogenous substances (usually not prescribed) which may cause a rise in blood pressure**
  Anabolic steroids
  Cocaine
  Ethanol

*Drugs which may antagonize the therapeutic effects of antihypertensive agents or which may raise blood pressure themselves.*

the management of a patient whose blood pressure is difficult to control, a routine check should be run for possible drug-induced hypertension and appropriate action taken where possible. Implicit in any plan for hypertension therapy is that the physician has prescribed adequately. The unwillingness of some doctors to increase drug doses and thus gain the benefit of dose–response relationships (where these exist) underlies much poor antihypertensive management. It is frequently better to increase drug doses to gain control of blood pressure than to add in different agents, provided unacceptable adverse effects can be avoided. It is, however, often of little value to modify doses of ACE inhibitors and thiazide diuretics. It is not the purpose of this chapter to spell out what are maximal doses of commonly used antihypertensive drugs, but it behoves any physician treating hypertension to be aware of this information and to use it with maximum benefit for the patient. Equally important is that the prescribed regime should be acceptable to the patient. In general, thrice-daily drug dosing will lead to poorer adherence to instructions than once- or twice-daily dosing; if more frequent dosing is required then the reasons must be clearly explained to the patient and agreed with him. Similarly, the use of socially inconvenient agents (e.g. loop diuretics) at difficult times (e.g. when travelling) must be carefully considered by the doctor and if necessary agreed as part of the contract with the patient.

## Patient-resistant hypertension

Failure by the patient to adhere to an agreed therapeutic programme underlies many cases of apparent resistant hypertension. This failure may refer to dietary items (excess alcohol intake is now widely recognized as an important aetiological factor in many hypertensive patients although its basis is not entirely clear). Weight reduction is an important stratagem in patients whose hypertension is difficult to control. Significant reduction may be a useful method, albeit difficult to achieve, to regain control of blood pressure which has become difficult. The basis of the relationship between weight loss and blood pressure control is uncertain. One aspect of the problem of weight and blood pressure may be the failure by the doctor or nurse to use an adequately sized cuff on an overweight arm.

The failure of patients to adhere to a prescribed drug regime (often referred to as failure of compliance) is a most important cause of resistant hypertension. This failure may take several forms—total failure to take any medication, missing several doses at socially inconvenient times, failing to take medication when adverse effects intervene. The psychology of non-compliance with drug therapy is a jungle; but for patients with conditions such as hypertension or epilepsy the importance of maintaining agreed therapy, or failing to disclose this poor compliance to doctors, is of the utmost importance. One stratagem of managing resistant hypertension where poor compliance is suspected is to admit the patient to hospital, where measures are taken to ensure that he does take his medication in the dose which he was allegedly taking as an outpatient, and observing the outcome. This is discussed further below.

Patients' reasons for discontinuing medication abound; one problem is that the care of many patients with hypertension which is difficult to control is shared between a general practitioner and a hospital specialist. Unless there is clear and frequent communication between these parties, working to an agreed protocol (agreed by the three parties), there are many possibilities for mutual confusion. At its most extreme, the patient may end up attending neither doctor and discontinuing all medication.

Failure to follow a prescribed regime has been cited as a cause of up to 50 per cent of cases of resistant hypertension.[3] Issues of cost (not only drugs but travelling), patients' level of literacy, complexity of the regime and nature of adverse effects of the various drugs are all contributing factors. Non-compliance should be suspected in every patient with resistant hypertension, irrespective of social, educational or economic background. Markers of drug consumption or their absence (bradycardia with beta-blocker, hypokalaemia or hyperuricaemia with diuretics) may be useful pointers to the fact that the problem of poorly controlled blood pressure may lie with failure to take appropriate drugs.

## Resistant hypertensive disease

So-called 'white coat hypertension' implies that the blood pressure is higher when measured by a doctor (or more rarely, nurse) than at other times. This can be ascertained by arranging for the patient to measure his blood pressure using appropriate apparatus at home. If this is embarked on, he should check his blood pressure measuring technique when he is seen by his doctor (with both parties making the measurement). This problem can often be suspected if blood pressure readings are consistently high in the surgery or clinic, yet there is no objective evidence of end-organ damage (retinal changes, ECG and chest X-ray and renal monitoring).

- **Commoner**
  Renal vascular disease
  Renal parenchymal disease
  Phaeochromocytoma
  Adrenal adenoma
  Coarctation of aorta
- **Rarer**
  Sleep apnoea
  Acromegaly
  Porphyria

*Causes of secondary hypertension.*

The importance of failure to recognize an underlying and potentially remediable cause for hypertension is probably overemphasized. Implicit in our working definition of resistant hypertension (see above) is that routine evaluation does not suggest an underlying cause. Two questions which must be asked are, firstly, what is meant by routine evaluation, and, secondly, even if a secondary cause were ascertained, to what extent does this usually contribute to the poor blood pressure control?

All newly diagnosed hypertensive patients should have renal function monitored (urine examination, measurement of serum creatinine and urea) and measurement of serum potassium (screening for hyperaldosteronism). Those referred to hospital because of management problems should also have urine or serum catecholamines or their metabolites assayed (screening for phaeochromocytoma). Clinical examination, ECG and chest X-ray are also routine procedures and should detect any patient with coarctation of the aorta. Thus most common secondary causes of hypertension should be detected early in the course of management.

In patients with resistant hypertension, more detailed investigation of renal structure and function may be advisable, especially as this can now be done using techniques such as isotope renal scanning, preserving intravenous urography and renal arteriography for more complex cases.

Sleep apnoea and its association with hypertension has been recently advanced as a cause of secondary hypertension. Its prevalence is unknown; while it may lead to raised blood pressure at night, its relationship to daytime hypertension is unknown. At present, we would not recommend investigation of this as a cause of resistant hypertension, even if this type of investigation were widely accessible.

The finding of a structural abnormality such as unilateral renal artery stenosis in a patient with resistant hypertension begs the question of whether reversal (by open surgery or angioplasty) will lead to permanent cure of hypertension or even to a decrease in required drug dose. Poor overall renal function and the presence of widespread vascular changes (including those in the contralateral kidney) may turn the physician against intervention; transluminal angioplasty for accessible and appropriate renal arterial lesions has made such decisions easier. The possibility of bilateral renal artery stenosis, especially in the arteriosclerotic elderly patient, as a cause for resistant hypertension may pose both diagnostic and therapeutic problems. Other unusual causes of renal hypertension include vasculitis (e.g. polyarteritis) and tuberculosis and require specific therapy.

Some sources claim that as many as 10 per cent of cases of resistant hypertension have been attributed to secondary causes which have eluded routine evaluation; what these sources do not quote is the success rate obtained by treating these lesions.

## Prevalence of resistant hypertension

The prevalence of hypertension which is deemed resistant is predicated by the definition. In a recent review[4] Alderman and his colleagues review some 37 articles dealing with the problem of resistant hypertension which appeared between 1975 and 1985 (i.e. when effective antihypertensive drugs were available). Some 15 of these articles utilized quantitative definitions of resistance, yet only two addressed the issue of prevalence. The first, a study by Andersson and colleagues from Sweden in 1977,[5] found that 20 of 589 patients (3 per cent) had blood pressures in excess of 200/100 mm Hg after 2 years of 'adequate' therapy. Swales and colleagues[6] reviewed the experience of the University of Leicester hypertension clinic from 1974 to 1981. Of 957 patients, 126 (13 per cent) failed to reduce diastolic pressure to 100 mm Hg over some unspecified time. These 126 patients were then allocated to subsequent therapy with one of four regimes using diazoxide, minoxidil or captopril, or to quadruple therapy with prazosin, hydralazine, a beta-blocker and diuretic. Within weeks, the blood pressure in virtually all patients was satisfactorily controlled. Alderman and colleagues[4] reviewed some 1781 hypertensive patients drawn from seven large employee groups in New York in order to determine the prevalence of resistant hypertension. Criteria for resistance was failure to reach and maintain a blood pressure of 160/95 mm Hg on two separate occasions during a 1-year follow-up. Using these criteria, some 75 (4.2 per cent) were classified as resistant. When the additional criterion of blood pressure not being controlled despite prescribing at least two antihypertensive drugs simultaneously, the prevalence fell to 2.9 per cent (52 patients). Of these 52 patients, 33 achieved control in subsequent years. Alderman and colleagues conclude that genuine resistance in the hypertensive population is extremely rare.

## Risks of resistant hypertension

The risks of resistant hypertension are largely those to which any patient with the disease is exposed.

Data on outcome in patients with hypertension are still largely based on data gathered in the 1940s and 1950s, mostly from life insurance statistics. The advent of antihypertensive drugs with their widespread and successful use in patients with moderate and severe hypertension has made it ethically impossible to gather corresponding data today. These data are well known and widely quoted. The risks of hypertension are not only those associated with elevation of blood pressure itself but also the vascular and cardiac damage caused. The information on which we rely for prognosis in hypertension were obtained casually (i.e. under conditions of a single medical examination) and outcome is usually related to this one reading of blood pressure. Untreated patients with diastolic blood pressure of between 110 and 120 mm Hg have an 80 per cent 2-year survival rate; those with diastolic blood pressures of 130 mm Hg and above have a 40 per cent 2-year survival rate. There is no reason why these figures should not also apply to patients with resistant hypertension if one accepts that the risks of the disease are related to blood pressure and its attendant changes.

The cardiac, vascular, brain and renal changes in hypertension have been described very adequately elsewhere; there are no additional problems in resistant hypertension.

# Pathophysiological considerations in resistant hypertension

We have described above possible contributory factors in resistant hypertension. Many of these relate to educational or attitudinal problems in either the physician or patient, or to substandard medical practice. When such issues have been addressed, are there any pathophysiological characteristics which are common to patients who fulfil the criteria used in this chapter for resistant hypertension? In this context, it should be remembered that the resistant hypertensive patient may not necessarily have very high levels of pressure; these pressures are merely refractory to conventional drug treatment given for a reasonable time.

## Cardiac considerations

In most patients with hypertension, adequate therapy which produces a satisfactory fall in blood pressure also results in a decrease in cardiac size (when this is increased) and an improvement in cardiac function (where this is impaired). It has been suggested that in some instances the heart itself may interfere with blood pressure control because of increased cardiac output or because of cardiogenic reflexes that could conceivably not only initiate but also perpetuate peripheral vasoconstriction, thus resulting in resistant hypertension.

### Increased cardiac output
The late Robert Tarazi[7] suggested that the initial reduction in total peripheral resistance induced by powerful peripheral vasodilators such as minoxidil may produce countereffects thwarting their antihypertensive effectiveness.

Selective arteriolar without accompanying venous vasodilatation (e.g. as found with minoxidil) produces a marked increase in cardiac output because of the decreased aferload and reflex increase in sympathetic activity. The resulting increase in cardiac output, in Tarazi's extensive experience, was enough to compensate for the reduction in peripheral resistance so that blood pressure remains unchanged. Further, vasodilatation induces renin release with its attendant activation of the renin–angiotensin–aldosterone system and blunting of the desired vasodilator response. Both these effects can be overcome by simultaneous administration of a beta-adrenoceptor blocking agent; in practice this is largely how powerful vasodilators are used—as part of combination therapy.

### Role of cardiogenic reflexes
Powerful pressor reflexes originate from the heart, triggered by distension of coronary vessels, or specific receptors within the myocardium.[8] These are characteristically described as paroxysmal but in experimental animal studies, the resulting rise in blood pressure has been shown to persist for up to 7 days. In man, in cases of borderline hypertension, cardiac receptors are thought to be hyperactive and thus maintain net sympathetic activity. It has been postulated that in resistant hypertension, an exaggeration of this activity occurs, triggered by abnormal left ventricular diastolic function (LVDF). This is supported by studies in hypertensive patients with and without abnormal LVDF. In the former, head-up tilt resulted in a predictable response in total peripheral resistance, whereas this was very abnormal in the latter.[9] These observations suggest that persistence of hypertension may induce further cardiac changes which will in turn perpetuate the rise in blood pressure. Which, if any,

antihypertensive drugs will modify these responses is not known.

## Renal considerations

Williams and Hollenberg have identified a group of sodium-sensitive hypertensive patients, whom they have termed 'non-modulators',[10] who have a defective ability to suppress renin and aldosterone in response to angiotensin II. In these patients, sodium does not modulate renal and adrenal responsiveness to angiotensin II. Non-modulators exhibit a rise in blood pressure after an acute sodium load, whereas normotensives and hypertensive controls do not. A sodium load does not cause an increase in renal bloodflow in non-modulators and their ability to excrete the sodium load is impaired. Saline infusion or angiotensin II fails to suppress renin activity in non-modulators. Administration of ACE inhibitors corrects all these abnormalities except the last. Thus these hypertensive patients are readily controlled with ACE inhibitors but appear resistant to treatment when inappropriate drugs are given.

The relationship between renal disease and hypertension is complex and outside the scope of this chapter. Hypertension which may be resistant to therapy develops in most patients with renal parenchymal disease and often does so many months or even years before renal function deteriorates to a level where dialysis or transplantation is needed. Volume expansion appears to be the commonest pathophysiological factor underlying this. Both blood volume and total body sodium are increased early in renal insufficiency, and early expansion in blood volume may lead to rises in cardiac output and renal bloodflow. In time, autoregulatory processes return bloodflow towards normal but at the expense of increases in total peripheral vascular resistance.

# Management of the resistant hypertensive patient

Figure 14.1 is an algorithm for the management of the resistant hypertensive patient. Each of these steps in the process will be considered. The issue of which drugs may be used will be considered in the next section.

## Step 1   Does the patient understand the therapeutic stratagem?

As discussed above, the understanding of many patients about antihypertensive therapy is fragmentary. Either this has never been explained to the patient, or it has been put in terms which he cannot understand. Thus the first step in managing any resistant hypertensive patient is to explain in the simplest terms what the doctor's aim is; that treatment regimes must be agreed between the two parties, i.e. a 'contract' must be drawn up.

## Step 2   Is the patient adhering to the overall therapeutic regime?

The most important part of this exercise is to ascertain if the patient is taking the prescribed drug at the agreed dosing schedule. There are few methods of checking for compliance which are completely foolproof. Subjectively one can ask the patient or a relative about times at which medication is not taken; objectively one can count tablets returned, monitor drug levels in blood or measure physiological indices compatible with drug consumption (e.g. exercise tachycardia or the lack of it when the patient is on a beta-blocker, hypokalaemia when a patient is on a diuretic). Once one suspects non-compliance with drug therapy, there are various procedures which can be set

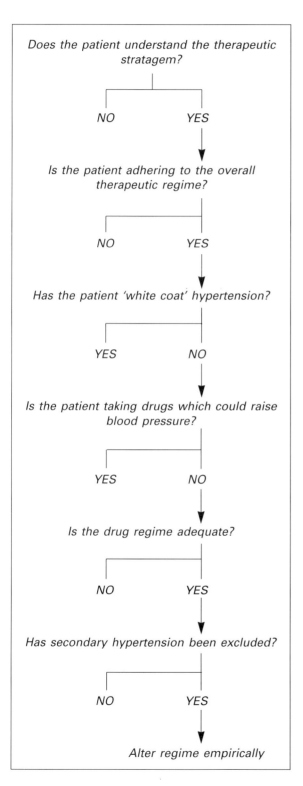

in motion. First, one can examine the drug regime and see if it can be simplified. Second, one can attempt to improve the doctor–patient relationship by explaining the regime (see above), paying especial attention to reasons for possible poor compliance, e.g. adverse effects, cost or inconvenience. Third, one can admit the patient to hospital, administer the drugs in the agreed dose, while maintaining his ambulatory status, and after taking measures to ensure that the patient does take his medication, observe the blood pressure response. If the blood pressure falls rapidly to achieve good control (and often in these situations the patient may become hypotensive, since doses may have been 'increased' as an outpatient to counteract poor blood pressure control) then one can be reasonably certain that poor compliance is the basis for poor blood pressure control although its reasons remain to be ascertained.

Inadequate adherence to the therapeutic regime includes excess sodium or alcohol intake, or failure to lose weight. Each must be dealt with in the appropriate manner, although no one should be under any illusion about the difficulties that can be encountered in dealing with these problems.

## Step 3 Has the patient 'white coat' hypertension?

As discussed above, this is suspected if the levels of pressure are persistently high in the surgery or clinic, yet there are few objective measures of end-organ damage.

Two strategies have been suggested to deal with this situation. The most satisfactory is to invite the patient (or a near relative) to measure his blood pressure at home, after suitable training. When the patient attends the doctor, both parties will check the blood pressure. A second stratagem is to measure blood pressure over 24 h using one of the commercially available portable machines. Most of these are still cumbersome, and many patients find them disturbing. If 'white coat' hypertension is proven, then less frequent visits to clinic or surgery are needed.

One other form of 'non-hypertension' which is discussed is given the name 'pseudohypertension'.[1] This implies that the intra-arterial pressure is within acceptable limits but, due to rigidity of the blood vessel wall (because of aging and atherosclerosis), its compression by the cuff of the sphygmomanometer is difficult and a falsely high level of systolic pressure is recorded. If such a diagnosis is thought likely, the direct intravascular pressure can be checked.

## Step 4   Is the patient taking drugs which could raise the pressure or is the high level of pressure caused by drug interactions?

Here the doctor must become a detective. First, he must review the prescribed drugs to see if there are any incompatibilities. Second, he must, by whatever means he can, detect any other substances which the patient may be taking and which may raise the pressure. Alcohol in excess is probably the commonest of these and is certainly a more frequent cause of resistant hypertension than cocaine or anabolic steroids.

## Step 5   Is the drug regime adequate?

Once steps 1–4 have been taken and appropriate measures adopted, the practitioner should review critically the therapeutic advice he has given the patient. He (the doctor) may wish to seek a second opinion at this stage, but he should not do so before the preceding steps have been taken. Merely increasing the drug doses, or adjusting their frequency, may be sufficient to achieve blood pressure control.

## Step 6   Has secondary hypertension been excluded?

The doctor will wish, as part of step 4, to consider whether any underlying cause for hypertension has slipped his attention. It may be, of course, that a patient may, over the years, have acquired a new renal artery stenosis or other form of kidney disease and in our experience this may be a cause of loss of control of blood pressure in patients at risk of atheromatous disease. Thus the doctor must consider all the common secondary causes for hypertension and decide whether to embark on the sometimes complex and expensive investigations for phaeochromocytoma, adrenal adenoma, and renovascular hypertension.

## Step 7   Alter regime empirically

When steps 1–6 have been taken, it is quite justified to alter the therapeutic regime empirically. We still know remarkably little of why hypertensive patients fail to respond to a specific drug but perfectly well to another. While it is commonly said that beta-blocking drugs are not effective in the black population, and that the elderly respond preferentially to diuretics (and perhaps calcium antagonists), these group aphorisms have little or no relevance in the individual patient. Each patient must be considered individually at this stage of management of resistant hypertension and if the blood pressure can be lowered without causing unacceptable adverse effects any drug regime is worth a trial.

# Drugs used in resistant hypertension

This section is brief, and will merely describe the types of regime which a patient with resistant hypertension may be prescribed, once the stages of management described above have been successively undertaken. The pharmacology of individual agents is not discussed, as accounts of these are given in formal textbooks of clinical pharmacology. Thus, if failure to adhere to a prescribed regime is the underlying problem in the resistant hypertensive patient, then the solution is to ascertain, where possible, why the non-adherence has occurred, and prescribe a drug or regime which is appropriate for the patient (e.g. less frequent dosage or one with different but acceptable side-effects).

Many reviewers of the therapy for resistant hypertension in the 1970s and even 1980s describe complex therapeutic regimes which are out of date in the 1990s. The essence of a therapeutic regime for any hypertensive patient is as follows: firstly, it must be acceptable to the patient and the doctor; secondly, it must allow adequate control of blood pressure while allowing the patient to lead an optimal existence; and thirdly, it must be as simple as is compatible with the first two objectives. Exactly the same principles apply—if anything more so—to the resistant patient.

Antihypertensive drug therapy in the 1990s is based on four drug groups—diuretics, beta-adrenoceptor blocking agents, calcium channel antagonists and ACE inhibitors. These drugs may be given separately or in combination, depending on efficacy and adverse effects.

In a recent (unpublished) review of patients attending the Hypertension Clinic at Royal Liverpool University Hospital because of blood pressure being difficult to control, the commonest drug regime was ACE inhibitor plus diuretic (usually frusemide) plus calcium channel antagonist (usually nifedipine). The second most common regime was a traditional stepped care type approach, with a beta-blocker, thiazide and calcium channel antagonist.

Brief notes on the use of these four drugs are given, together with comments on other agents used by other workers in this area.

## ACE inhibitors

Captopril, enalapril and lisinopril are the three agents in this group with which there is most experience in resistant hypertension. The important issues concerning their usage are:

1 Check the renal function of the patient before and at regular intervals during usage because of their propensity to exacerbate renal failure in patients with renal impairment.
2 Use as small a dose as is compatible with the risk/benefit ratio.

## Diuretics

We consider that diuretics, usually thiazides, should be part of the initial regime in any resistant patient. Especially when given with ACE inhibitors, loop diuretics such as frusemide may be found superior to thiazide diuretics. The important issues here are:

1 Check renal function before and at regular intervals during usage. It is frequently necessary to adjust the dose of both the ACE inhibitor and diuretic to prevent undue deterioration in renal function.

2 Utilize the range of the dose–response curve of the loop diuretic (which is large, in contrast to the thiazide diuretics).

## Beta-blockers

1 The first important point to remember is that water-soluble beta-blockers such as atenolol tend to be excreted by the kidney, whereas lipid-soluble agents such as propranolol are eliminated by hepatic metabolism. This may predicate their use in patients with hypertension and renal impairment.
2 Cardioselective beta-blockers (such as atenolol) have been found to be more effective in resistant hypertension than non-selective beta-blockers (such as propranolol) because the latter beta$_2$-adrenoceptor blocking action tends to inhibit beta$_2$-mediated vasodilatation.
3 The usual precautions with respect to use of beta-blockers should be observed in patients with asthma or heart failure, i.e. not to use them wherever possible.

## Calcium channel antagonist

The usual choice lies between a dihydropyridine compound, such as nifedipine, or verapamil. The practical points are:

1 Nifedipine tends to cause vasodilatation and fluid retention, and thus is probably best used in combination with beta-blockers and diuretics.
2 Verapamil tends to cause constipation and thus should be used with care in the elderly.
3 There is no evidence of increased efficacy of one over the other in resistant hypertension, and choice is often by patient tolerability.

## Other regimes used

Previously recommended regimes have frequently included vasodilators such as minoxidil and oral diazoxide. In our experience it is rare to require these today and their attendant adverse effects usually cause unacceptable problems. It may be necessary to 'buy time' in the very resistant hypertensive patient by lowering his blood pressure with systemically administered vasodilators such as nitroprusside or labetalol. In some patients, lowering the blood pressure by their use for a period of, say, 1 week will permit control to be re-achieved with oral regimes and may also allow time for other management procedures to be instituted.

# If I had ...

If my blood pressure was raised and I was on regular medication, I would have the pressure checked at regular (e.g. 3-monthly) intervals so that if the diagnosis of resistant hypertension were made, it would be made after the shortest possible time of appropriate treatment.

I would review all aspects of my management with my doctor. Our therapeutic contract would be carefully reviewed—had my weight or salt intake increased inappropriately, had my alcohol intake increased? I would review with honesty whether I had been remiss in taking medicines at the designated intervals. I would be surprised, as a wearer of a white coat myself, if the diagnosis of 'office' hypertension could be levelled at me, but a surreptitious measurement or two of blood pressure at home would not be out of order. I would be surprised to find any unplanned drug interaction. I would next check for evidence of end-organ damage—reviewing chest X-ray, ECG and echocardiographic evidence for changes in cardiac size, and serum creatinine and urine analysis for renal deterioration. Had a cause for secondary hypertension intervened? I would find this surprising, since my therapeutic contract would have entailed a reasonably detailed search for a secondary cause at the beginning of therapy. The decision to investigate further would not be made by me, but if my physician decided that a renal scan was required, I would submit without demur. If all these stages were passed satisfactorily and my blood pressure was still poorly controlled, I would expect advice on how to change my drug treatment. I would insist on as simple a regime as is compatible with controlling the pressure and allowing my normal lifestyle to continue. I would hope that a judicious mix of ACE inhibitor, beta-blocker, diuretic and calcium channel antagonist would keep my doctor at bay, and I would strongly resist any attempt to delve into therapeutic history.

# References

1 Setaro JF, Black HR, Refractory hypertension, *N Engl J Med* (1992) **327**:543–7.

2 Frohlich ED, Classification of resistant hypertension, *Hypertension* (1988) **11**(suppl 11):67–70.

3 Klein LE, Compliance and blood pressure control, *Hypertension* (1988) **11**(suppl 11):67–70.

4 Alderman M et al, Prevalence of drug resistant hypertension, *Hypertension* (1988) **11**(suppl 11):71–5.

5 Andersson O, Management of hypertension, *Acta Med Scand* (1977) **617**(suppl):3–62.

6 Swales JD et al, Treatment of refractory hypertension, *Lancet* (1982) **1**:894–6.

7 Abi-Samara F, Fouad FM, Tarazi RC, Determinants of left ventricular hypertrophy and function in hypertensive patients, *Am J Med* (1983) **75**(suppl 3A):26–33.

8 Fovad-Tarazi FM, Factors contributing to resistant hypertension—cardiac considerations, *Hypertension* (1988) **11**(suppl 11):84–7.

9 Fovad FM et al, Alteration in left ventricular filling with beta adrenoceptor blockade, *Am J Cardiol* (1983) **51**:161–4.

10 Williams GH, Hollenberg NK, Non-modulating essential hypertension. A subset particularly responsive to converting enzyme inhibitors, *J Hypertens* (1985) **3**(suppl 2):S81–S87.

# 15

# Hypertension in pregnancy
*James J Walker*

Hypertension in pregnancy (PIH) remains one of the main causes of maternal and perinatal mortality and morbidity throughout the world. The aetiology is still largely unknown. The diagnosis is often difficult. However, advances in management and understanding have led to improvements in outcome for the mother and baby.

## History

There is still much confusion concerning the conditions of hypertension and convulsions in pregnancy, although the association of seizures and maternal death has been known since ancient times. The word 'eclampsia' comes from the Greek verb 'eclamptien', meaning 'to flash out'. This relates either to its sudden onset or to the flashing hallucinations experienced in the prodromal phase. Hippocrates described the condition in 'On The Sacred Disease' and stated that 'it proves fatal to women in the state of pregnancy'.[1] In the sixteenth century, Gabelchoverus noted that pregnancy was a cause of epilepsy and described the epigastric pain associated with this. He felt that this pain was a sign that the cause of the convulsion came from the uterus.[1] Mauriceau[2] refers to eclampsia, as does Denman[3] in a book dedicated to the problem along with puerperal fever. He recognized eclampsia as a major cause of morbidity and mortality.

In 1843 Lever found that patients with eclampsia had proteinuria.[4] Although he realized that eclampsia was different from renal disease, since the proteinuria disappeared after delivery, others thought that the condition was very similar to that seen in glomerulonephritis. Simpson, who found proteinuria at about the same time, saw contracted kidneys in one of his patients and felt that this was the cause of the problem.[5] This became the popular opinion for some time. It was not until the development of methods of assessment of renal function and, finally, the renal histology studies of Sheehan[6] and McCartney[7] that the specific lesions of pre-eclampsia were described.

It was not until the late nineteenth century that hypertension was first noted to be associated with eclampsia.[8,9] In 1896, essential hypertension was first differentiated from renal hypertension. However, as it was originally called 'senile plethora', many obstetricians felt that none of their (mostly young) patients could have this condition.[1] It was not until the 1940s that the possibility of essential hypertension as a cause of hypertension in pregnancy was accepted. From this time, it was realized that renal disease was a relatively rare cause of hypertension in pregnancy. It was then realized that, although pregnancy could occur in a patient with pre-existing essential hypertension, renal disease or other hypertensive disorder, there was a specific hypertensive syndrome arising in pregnancy that disappeared when the pregnancy was over and apparently carried no long-term sequelae.[10]

The realization that this pregnancy-'associated' hypertension often antecedes convulsions led to the term 'pre-eclampsia'. This term was initially used for the immediate prodromal stage of eclampsia but now is applied to patients with milder forms of the disease. Although eclampsia is associated with hypertension it is not an obligatory end-point of the condition. Convulsions are independent of the severity of the disease. 'Mild' pre-eclampsia may be associated with convulsions and 'severe' may not. Between 15 and 20 per cent of the patients suffering from 'eclampsia' have no record of hypertension prior to the seizure.[11-13]

## Classification of the disease

It is obvious that there are two main groups with hypertension in pregnancy:

1 Hypertension occurring for the first time during the pregnancy, labour or puerperium and returning to normal after the end of the pregnancy.
2 Pregnancy occurring in patients with pre-existing essential hypertension, renal disease or other hypertensive disease diagnosed by a previous history prior to pregnancy, high blood pressure at the booking clinic or persistent hypertension after the pregnancy is over.

However, it is often not possible to be sure of which group a patient belongs to at the time of presentation. If hypertension was present before the pregnancy or prior to 20 weeks of gestation, a diagnosis of pre-existing disease is likely. Absence of evidence of hypertension at these times does not exclude this possibility. A rise of blood pressure to above the accepted cut-off level in late pregnancy may be due to an underlying latent hypertension rather than pre-eclampsia.[14] It is often after the pregnancy is over or even in the next pregnancy that evidence for the diagnosis of essential hypertension is found. If hypertension is thought to be pre-existing, the possibility of renal disease should be considered before any diagnosis of essential hypertension is made.

There are various markers of disease that can help in the attempt to get a 'true' diagnosis. In progressive PET, uric acid will rise[15] and platelet counts will fall.[16] Therefore, if there is hypertension without abnormalities in these parameters, the diagnosis of pre-eclampsia must be questioned. Proteinuria, although a sign of worsening pregnancy hypertension, can occur in essential hypertension and renal disease.[17] If the plasma urea or creatinine is elevated, especially in the presence of a relatively normal plasma uric acid, underlying renal disease is likely.

But does the accuracy of the diagnosis matter? It is advisable to manage the patients simply and assess the risks when the disease presents. The risks to the mother are largely related to the level of blood pressure and cardiac failure.[18] The risk to the fetus is due to failure of placental function and iatrogenic prematurity following delivery in the maternal interest.[19] These risks exist whether the hypertension is pregnancy related or not. Therefore, although it it safe to assume that a primigravida with no history of hypertension presenting at 30 weeks with a blood pressure of 140/90 mm Hg has pre-eclampsia and a parous patient with a known hypertensive tendency presenting in the same way has essential hypertension, the management of these two patients should be the same. Maternal death and eclampsia occur in both groups.[18]

# The pathophysiology of pre-eclampsia

In normal pregnancy, cardiac output increases by around 40 per cent during the first trimester and this increase is maintained throughout pregnancy. Blood pressure falls in the first trimester, reaches a nadir in mid-pregnancy, and then slowly rises during the third trimester to levels comparable with those in the non-pregnant state.[20] As arterial pressure is determined by cardiac output and total peripheral resistance, the decrease in blood pressure must be due to a fall in the latter. Since these changes occur early in pregnancy, they must reflect a change in systemic vascular resistance, as the uteroplacental circulation is not sufficiently large to account for such a reduction in peripheral resistance at this stage of pregnancy.

The fall in peripheral resistance in normal pregnancy is associated with a relative insensitivity to the pressor effects of exogenous angiotensin II (AII),[21] which is detectable as early as 8 weeks of gestation and reaches a peak in mid-pregnancy. The mechanism underlying this insensitivity is unknown but is probably due to increased vasodilator substances. Changes in vascular reactivity may be the cause of the hypertension in pre-eclampsia. Gant et al,[21] Wallenburg et al[22] and Dekker et al[23] have all shown that an increased sensitivity to angiotensin infusion can select out patients who are destined to develop pre-eclampsia as early as 16–18 weeks. This suggests that the sensitivity is present prior to the disease presentation, implying susceptibility to the condition. A further stimulus would then be required and the vasoconstriction would be a secondary effect of this stimulus.

The susceptibility of the patient to respond to this stimulation may be related to vascular endothelial dysfunction. This could be due to alterations in the local effects of the vasodilators prostacyclin ($PGI_2$) and endothelial derived relaxing factor (EDRF), or the vasoconstrictors thromboxane and endothelin. In pre-eclampsia, production of $PGI_2$ from both maternal and fetal vascular tissue has been shown to be reduced.[24–26]

Increased thromboxane $A_2$ ($TxA_2$) production from the placenta and platelets has been shown to occur in pre-eclampsia.[27–29] Raised levels of endothelin have also been found[30,31] and the levels correlate with other markers of disease severity.[32]

EDRF can attenuate the effects of thromboxane and endothelin.[33] Deficiency of EDRF and prostacyclin could be due to damage to the vascular endothelium.[34] It is thought that this damage is secondary to increased free radical activity[35,36] and can lead to increased platelet activity and placental vascular damage.

In normal pregnancy, there is a significant drop in platelet numbers with a rise in the MPV in the last weeks of normal gestation.[37–39] Many studies in women with pre-eclampsia have reported changes in platelet numbers, platelet survival and MPV which have been interpreted as evidence of increased platelet consumption.[39–43] Thrombocytopenia is a common finding,[44] is associated with progressive disease[16,40,45] and has been shown to be related to disease severity.[46] Platelet lifespan is known to be reduced in pre-eclampsia,[47] and this is thought to be secondary to intravascular platelet aggregation and increased adhesion to damaged vascular endothelium. The primary site for this vascular damage is in the placental vascular bed.

The fetus depends on the placenta for its survival. The ability of the placenta to exchange nutrients and gases with the fetus is largely dependent on bloodflow, both in the mother and in the fetus. It has been known for some years that the bloodflow to the placenta is reduced in maternal hypertension.[48–50] Campbell[51] has shown abnormalities in the uterine artery velocity waveform as early as 18

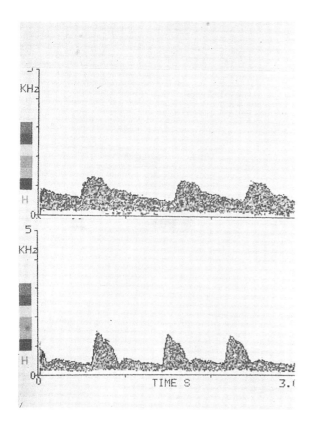

**Figure 15.1**
Doppler velocity waveforms from the uterine artery. The top trace is normal, showing good end-diastolic flow. The lower trace is from a patient with severe pre-eclampsia. It shows diminished diastolic flow velocity and the characteristic notch.

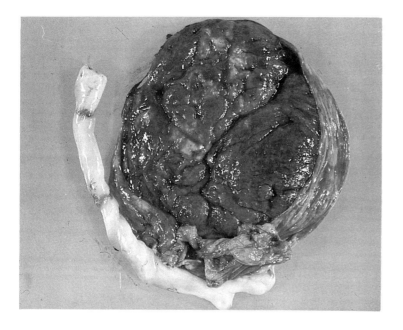

**Figure 15.2**
A placenta from a patient delivered at 29 weeks gestation because of severe proteinuric pre-eclampsia. Large areas of infarction and calcification can be seen. Other parts show some compensatory hypertrophy.

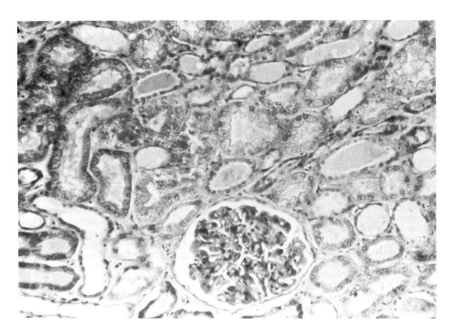

**Figure 15.3**
*A section from a kidney of a patient with severe proteinuric pre-eclampsia. It is stained with Orange G (an acid stain) and Light Green (a basic stain). There is thickening of the basement membrane of the glomerulus, and protein, staining red, can be seen in the endothelial cells of the tubules in an attempt at reabsorption.*

weeks in patients who are destined to develop pre-eclampsia and intrauterine growth retardation (IUGR) (Figure 15.1).

Within the placenta, the terminal segments of the uterine spiral arteries become obstructed by fibrin and platelet aggregates.[52] Placental infarctions and ischaemic villus necrosis are also found[53] (Figure 15.2). There is a failure of the normal invasion of the maternal spiral arteries by the trophoblastic cells. This invasion is necessary to destroy the musculoelastic tissue in the media to allow vasodilatation of the spiral arteries. In pre-eclampsia, there is failure of the normal spiral artery vasodilatation, leading to a reduced placental bloodflow.

Therefore, the maternal changes seen in pre-eclampsia may be secondary to placental ischaemia.[54] Animal models of the disease depend on procedures which cause this.[55] Symonds believes that uteroplacental stimulation of the renin–angiotensin system secondary to placental ischaemia plays a central role in the development of hypertension.[56]

The classic pathological change in pre-eclampsia is in the kidney.[6,7] In normal pregnancy there is an increase in the glomerular filtration rate (GFR) of 50 per cent. This leads to a reduction in the plasma urea and creatinine concentrations. In pre-eclampsia, there is a reduction in the GFR, leading to a rise in plasma creatinine and urea and a fall in the creatinine clearance rate. In severe pre-eclampsia, there is a characteristic increase in the amount of protein excreted by the kidney into the measurable range (above 300 mg/l). In the presence of proteinuria, the renal lesions are usually found.[7,57] Glomeruli are enlarged by 20 per cent, with cellular swelling and glomerular capillary endotheliosis (Figure 15.3). Deposition of fibrin protein strands is seen within Bowman's capsule. Chesley[58] showed that the kidney has a decreased ability to secrete uric acid in pre-eclampsia; hence the increase in the concentration of uric acid and the fall in bicarbonate concentration. Altchek et al[59] have reported a lesion in the loop of Henle, the severity of which is related to the level of uric acid. Sheehan showed that the renal changes regress quickly after delivery.[6]

## Hereditary influences

There is increasing evidence that severe pre-eclampsia is a familial disease.[60–63] Chesley, and Cooper[64] traced 96 per cent of the grown daughters of the women who had had eclampsia at the Margaret Hague Maternity Hospital. The incidence of pre-eclampsia in daughters was 26 per cent. It was 32 per cent in sisters and 16 per cent in granddaughters. Sutherland et al[65] studied the mothers and mothers-in-law of patients with severe pre-eclampsia. The study showed that mothers-in-law did not have an incidence higher than expected (4 per cent) but mothers did (14 per cent). This could be due to a single recessive gene.[62] This is unlikely, as other factors are undoubtedly involved. In a large study through four generations in Iceland, similar results of inheritance were found and the condition was manifest in most generations.[63] It is more likely that the inheritance is dominant in nature with reduced penetrance. This would allow for the other factors to influence the disease penetration and reduce the incidence of the carrier gene required in the population to support the single recessive gene theory. Incomplete penetrance is very difficult to distinguish from multifactorial inheritance.

## The risks of pregnancy hypertension to the mother and baby

Hypertension in pregnancy is not a disease in itself but a reflection of a maternal response to the underlying disease. Since pre-eclampsia is a multisystem disorder, blood pressure alone may be inadequate for assessing absolute risk. The disease affects different organs in different ways and to different degrees. The risks to the mother and baby depend on how the disease affects the patient and which organs are involved. Not all patients with the same abnormalities of disease parameter will necessarily have the same risks. The problems for the mother and the baby are different and they will be treated separately.

### Risks to the mother

Pregnancy hypertension has been the largest cause of maternal death in England and Wales in the last 30 years. Cerebral vascular accident (CVA) was the commonest mode of death in this group[18] (Table 15.1). Even if patients with eclampsia are studied, cerebral haemorrhage still appears to be the main cause of mortality. The risk to both mother and baby appears to relate to the degree of pre-eclampsia preceding the seizure, rather than the seizure itself. Therefore, in the UK, although eclampsia is the main preoccupation of therapeutic approach, CVA is the main maternal risk of hypertension in pregnancy. Blood pressures of 170–180/110–120 mm Hg or greater are equivalent levels to those that produce vascular damage in experimental animals.[66] Therefore diastolic blood pressure of above 110 mm Hg appear to increase the risks of morbidity and mortality to the mother and can be taken as abnormal, meriting some form of management

| Causes | Eclampsia | Pre-eclampsia | Total |
|---|---|---|---|
| Cerebral haemorrhage | 11 | 13 | 24 |
| Cerebral oedema | 3 | 1 | 4 |
| Cerebral infarction | 0 | 2 | 2 |
| Cerebral cortical necrosis | 1 | 0 | 1 |
| Cerebral softening | 1 | 0 | 1 |
| Pulmonary complication | 10 | 4 | 14 |
| Hepatic necrosis | 0 | 2 | 2 |
| Other | 0 | 3 | 3 |
| Total | 24 | 17 | 51 |

**Table 15.1**
*The causes of the 54 maternal deaths associated with eclampsia or pre-eclampsia in England and Wales in years 1982–1987. One of the patients with pre-eclampsia in the triennium 1982–1984 did not have a post mortem and is not included in the figures. Thirty-two of the 51 patients had evidence of cerebral lesions.*

decision. However, the absolute level of blood pressure measured may be less important than the rise and the temporal aspect of that rise.[67–69] If CVA does occur, it generally occurs early in the disease presentation.[70]

Pulmonary oedema has always been a major contributor to maternal mortality.[70] When cardiac failure occurs, it is most common between 24 and 48 h post-delivery. It is not due to modern fluid management but is a risk of the disease itself. Obviously, excessive fluid replacement can contribute to the problem.[71] Although there may be depletion of the plasma volume, the vascular tree is contracted, reducing the capacity for fluid replacement.

Other problems are relatively uncommon. Renal failure has always been a rare cause of maternal death, responsible for less than 5 per cent of cases of maternal mortality.[70] If it does occur, it is usually due to acute tubular necrosis and can be easily managed.

Coagulation abnormalities associated with elevated liver enzymes and haemolysis have recently been described and termed the HELLP syndrome.[72] This may not be anything new, as low platelets, liver problems and haemolysis are well-recognized complications of pre-eclampsia.[73] However, these signs do highlight the high-risk patient.

Eclampsia is now uncommon in the UK. There has never been an absolute correlation between blood pressure level and eclampsia. Cruickshank,[12] in a review of patients in the Glasgow Royal Maternity Hospital, showed that 18.5 per cent of the eclamptics had a systolic blood pressure below 140 mm Hg. In the John Hopkins Hospital between 1924 and 1943, in 2418 cases of pre-eclampsia only 92 (3.8 per cent) of the patients developed eclampsia.[74] The chances of eclampsia occurring may be more related to the patient's seizure threshold than to the level of blood pressure.[14] In

Scotland, the incidence of eclampsia is now 1 in 300 of the total of the pre-eclamptic/eclamptic patients.[75] Since many of the eclamptics are acute onset or occur in intrapartum/postpartum patients with no prodromal pre-eclampsia, the incidence of eclampsia occurring in any hypertensive patient must be even lower than 1/300. Therefore, eclampsia is not an inevitable progression of pre-eclampsia and the risk of eclampsia for the average hypertensive patient is low. The main risk of mortality is from the hypertension itself leading to CVA and pulmonary oedema.

In the 1930s, over 75 per cent of all cases of abruptio placenta were associated with pre-eclampsia.[76] Recent studies show that two-thirds of the cases now occur in patients with normal blood pressure.[77] Although the British Birth Survey 1970 shows a slight increase of abruption in hypertensive patients (1.38 per cent) compared with normotensive patients (1.05 per cent),[78] there was no increase in the perinatal mortality rate unless the abruption accompanied severe hypertension. Hypertension should not be classified as a risk factor for abruption.

A common belief is that delivery cures the patient with pre-eclampsia. In Scotland, all the women that died did so after delivery.[75] Although the removal of the trophoblast removes the stimulus to the disease, this is not immediate and continued vigilance is required after delivery.

## Risks to the fetus and neonate

The risks to the fetus depend on the degree of placental involvement and the gestation time at delivery.[75,79] Although pre-eclampsia is thought to be a placental disease,[80] not all the pregnancies are equally badly affected. The occurrence of intrauterine growth retardation is not absolute and many babies are well grown with no apparent placental insufficiency.[81]

Older studies showed that a diastolic blood pressure above 90–95 mm Hg is associated with an increased perinatal mortality[82–85] (Table 15.2). The more recent British Births Survey[78] did not demonstrate this. The perinatal mortality rate did not rise until the diastolic blood pressure was either above 110 mm Hg, or above 90 mm Hg with significant proteinuria (Table 15.3). Similar findings were seen if the end-point was neonatal neurological complications. The report concluded that raised arterial pressure in pregnancy, whether due to pre-existing hypertension or to pre-eclampsia, increases the risks that the fetus will grow poorly, die in utero or be delivered prematurely.[78]

If blood pressure is not accurate in predicting perinatal outcome, is there anything that is better? Nelson[81] used the presence of proteinuria as his main differentiating factor between mild and severe disease. Friedman and Neff,[82] in their study of over 32 000 pregnancies, showed that, in combination with hypertension, proteinuria increases the risk of perinatal loss, neonatal cerebral signs and intrauterine growth retardation (Table 15.2). It is difficult to explain why proteinuria is associated with this increased risk to the fetus. It is almost always associated with the 'pathognomonic' pre-eclamptic glomerular lesions.[86] Rather than being associated with a worsening disease risk, it may be that the presence of proteinuria increases the probability of the patient having 'true' pre-eclampsia. The risk to the fetus is therefore higher because the pregnancy is complicated by pre-eclampsia rather than 'simple' hypertension.

Redman[15] showed that uric acid was a better predictor of poor perinatal outcome than blood pressure. The increasing uric acid level is thought to be a sign of the renal involvement in the disease. It also increases the likelihood

| Diastolic blood pressure mm Hg | None | Trace | Proteinuria + | ++ | +++ | ++++ | Total |
|---|---|---|---|---|---|---|---|
| <65 | 15.5 | 13.64 | 6.20 | – | – | – | 13.60 |
| 65–74 | 9.30 | 8.06 | 5.58 | 32.86 | 41.54 | – | 8.84 |
| 75–84 | 6.20 | 7.44 | 6.20 | 19.22 | – | – | 6.80 |
| 85–94 | 8.68 | 9.30 | 23.56 | – | 22.32 | – | 10.20 |
| 95–104 | 19.22 | 17.36 | 26.66 | 55.80 | 115.32 | 143.22 | 25.16 |
| 105+ | 20.46 | 27.90 | 62.62 | 68.82 | 125.24 | 110.98 | 41.48 |
| Total | 8.60 | 9.46 | 12.94 | 23.22 | 41.96 | 56.76 | – |

*Source:* Friedman, Neff[82]

**Table 15.2**
Stillbirth rate per 1000 births by diastolic blood pressure and proteinuria.
It can be seen that each parameter appears to exert an independent
factor affecting fetal outcome. A diastolic blood pressure of 95 mm Hg
and proteinuria of 2+'s appear to be the cut-off points of increased risk.
However, 1+ does increase the risk further when the diastolic is above 85
mm Hg.

| | No. women | No. of perinatal deaths | Perinatal mortality rate/1000 |
|---|---|---|---|
| Normotensive | 10 787 | 207 | 19.2 |
| Pre-eclampsia | | | |
|     Mild | 2 459 | 48 | 19.5 |
|     Moderate | 610 | 11 | 18.1 |
|     Severe | 830 | 28 | 33.7 |
| Total | 14 686 | 294 | 20.0 |

**Table 15.3**
Data from the British Birth Survey 1970 showing that the perinatal
mortality is only increased in association with severe proteinuric pre-
eclampsia. It is important to note that even in these patients the perinatal
mortality is only 175 per cent of normal and the vast majority of the
pregnancies do well.

of the disease being pre-eclampsia. It is associated with IUGR and fetal distress.[87]

The platelet count also falls in patients with progressive disease before the increasing severity becomes apparent.[16,40] Platelet consumption is thought to be associated with placental deposition and fibrin formation.[80] This could be a sign of impending placental insufficiency. There is a higher incidence of IUGR in cases of perinatal mortality associated with hypertension compared to the other causes of perinatal mortality.[75,88,89]

Therefore, the risks to the fetus are associated with changes found in placental function. In the presence of a normally functioning placenta and when the hypertension remains mild or moderate, the risk to the fetus appears to be less than normal.[14]

The other significant cause of perinatal mortality in pregnancies complicated by pregnancy hypertension is prematurity. Many workers have shown the poor outcome of pre-eclamptic pregnancies in the second and early third trimesters.[79,90] Some have suggested that it is a different disease.[91]

The reason for this is obvious. If the patient has severe disease in the early gestations, delivery of the fetus carries a poor outcome, whereas severe pre-eclampsia occurring at 34 weeks can easily be treated by delivery with an excellent prospect of a satisfactory fetal outcome. Therefore, the need to deliver the baby in the maternal interest is only a risk to the fetus in the earlier trimesters when, despite good growth and wellbeing, the fetus may well die because of prematurity. Placental insufficiency and IUGR can cause problems at any stage of gestation and with any severity of hypertension. The Scottish perinatal mortality figures show that the perinatal loss associated with PET is mostly postnatal prior to 32 weeks and antenatal after 32 weeks.[75]

# Management of pregnancy hypertension

Hypertension in pregnancy is a major contributor to the workload and anxiety in the practice of obstetrics. It produces a management dilemma and is responsible for a large percentage of the admissions.[92] The management of the condition is based on an accurate diagnosis, risk assessment for the mother and baby, accepted treatment regimes, and appropriate timing of delivery and postpartum care.

## The diagnosis of pregnancy hypertension

The measurement of blood pressure is inherently inaccurate. Blood pressure varies widely,[76,93,94] and methodology is not standardized.[95] In the non-pregnant patient the fifth Korotkoff sound corresponds to the intra-arterial measurement.[96] However, in pregnancy, the fifth sound may continue down to zero because of the hyperdynamic circulation, and the fourth Korotkoff sound is more reproducible.[20] This is used in the UK to measure the diastolic blood pressure in the pregnant woman. The blood pressure should be taken in the right arm with the sphygmomanometer at the level of the heart after a period of rest.

Most workers use a single diastolic blood pressure reading above 110 mm Hg as being adequate for a diagnosis of severe pre-eclampsia.[81,97,98] For the diagnosis of mild or moderate hypertension, two readings above 90 mm Hg diastolic at least 6 h apart are accepted. It is important that these readings are close enough together to imply a definite relationship.[81]

## Proteinuria

The definition of 'proteinuria' depends on the methods used. Protein excretion goes up in pregnancy from around 18 mg in 24 h in the non-pregnant to over 300 mg total protein. Albumin represents about 55 per cent of this. A total daily protein excretion over 300 mg is taken as abnormal.[97] When 'dip' sticks are used, the false positive rate is around 25 per cent with 'a trace' and 6 per cent with '1+'. This is probably due to the fluctuation in the concentration of protein in the urine and the presence of vaginal contamination. Therefore, if proteinuria is suspected, 24-h urine collections should be made.

## Oedema

Oedema is a common finding in normal pregnancy. Sixty-four per cent of normal women have oedema of the face and hands,[99] and this is associated with no adverse effects.[78,99] Although Hamlin[100] reported oedema in the fingers of almost every primigravida who developed PIH 6 weeks later, the additional presence of oedema does not increase the risk of hypertension to the mother or baby.[101]

## Parity

'Pure' pre-eclampsia is defined by Nelson as a diastolic blood pressure over 90 mm Hg with proteinuria of over 300 mg in 24 h occurring in a primigravid patient where there is no evidence of pre-existing hypertensive disease.[81] This definition is widely accepted and was validated by the biopsy studies of McCartney.[7] This study showed that the majority of primigravid patients with proteinuric hypertension had the pathognomonic renal lesion of pre-eclampsia. However, the results also showed that although most of the multigravid patients with proteinuric hypertension had underlying renal disease, some patients did have the classic renal lesions. Therefore, the diagnosis of pure pre-eclampsia is more likely in primigravidae but it cannot be excluded in a multigravida.[7] If a patient has pre-eclampsia in her first pregnancy, she is more likely to have problems in her next pregnancy. However, if apparent 'mild pre-eclampsia' is found in a multigravid patient, the patient may be demonstrating a tendency towards 'latent' hypertension which recurs in subsequent pregnancies and she will have an increased chance of developing hypertension in later life. Such women often have a strong family history of essential hypertension.[1,67,81,102]

Therefore, although hypertension in pregnancy is indeed polysymptomatic, high blood pressure is the primary sign of danger to the mother. Proteinuria is significant as a risk marker for the fetus and oedema appears to have no significance at all. It would seem reasonable to classify the problem for the mother on the basis of hypertension and the fetal risk on the presence of proteinuria or some more specific method of fetal monitoring.

## Assessment of risk

Maternal mortality is associated with poor antenatal care and unbooked patients.[103] It is through the antenatal screening process that most of the hypertensive patients will be found. Therefore, the basis of management of hypertensive diseases is comprehensive antenatal care.

The hypertensive patient can present in various ways. The hypertension may be an incidental finding at routine antenatal examination. There may be no symptoms and the diagnosis of a 'disease' with serious implications is difficult for the patient to accept. Many

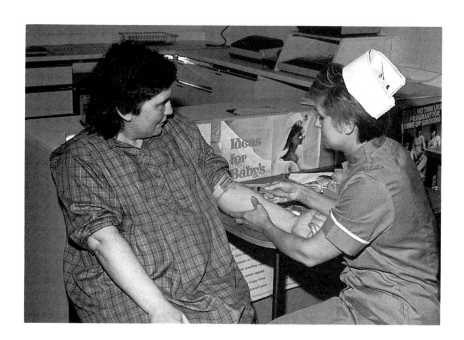

**Figure 15.4**
*The daycare unit where patients have full access to inpatient facilities on an outpatient basis.*

obstetricians would favour admission for assessment and/or observation once hypertension has been found.[104] The patient may find this unacceptable and invoke a conflict between her and her doctor. More unusually, she may present herself at the hospital with headache, increasing oedema or convulsion.

Assessment of the risk for the mother and baby is the initial stage of the management process. In the Glasgow Royal Maternity Hospital (GRMH), this is performed through the Daycare Assessment Unit[105] (Figure 15.4). This provides an inpatient monitoring system on an outpatient basis. The degree of blood pressure problem can be assessed and the need for admission decided. Daycare increases the access to full monitoring but has reduced the number of admissions for hypertension by 60 per cent.[106] This has allowed the targeting of inpatient care to the patients who most benefit from it with the potential reduction in costs.[106,107]

In any pregnancy condition, there are two patients to consider, the mother and her fetus. Pre-eclampsia affects them in different ways. The aim is to differentiate the patient with transient hypertension from those with a progressive disease who require continuing monitoring. A protocol was developed.

All results are available by 12.30 p.m. The patient is interviewed and the further management is discussed. Patients are classified as

Attendance between 9.00 and 9.30 a.m.
Clinical examination
Confirmatory tests performed on arrival
All results available at 12.30 p.m.
Medical staff assessment of risk
Future plan set out

*Plan of daycare attendance*

- **Routine**
  Five blood pressure readings at hourly intervals
  Abdominal palpation
  Serum uric acid
  Haemoglobin
  Platelet count
  Cardiotocograph

- **Follow-up**
  Ultrasound assessment
  Estimation of fetal weight
  Liquor volume estimation
  Biophysical profile

being of normal/low risk, mild/moderate risk or of high risk of blood pressure-related problems using the four main parameters: blood pressure (average of five readings), platelet count, uric acid and urinalysis.

The choices of management are based on these three risk categories, provided fetal wellbeing is confirmed by cardiotocograph and/or ultrasound. If normal or low risk (60 per cent of the referrals), the patient is referred

*The monitoring tests carried out at the daycare unit on the day of attendance. The follow-up assessments are carried out in those patients returning to daycare for a second attendance or if there is a particular risk to the pregnancy.*

- **Low risk**
  Average diastolic blood pressure<90 mm Hg
  Uric acid <350 mmol/l
  Platelet count >200 × $10^9$
  Absence of proteinuria
  Reactive cardiotocograph
  Absence of IUGR

- **Moderate risk**
  Average diastolic blood pressure >90 but <100 mm Hg
  Uric acid >350 but <450 mmol/l
  Platelet count <200 but >100 × $10^9$ proteinuria <++ or <1.5 g/24 h
  Reactive cardiotocograph
  Signs of IUGR but adequate liquor volume

- **High risk**
  Average diastolic blood pressure >100 mm Hg
  Uric acid >450 mmol/l
  Platelet count <100 × $10^9$ proteinuria >++ or >1.5 g/24 h
  Non-reactive cardiotocograph
  Signs of IUGR reduced liquor volume

*Risk categories used at daycare for the assessment of the patients. To be low risk, all the parameters must be met. If any of the parameters in the moderate- or high-risk category were met, that classified the patient into that group.*

back to the antenatal clinic within 10 days of their daycare appointment.[105] If moderate risk (20 per cent), the patient is brought back for a return visit at the daycare unit, either the same or the following week, to assess any progression of the disease. If the risk is high (10 per cent), the patient is admitted to hospital the same day or the next when further observation and management is carried out. A further 10 per cent of patients are approaching term and are admitted for induction of labour. At all times, the system allows flexibility to overrule the protocol and bring the patient back to daycare, or to admit them to hospital if there is any doubt about the safety of the mother or the fetus. Any clinical symptoms are considered worrying, particularly headache, visual disturbances and abdominal pain.

## Treatment

The routine admission of patients with hypertension has been challenged[108] and there appears to be no evidence that bedrest is of benefit.[109,110] Admission to hospital should be reserved for those requiring observation, treatment and/or delivery. After admission, the trend of blood pressure levels should be observed. The average of the daily readings should be taken for this assessment. Single or sporadic rises are common and are not of concern. Since the evidence suggests that a diastolic blood pressure of 110 mm Hg may cause vascular damage, it would seem logical to give antihypertensive drugs if the average daily diastolic blood pressure is over 100 mm Hg.[111] But is antihypertensive therapy of value?

Antihypertensive drugs lower blood pressure. They should not be expected to do anything else. They all act in different ways and have different benefits and side-effects.[111] The aim of therapy is to reduce the risk to the mother by preventing progressive vascular damage and cerebral vascular accident. By lowering the perceived risk, it may be possible to allow the pregnancy to continue to the benefit of the fetus by increasing maturity. This is the only way that antihypertensive therapy can improve the outcome for the baby. Lowering blood pressure will not improve the fetal state, although it may reduce the chance of a further deterioration.

Some obstetricians feel that lowering blood pressure will mask the symptoms of the hypertension and make management of the condition more difficult. The hypertension is a symptom of the underlying problem. The level of blood pressure should not be used as the sole parameter for evaluation of maternal or fetal risk. Just as additional monitoring of blood parameters are used when the patient first presents with hypertension, continuing monitoring of both mother and baby is used to assess the progression of the condition and the timing of delivery after lowering the blood pressure with medication.

Antihypertensive drugs appear to be safe for use in pregnancy but if they are used inappropriately there can be side-effects. These vary with drugs used. Vasodilators given intravenously can cause a sudden drop in blood pressure and can be related to signs of fetal and maternal distress[111] and should be used with care.

Methyldopa and atenolol, the two drugs commonly used in the non-pregnant situation, have been associated with growth retardation. However, methyldopa has been studied extensively in pregnancy, with extended follow-up, demonstrating apparent safety.[112,113] The 'vasodilator' beta-blockers, oxprenolol, pindolol and labetalol, would appear to have some advantages.[111] Labetalol has now become widely accepted as first-line treatment in this condition. This preparation has the advantage

- **Prepregnancy**
  If patient is normotensive, consider stopping all antihypertensive drugs.
  Aim to stop ACE inhibitors and diuretics if at all possible.

- **Less than 20 weeks**
  If the patient is normotensive, stop antihypertensive medication.
  If presenting for the first time, investigate for renal disease.
  For both—refer to the outpatient daycare assessment unit for follow-up.

- **After 20 weeks**
  A patient presenting for the first time or with worsening blood pressure after 20 weeks is presumed to have pre-eclampsia until monitoring suggests otherwise.
  Criteria for antihypertensive usage:
  (a) If BP is persistently elevated above 150/100 mm Hg, start labetalol 200 mg three times a day.
  (b) If BP not controlled, increase to 200 mg four times a day, and then increase dosage up to 1200 mg a day.
  (c) If BP not controlled, add in nifedipine 10 mg twice a day, and then increase up to 40 mg a day.

- **Hypertensive crisis**
  If BP greater than 160/110 mm Hg, give 200 mg oral labetalol
  > or 50 mg i.v. labetalol
  > or 10 mg oral nifedipine
  > or 20 mg i.v. hydralazine.
  Repeated oral doses or an infusion of labetalol can then be used.

- **Labetalol infusion**
  A solution containing 300 mg of labetalol in 60 ml, or 5 mg/ml.
  Infusion started at 12 ml/h and increased/decreased depending on the blood pressure response.
  Control is normally achieved at a rate of between 24 and 48 ml/h.

- **Anticonvulsant protocol**
  Valium 5 mg i.v. in repeated doses to help stop convulsions.
  Phenytoin is used to prevent further seizures.
  A loading dose of 10 mg/kg pregnant weight followed by 5 mg/kg pregnant weight 2 h later.
  Oral phenytoin 200 mg is given after 12 h.
  Phenytoin is continued until 48 h after delivery.

*Management protocol for the use of antihypertensive drugs in the Glasgow Royal Maternity Hospital.*

that it can be used in the acute situation as well as the chronic setting. It can be given by the intravenous route as well as orally. This means that medical staff only require to learn one regime for all patient groups. How any given patient is treated depends on the gestation of presentation and the severity of disease.

## Essential hypertension

Patients with known chronic hypertension should be assessed prior to pregnancy concerning the need for medication. The risks and probable outcome of the pregnancy should be discussed at this time. If the patient is on acceptable therapy and her blood pressure is stable, she should be continued on her medication and then reassessed in the first trimester. Although there are some drugs, such as ACE inhibitors, which are contraindicated,[114,115] any change of therapy should be balanced against the need for that medication. If enalapril is the only method of controlling blood pressure, then it may be better to continue this therapy even with the knowledge that it may cause problems.[111] If the blood pressure falls below 140/90 mm Hg, the therapy can be stopped and restarted only if the blood pressure rises again to over 150/100 mm Hg.

If a patient presents with hypertension for the first time before 20 weeks, she may not require therapy[116] but should be investigated for renal disease, as this is often initially discovered during pregnancy.[70] As long as the blood pressure remains below 150/100 mm Hg, the patient is observed through daycare, as it will normally drop by 18–20 weeks. If the blood pressure is higher than this or rises later in the pregnancy, antihypertensive therapy is commenced. When treating essential hypertension, the drug used probably does not matter very much. Labetalol is the drug of choice in the GRMH. After therapy is commenced, close

monitoring of maternal and fetal wellbeing must be continued. The patient can remain as an outpatient as long as adequate blood pressure control is maintained.

## Mild/moderate PIH

If patients present with hypertension after 20 weeks of gestation, the protocol is principally the same. After initial daycare assessment, the patients with mild to moderate disease are followed for evidence of disease progression. If the average diastolic blood pressure rises above 100 mm Hg, antihypertensive therapy is started. Again, labetalol is the drug of choice. Close monitoring is continued and the hypertensive drugs are increased as outlined if the blood pressure rises again. PET is largely a progressive disease. Increasing requirements of labetalol and the addition of nifedipine are to be expected in nearly 50 per cent of the patients. Delivery is planned when a reasonable gestation has been reached or there are signs of maternal or fetal deterioration. If blood pressure is controlled well and the fetus is not compromised, management can be carried out as an outpatient through daycare.

## The hypertensive crisis

Severe hypertension is a crisis for the mother, fetus, paediatrician and obstetrician. The aim of therapy is to stabilize the mother to reduce risks and allow either prolongation of the pregnancy or delivery of the fetus in a controlled way. Any patient with a blood pressure above 160/110 mm Hg is given 200 mg of oral labetalol. A fall of around 10/20 mm Hg should be achieved within 60 min. There is no need to reduce the blood pressure quickly. An acute drop in blood pressure is dangerous to both mother and fetus.[111] A further 200 mg of labetalol is given as required.

If oral therapy is not effective, a slow intra-venous injection of 50 mg labetalol is almost always successful in reducing blood pressure. This can be followed by a slow infusion of a solution containing 300 mg of labetalol in 60 ml, or 5 mg/ml. The infusion is started at 12 ml/h and increased or decreased depending on the blood pressure response. Control is normally achieved at a rate of between 24 and 48 ml/h. There has been no evidence of fetal distress in response to this regime. It is the author's experience that once a patient is started on an intravenous infusion to control the blood pressure, delivery is required, as it is rare to transfer control to oral therapy.

It is important to stabilize all patients with blood pressures above 160/110 mm Hg prior to delivery or patient transfer as these are the times of greatest risk to the mother.

## Anticonvulsant therapy

The use of anticonvulsant drugs is more controversial. The risk of eclampsia in estab-lished pre-eclampsia is now small. In North America, the use of magnesium sulphate to prevent convulsions is routine[117] although it has never been subjected to a randomized, placebo-controlled trial. Different anticonvul-sant therapies have been compared.[118,119] It is clear that patients may convulse on any therapy. It can be concluded that the need for prophylactic therapy is unproven. It is not our practice to use anticonvulsant therapy in the patient who has not seized. Clinical signs such as hyperreflexia and clonus are not good predictors of eclampsia and should not be used as justification for anticonvulsant therapy. There are rarely abnormalities in the ophthalmic fundus and their presence would suggest pre-existing hypertension. The prime approach to therapy in the acute situation should be to reduce the blood pressure.[111]

If a convulsion has already occurred, valium can be used in repeated 5-mg boluses until the convulsions stop. Following this, phenytoin is used to prevent further seizures.[120] This regime uses a loading dose of 10 mg/kg pregnant weight followed by 5 mg/kg pregnant weight 2 h later. Oral phenytoin 200 mg is given after 12 h. Phenytoin is continued until 48 h after delivery.

Once the patient has been stabilized, it is important to reassess the situation. Is the condition as bad as originally thought? If the mother and baby are well, would it be possible to prolong the pregnancy? Should the patient be transferred to a specialist unit to provide the necessary back-up for both the mother and the baby?

## Delivery

Delivery will lead to resolution of the symptoms over time. It is the only ultimate cure of the condition. However, it is important to remember that many of the maternal deaths occur after delivery. Continuing vigilance is required. Delivery is not always a simple solution and can be a procedure of great risk. It should be carried out on the best day, in the best place, in the best way, by the best team.

The timing of the delivery will affect the outcome for both mother and baby. If the mother is unstable, a rushed delivery may add to her risk, but delay in delivery can be equally treacherous. As far as the mother is concerned, it is stabilization of her blood pressure and/or convulsions that is paramount. Once this is achieved, a decision of when to deliver can be made in a calm and considered way. In the presence of eclampsia, delay in delivery after stabilization of the mother cannot be justified. However, in the absence of convulsions, prolongation of the pregnancy may lead to an improved outcome in the premature fetus. This may only be for a few hours. This may allow the paediatric unit to prepare for the delivery or to transfer the patient to a unit with more experience and equipment to look after the patient to a unit with more experience and equipment to look after the premature infant. A delay of a few days may allow the use of steroids to increase lung maturity. A delay of a week or more would allow an increasing chance of fetal survival. However, a full assessment of fetal wellbeing is required before this management is carried out. If there is any sign of fetal compromise, excessive prolongation of the pregnancy can lead to intrauterine death. It is better to deliver a small but healthy baby than a slightly bigger but compromised one.

If delivery of a baby is thought likely under 32 weeks, the mother should be given betamethasone 12 mg on two occasions 12 h apart. This has been shown to improve fetal lung maturity. If the patient has not been delivered 1 week later, the steroids should be repeated weekly until delivery or 32 weeks has been reached.

Once the patient is stable, the transfer to a more specialized unit may be prudent. Facilities should be available for the intensive care of the mother as well as the neonate. This transfer should be at an early stage after communication with the relevant paediatric and obstetric consultants, not with junior staff.

When elective delivery is to be carried out, a decision is required regarding the mode. In pregnancies less than 32 weeks, a caesarean section is advisable, to allow a controlled delivery for the mother and baby. After 34 weeks, a vaginal delivery can be attempted, as long as the fetus is in good condition. The use of vaginal prostaglandins has increased the likelihood of success. With caesarean section, problems can arise with the need of analgesia and anaesthesia. Intubation causes a further

rise in blood pressure of between 20 and 30 mm Hg in both systolic and diastolic pressure.[121,122] This is associated with CVAs occurring under anaesthetic leading to postpartum death. The acute rise in blood pressure, seen with intubation, can be attenuated by using intravenous labetalol 50 mg or concomitant narcotic drugs.[122] Local analgesia is preferred. Spinal analgesia has the advantage that it can be used in the presence of a reduced platelet count. However, coagulation defects are a rare complication of pre-eclampsia and epidural analgesia can be used safely in most cases.

Care has to be taken with fluid management. It should be remembered that although patients with pre-eclampsia can be hypovolaemic their tissues are fluid overloaded.[123] They cannot tolerate fluid 'loads' or 'challenges'. Dextrose or crystalline solutions should be used with great care, as they will accentuate the tissue overload. This increases the chance of development of pulmonary oedema and adult respiratory distress syndrome. If colloid solutions are used, the cardiovascular system may not tolerate the plasma expansion. It is rarely necessary to give routine fluid replacement to the pre-eclamptic patient. Renal failure is a rare complication and is usually associated with abruption, coagulation disorders or sepsis. If it does occur, it is easily managed and it is not associated with long-term sequelae. There is no need to maintain urine volume above a certain flow rate to 'protect the kidneys' and intravenous fluids should be used with caution. In the USA, it is common for patients to have a Swan–Ganz catheter inserted. This is invasive and not necessary in most cases. If a central venous pressure (CVP) line is used, it can be misleading and is often not sited properly or misread. When it is used, it should be to make sure that the CVP does not rise above 5 mm Hg. It is far safer and sensible to run the patient 'dry' by reducing the intravenous fluids to a minimum. This will help reduce the chances of pulmonary oedema without increasing the risks to the mother. A good monitor of pulmonary oedema is the measurement of blood gases. This can be carried out simply and continuously using a pulse oximeter. Cardiovascular problems usually occur at around 24–48 h after delivery.[70] This is associated with a failure of the postpartum diuresis seen with resolving pre-eclampsia. In the oedematous patient, or when the patient is in a positive balance, a forced diuresis can help to remove the excess fluid. This is done by using intravenous frusemide 40 mg followed by 20 g of intravenous mannitol. This helps to reduce the pulmonary oedema, increase oxygen saturation, reduce cerebral oedema and improve the blood pressure control. If a diuresis occurs, the patient's condition normally improves steadily.

## Postpartum management

Many of the maternal deaths associated with this condition occur postpartum. The fluid management is the most crucial part of the care at this time. The dosage of hypertensive drug can usually be reduced in a stepwise process until it can be stopped. If the drugs are stopped suddenly, rebound hypertension can occur with the concomitant risks to the mother. Most of the drugs used are excreted in the breast milk but appear to be safe to use in breast-feeding mothers.

Some patients become more hypertensive after delivery or are more difficult to control. In these situations, enalapril can be useful. The starting dose is 2.5 mg twice a day, increasing in steps until control is achieved. When enalapril is started, any other therapy can be reduced and stopped. All patients that remain hypertensive are followed at the daycare unit. If patients do not settle within weeks of delivery, the diagnosis should be reconsidered and the patient referred for further investigation and management. If severe disease had occurred, the implications for any subsequent pregnancy should be discussed.

## If my wife had ...

If my wife developed high blood pressure in pregnancy, I would want a full and proper assessment of the situation. This would include haematological and biochemical testing and ultrasound estimation of fetal wellbeing. A Doppler estimation of bloodflow in the fetal umbilical artery demonstrating end-diastolic flow would reassure me that the baby would probably do well.

If her diastolic blood pressure remained above 100 mm Hg, I would want this reduced using labetalol as previously described. The uric acid and platelet count should be carried out twice a week, as should fetal monitoring by cardiotocograph and liquor volume estimation.

If she was not already attending a specialized unit I would want her care transferred to a unit with experience to manage this problem and which possesses a special baby care unit and an adult intensive care area. If she was less than 32 weeks, I would wish betamethasone to be administered on a weekly basis until delivery or 32 weeks of gestation.

Close monitoring of the mother and the baby should continue to allow the decision concerning delivery to be made at the optimum time. If it is required, I would wish the caesarean section to be carried out by an experienced obstetrician still commonly performing these procedures. I would wish an experienced paediatrician present to resuscitate my baby.

Post-delivery I would want my wife's fluid management to be carefully monitored. If there are signs of positive balance or oedema, I would wish the liberal use of diuretics to increase the removal of her excessive interstitial fluid, which I consider to be the main risk to her life.

If the hypertension persisted following delivery, I would want her fully assessed by a renal physician for any underlying problems.

# References

1   Chesley LC, Evolution of concepts of eclampsia. In: Bonnar J, MacGillivary I, Symonds EM, eds. *Pregnancy hypertension* (MTP Press: Lancaster 1980) 1–4.

2   Mauriceau F, Desmaladies DES, Fennes Grosses ET, *Accouches avec la bonne et veritable* (Cercle du Livre Precieux: Paris 1668).

3   Denman T, *Essays on the puerperal fever and on puerperal convulsions* (Waller: London 1768).

4   Lever JCW, Cases of puerperal convulsions with remarks. In: Barlow GH, ed. *Guys Hospital Reports*, Vol. 1 (Samuel Highley: London 1843) 495–506.

5   Simpson JY, Contributions to the pathology and treatment of diseases of the uterus, *Edinburgh Monthly J Med Sci* (1843) **3**:1009–13.

6   Sheehan HL, Pathological lesions in the hypertensive toxaemias of pregnancy. In: Hammond J, Browne FJ, Wolstenholme GEW, eds. *Toxaemias of pregnancy* (J & A Churchill: London 1950).

7   McCartney CP, Pathological anatomy of acute hypertension of pregnancy, *Circulation* (1964) **30**:37–41.

8   Ballantyne JW, Sphygmographic tracings in puerperal eclampsia, *Edinburgh Med J* (1885) **30**:1007–11.

9   Cook HW, Briggs JC, Clinical observations on blood pressure, *John Hopkins Hosp Rep* (1903) **11**:451–5.

10  Chesley LC, Annitto JE, Cosgrove RA, The remote prognosis of eclamptic women. Sixth periodic report, *Am J Obstet Gynecol* (1976) **124**:446–50.

11  Cruickshank JM, Studies of the toxaemias of pregnancy as they occur in Glasgow, *J Obstet Gynaecol Br Emp* (1923) **30**:541–5.

12  Cruickshank JM, Hewitt R, Couper J, The toxaemias of pregnancy: a clinical and biochemical study. In: *Medical Research Council, Special Report Series* (Medical Research Council: London 1927) 47–51.

13  Sibai BM et al, Eclampsia. 1 Observations from 67 recent cases, *Obstet Gynecol* (1981) **58**:609–13.

14  Nelson TR, A clinical study of preeclampsia. Part 2, *J Obstet Gynaecol Br Emp* (1955) **62**:58–62.

15  Redman CW, Beilin LJB, Wilkinson BH, Plasma urate measurements in predicting fetal death in hypertensive pregnancy, *Lancet* (1976) **1**:1370–4.

16  Walker JJ et al, Can platelet volume predict progressive hypertensive disease in pregnancy? *Am J Obstet Gynecol* (1989) **161**:676–9.

17  Ferrazzani S et al, Proteinuria and outcome of 444 pregnancies complicated by hypertension, *Am J Obstet Gynecol* (1990) **162**:366–71.

18  Turnbull A et al, Report on Confidential Enquiries into Maternal Deaths in England and Wales 1982–1984, *Rep Health Soc Subj Lond* (1989) **34**:1–166.

19  Common Services Agency, *Scottish Stillbirth and Neonatal Death Report* (Scottish Home and Health Department: Edinburgh 1986).

20  MacGillivray I, Rose G, Rowe B, Blood pressure survey in pregnancy, *Clin Sci* (1969) **37**:395–9.

21  Gant N et al, A study of angiotensin II, pressor response throughout primigravida pregnancy, *J Clin Invest* (1973) **52**:2682–6.

22  Wallenburg HCS et al, Low dose aspirin prevents pregnancy induced hypertension and pre-eclampsia in angiotensin sensitive primigravidae, *Lancet* (1986) **1**:1–5.

23  Dekker GA, Makovitz JW, Wallenburg HC, Prediction of pregnancy-induced hypertensive disorders by angiotensin II sensitivity and supine pressor test, *Br J Obstet Gynaecol* (1990) **97**:817–21.

24  Downing I, Shepherd GL, Lewis PJ, Reduced prostacyclin production in pre-eclampsia, *Lancet* (1980) **2**:1374–8.

25 Remuzzi G et al, Reduced umbilical and placental vascular prostacyclin in severe pre-eclampsia, *Prostaglandins* (1980) **20**:105–9.

26 Jogee M, Myatt L, Elder MG, Decreased prostacyclin production by placental cells in culture from pregnancies complicated by fetal growth retardation, *Br J Obstet Gynaecol* (1983) **90**:247–51.

27 Makila UM, Viinikka L, Ylikorkala O, Increased thromboxane A2 production but normal prostacyclin by the placenta in hypertensive pregnancies, *Prostaglandins* (1984) **27**:87–91.

28 Fitzgerald DJ et al, Thromboxane A2 synthesis in pregnancy-induced hypertension, *Lancet* (1990) **335**:751–4.

29 Walsh SW, Thromboxane production in placentas of women with preeclampsia, *Am J Obstet Gynecol* (1989) **160**:1535–6.

30 Florijn KW et al, Elevated plasma levels of endothelin in pre-eclampsia, *J Hypertens Suppl* (1991) **9**:S166–S167.

31 Schiff E et al, Immunoreactive circulating endothelin-1 in normal and hypertensive pregnancies, *Am J Obstet Gynecol* (1992) **166**:624–8.

32 Clark BA et al, Plasma endothelin levels in preeclampsia: elevation and correlation with uric acid levels and renal impairment, *Am J Obstet Gynecol* (1992) **166**:962–8.

33 Myatt et al, Attenuation of the vasoconstrictor effects of thromboxane and endothelin by nitric oxide in the human fetal-placental circulation, *Am J Obstet Gynecol* (1992) **166**:224–30.

34 Roberts JM et al, Preeclampsia: an endothelial cell disorder, *Am J Obstet Gynecol* (1989) **161**:1200–4.

35 Zeeman GG et al, Endothelial function in normal and pre-eclamptic pregnancy: a hypothesis, *Eur J Obstet Gynecol Reprod Biol* (1992) **43**:113–22.

36 Wisdom SJ et al, Antioxidant systems in normal pregnancy and in pregnancy-induced hypertension, *Am J Obstet Gynecol* (1991) **165**:1701–4.

37 Sill PR, Lind T, Walker W, Platelet values during normal pregnancy, *Br J Obstet Gynaecol* (1985) **92**:480–3.

38 Fay RA, Hughes AO, Farron NT, Platelets in pregnancy. Hyperdestruction in pregnancy, *Obstet Gynecol* (1983) **61**:238–42.

39 Singer CRJ et al, Platelet studies in normal pregnancy and pregnancy-induced hypertension, *Clin Lab Haem* (1986) **8**:27–31.

40 Redman CW, Bonnar J, Beilin LJ, Early platelet consumption in pre-eclampsia, *Br Med J* (1978) **1**:146–50.

41 Wallenburg HCS, Rotmans N, Circulating large platelets and platelet turnover in normotensive and hypertensive pregnancies with insufficient fetal growth. In: Sammour MB et al, eds. *Pregnancy hypertension* (Aim Shams University Press: Cairo 1980).

42 Giles C, The platelet count and mean platelet volume, *Br J Haematol* (1981) **48**:31–7.

43 Hsieh C, Cauchi MN, Platelet and complement changes in preeclampsia, *J Obstet Gynaecol* (1983) **3**:165–96.

44 Birmingham Eclampsia Study Group, Intravascular coagulation and abnormal lung scans in pre-eclampsia and eclampsia, *Lancet* (1971) **2**:889–93.

45 Trudinger BJ, Platelets and intrauterine growth retardation in pre-eclampsia, *Br J Obstet Gynaecol* (1976) **83**:284–6.

46 Howie PW, Prentice CRM, McNicol GP, Coagulation fibrinolysis and platelet function in pre-eclampsia, essential hypertension and placental insufficiency, *J Obstet Gynaecol Br Com* (1971) **78**:992–6.

47 Rakoczi I et al, Platelet life-span in normal pregnancy and pre-eclampsia as determined by a non-radioisotope technique, *Thromb Res* (1979) **15**:553–6.

48 Browne JCM, Veall N, The maternal placental blood flow in normotensive and hypertensive women, *J Obstet Gynaecol Br Emp* (1953) **60**:141–5.

49 Dixon HG, Robertson WB, A study of the vessels of the placental bed in normotensive and hypertensive women, *J Obstet Gynaecol Br Emp* (1958) **65**:803–7.

50 Assali NS et al, Measurement of uterine blood flow and uterine metabolism with the N2O method in normotensive and toxemic pregnancies, *Clin Res Proc* (1954) **2**:102–6.

51 Campbell J et al, New doppler technique for assessing uteroplacental blood flow, *Lancet* (1983) **1**:675–9.

52 Robertsion WB, Utero-placental vasculature, *J Clin Path* (1976) **10**(suppl 29):9–1014.

53 Fox H, *Pathology of the placenta* (WB Saunders and Company Ltd: London 1978).

54 Bastiaanse NA, Mastboom JL, Ischaemia of the gravid uterus as a possible factor in the causation of toxaemia of pregnancy. In: Hammond J, Browne FJ, Wolstenholme GEW, eds. *Toxaemia of pregnancy, Human and Veterinary* (Churchill: London 1950) 182–91.

55 Cavanagh D et al, Experimental toxemia in the pregnant primate, *Am J Obstet Gynecol* (1977) **128**:75–85.

56 Symonds EM, The renin–angiotensin system in pregnancy, *Obstet Gynecol Annu* (1981) **10**:45–67.

57 Sheehan HL, Renal morphology in preeclampsia, *Kidney Int* (1980) **18**:241–52.

58 Chesley LC, Duffus GM, Preeclampsia, posture and renal function, *Obstet Gynecol* (1971) **38**:1–5.

59 Altchek A, Albright NL, Sommers SC, The renal pathology of toxaemia of pregnancy, *Obstet Gynecol* (1968) **31**:594–8.

60 Adams EM, Finlayson A, Familial aspects of pre-eclampsia and hypertension in pregnancy, *Lancet* (1961) **2**:1375–9.

61 Chesley LC, Annitto JE, Cosgrove RA, The familial factor in toxaemia of pregnancy, *Obstet Gynecol* (1968) **32**:303–7.

62 Cooper DW, Liston WA, Genetic control of severe pre-eclampsia, *J Med Genet* (1979) **16**:409–13.

63 Arngrimsson R et al, Genetic and familial predisposition to eclampsia and pre-eclampsia in a defined population, *Br J Obstet Gynaecol* (1990) **97**:762–9.

64 Chesley LC, Cooper DW, Genetics of hypertension in pregnancy: possible single gene control of pre-eclampsia and eclampsia in the descendants of eclamptic women, *Br J Obstet Gynaecol* (1986) **93**:898–908.

65 Sutherland A et al, Incidence of severe pre-eclampsia amongst mothers and mothers-in-law of pre-eclampsics and controls, *Br J Obstet Gynaecol* (1981) **88**:75–9.

66 Goldby FS, Beilin LJ, Relationship between arterial pressure and the permeability of arterioles to carbon particles in acute hypertension, *Cardiovasc Res* (1972) **6**:384–8.

67 Chesley LC, *Hypertensive disorders in pregnancy* (Appleton-Century-Crofts: New York 1978).

68 Zuspan FP, Treatment of severe preeclampsia and eclampsia, *Clin Obstet Gynecol* (1966) **9**:954–8.

69 Redman CW, Treatment of hypertension in pregnancy, *Kid Int* (1980) **18**:267–71.

70 Govan ADT, The pathogenesis of eclamptic lesions, *Pathol Microbiol* (1961) **24**:561–5.

71 Duncan SL, Does volume expansion in pre-eclampsia help or hinder? *Br J Obstet Gynaecol* (1989) **96**:631–3.

72 Weinstein L, Syndrome of hemolysis, elevated liver enzymes and low platelet count; a severe consequence of hypertension in pregnancy, *Am J Obstet Gynecol* (1982) **142**:159–63.

73 Pritchard JA, Cunningham FG, Mason RA, Coagulation changes in eclampsia: their frequency and pathogenesis, *Am J Obstet Gynecol* (1976) **124**:855–9.

74 Chesley LC, John Hopkins Hospital Figures. In: Hellman LM, Pritchard JA, eds. *Hypertensive disorders of pregnancy* (Appleton Century Crofts: New York 1971) 685–747.

75 Scottish Home and Health Department, *A report on an enquiry into maternal deaths in Scotland 1981–1986* (Her Majesty's Stationery Office: Edinburgh 1989).

76 Munro Kerr JM, *Maternal morbidity and mortality: a study of their problems* (ES Livingston: Edinburgh 1933).

77 Chamberlain GVP, Raised blood pressure in pregnancy. The fetus in hypertension, *Br J Hosp Med* (1981) **26**:127–31.

78 British Birth Survey et al, *British births 1970: a survey under the joint auspices of the National Birthday Trust Fund and the Royal College of Obstetricians and Gynaecologists.* (London: William Heinemann Medical Books, 1975).

79 Fairlie FM et al, Determinants of perinatal outcome in pregnancy-induced hypertension with absence of umbilical artery end-diastolic frequencies, *Am J Obstet Gynecol* (1991) **164**:1084–9.

80 Robertson WB, Brosens I, Dixon HG, The pathological response of the vessels of the placental bed to hypertensive pregnancy, *J Path Bact* (1967) **93**:581–5.

81   Nelson TR, A clinical study of pre-eclampsia. Part 1, *J Obstet Gynaecol Br Emp* (1955) **62**:48–52.

82   Friedman EA, Neff RK, Pregnancy outcome as related to hypertension, edema and proteinuria. In: Lindheimer MD, Katz AI, Zuspan FP, eds. *Hypertension in pregnancy* (J Wiley: New York 1975) 13–17.

83   Page EW, Christianson R, Influence of blood pressure changes with and without proteinuria upon outcome of pregnancy, *Am J Obstet Gynecol* (1976) **126**:821–5.

84   Butler NR, Bonham DG, *First Report of the British Perinatal Mortality Survey, 1958* (ES Livingston: Edinburgh 1963).

85   Butler NR, Alberman ED, Perinatal problems. In: Butler NR, Bonham DG, eds. *Second Report of the British Perinatal Mortality Survey, 1958* (ES Livingston: Edinburgh 1969).

86   Sheehan HL, Lynch JB, *Pathology of toxaemia of pregnancy* (Churchill Livingston: London 1973).

87   Harkness RA, Geirsson RT, McFadyen IR, Concentrations of hypoxanthine, xanthine, uridine and urate in amniotic fluid at caesarean section and the association of raised levels with prenatal risk factors and fetal distress, *Br J Obstet Gynaecol* (1983) **90**:815–20.

88   Scottish Home and Health Department, *A report on an enquiry into maternal deaths in Scotland, 1972–1975* (Her Majesty's Stationery Office: Edinburgh 1978).

89   Scottish Home and Health Department, *A report on an enquiry into maternal deaths in Scotland 1976–1980* (Her Majesty's Stationery Office: Edinburgh 1987).

90   Sibai BM et al, Maternal and perinatal outcome of conservative management of severe preeclampsia in midtrimester, *Am J Obstet Gynecol* (1985) **152**:32–7.

91   Moore MP, Redman CW, Case control study of severe pre-eclampsia of early onset, *Br Med J* (1983) **2**:580–4.

92   Hall M, Chang PK, MacGillivray I, Is routine antenatal care worthwhile? *Lancet* (1980) **2**:78–80.

93   Pickering G, *High blood pressure* (Grune & Stratton: New York 1968).

94   Redman CW, Beilin LJ, Bonnar J. Variability of blood pressure in normal and abnormal pregnancy. In: Lindheimer MD, Katz AI, Zuspan FP, eds. *Hypertension in pregnancy* (J. Wiley & Sons: New York 1977) 53–7.

95   O'Brien ET, O'Malley K, ABC of blood pressure measurement, *Br Med J* (1979) **2**:982–6.

96   Kirkendall WM, Recommendations for human blood pressure determination by sphygmomanometers, *Circulation* (1967) **36**:980–3.

97   Hughes EC, *Obstetrics—gynecological terminology* (Davis: Philadelphia 1972) 422–3.

98   Gant NF et al, Control of vascular responsiveness during human pregnancy, *Kid Int* (1980) **18**:253–7.

99   Dexter L, Weiss S, *Preeclamptic and eclamptic toxaemia of pregnancy* (Little Brown & Company: Boston 1941).

100  Hamlin RHJ, The prevention of eclampsia and pre-eclampsia, *Lancet* (1952) **1**:64–8.

101  MacGillivray I, Campbell DM, The effect of hypertension and oedema on birth weight. In: Bonnar J, MacGillivary I, Symonds EM, eds. *Pregnancy hypertension* (University Park Press: Baltimore 1980) 307–11.

102  Gibberd GF, Consideration of results of albuminuria occurring during pregnancy with special reference to the relationship between pregnant kidney and chronic nephritis, *Proc R Soc Med* (1928) **21**:39–43.

103  Turnbull AC, Maternal mortality and present trends. In: Sharp F, Symonds EM, eds. *Hypertension in pregnancy*. Proceedings of the Sixteenth Study Group of the Royal College of Obstetricians and Gynaecologists (Perinatology Press: New York 1987) 135–44.

104  Chamberlain GVP et al, How obstetricians manage hypertension in pregnancy, *Br Med J* (1978) **1**:626–30.

105  Walker JJ, The case fo early recognition and intervention in pregnancy induced hypertension. In: Sharp F, Symonds EM, eds. *Hypertension in pregnancy*. Proceedings of the Sixteenth Study Group of the Royal College of Obstetricians and Gynaecologists (Perinatology Press: New York 1987) 289–99.

106 Rosenberg K, Twaddle S, Screening and surveillance of pregnancy hypertension—an economic approach to the use of daycare. In: Hall M, ed. *Baillieres Clinical Obstetrics and Gynaecology*, Vol. 4. *Antenatal Care* (Bailliere-Tindall: London 1990) 89–107.

107 Twaddle S, Harper V, Day care and pregnancy hypertension, *Lancet* (1992) **339**:813–14.

108 Matthews DD, Patel IE, Sengupta SM, Outpatient management of toxaemia, *J Obstet Gynaecol Br Com* (1971) **78**:610–14.

109 Matthews DD, A randomised controlled trial of bed rest and sedation or normal activity and non-sedation in the management of non-albuminuric hypertension in late pregnancy, *Br J Obstet Gynaecol* (1977) **84**:108–14.

110 Crowther CA, Chalmers I, Bed rest and hospitalisation during pregnancy. In: Chalmers I, Enkin M, Kerse MJNC, eds. *The Effective care in pregnancy and childbirth*, Vol. 1 (Oxford University Press: Oxford 1989) 624–32.

111 Walker JJ, Hypertensive drugs in pregnancy. Antihypertension therapy in pregnancy, preeclampsia, and eclampsia, *Clin Perinatol* (1991) **18**:845–73.

112 Cockburn J et al, Final report of study on hypertension during pregnancy: the effects of specific treatment on the growth and development of the children, *Lancet* (1982) **1**:647–9.

113 Redman CW, Controlled trials of antihypertensive drugs in pregnancy, *Am J Kidney Dis* (1991) **17**:149–53.

114 Broughton Pipkin F, Symonds EM, Turner SR, The effect of captopril (SQ14,225) upon mother and fetus in the chronically cannulated ewe and in the pregnant rabbit, *J Physiol Lond* (1982) **323**:415–22.

115 Boutroy MJ et al, Captopril administration in pregnancy impairs fetal angiotensin converting enzyme activity and neonatal adaptation, *Lancet* (1984) **2**:935–6.

116 Sibai BM, Abdella TN, Anderson GD, Pregnancy outcome in 211 patients with mild chronic hypertension, *Obstet Gynecol* (1983) **61**:571–6.

117 Sibai BM, Magnesium sulfate is the ideal anticonvulsant in preeclampsia-eclampsia, *Am J Obstet Gynecol* (1990) **162**:1141–5.

118 Dommisse J, Phenytoin sodium and magnesium sulphate in the management of eclampsia, *Br J Obstet Gynaecol* (1990) **97**:104–9.

119 Crowther C, Magnesium sulphate versus diazepam in the management of eclampsia: a randomized controlled trial, *Br J Obstet Gynaecol* (1990) **97**:110–17.

120 Ryan G, Lange IR, Naugler MA, Clinical experience with phenytoin prophylaxis in severe preeclampsia, *Am J Obstet Gynecol* (1989) **161**:1297–304.

121 Lavies NG et al, Hypertensive and catecholamine response to tracheal intubation in patients with pregnancy-induced hypertension, *Br J Anaesthesiol* (1989) **63**:429–34.

122 Ramanathan J et al, The use of labetalol for attenuation of the hypertensive response to endotracheal intubation in preeclampsia, *Am J Obstet Gynecol* (1988) **159**:650–4.

123 Brown MA, Zammit VC, Lowe SA, Capillary permeability and extracellular fluid volumes in pregnancy-induced hypertension, *Clin Sci* (1989) **77**:599–604.

# 16

## Difficulties in the management of hypertrophic cardiomyopathy

*Alistair KB Slade and William J McKenna*

## Introduction

Hypertrophic cardiomyopathy has fascinated clinicians since its first description over 30 years ago by Teare.[1] Whilst initially studies focused on the classic variant of hypertrophic cardiomyopathy with asymmetrical septal hypertrophy, it has become clear from extensive family studies and routine health screening that the condition exists in a spectrum of morphological forms. Patients may be profoundly disabled or completely asymptomatic. Presentation may be in early infancy or be in old age. Whilst this broad spectrum of morphological and symptomatic presentations has altered the initial belief that hypertrophic cardiomyopathy carried a uniformly poor prognosis, considerable diagnostic difficulty may arise.[2,3]

The hereditary nature of the condition became apparent early on in studies of the condition[4] but it is only recently that advances in molecular genetics have allowed identification of the molecular abnormalities associated with hypertrophic cardiomyopathy.[5,6] This major advance may allow accurate diagnosis in previously borderline cases and enable a more accurate prediction of the course of the disease.

Therapy in patients with hypertrophic cardiomyopathy is aimed at reducing symptoms of dyspnoea, angina pectoris and syncope. Symptomatic improvement may be gained pharmacologically with beta-blockers, calcium antagonists and amiodarone or surgically with myectomy or mitral valve replacement.[7–10] Because of drug side-effects and surgical mortality/morbidity, other treatment modalities continue to be sought. The multiprogrammability of modern pacemaker generators has allowed investigation of atrioventricular sequential pacing with short non-physiological AV delays providing abnormal ventricular activation. This has been reported to be an effective treatment modality although the precise mechanisms for this remain unclear.[11–13]

Hypertrophic cardiomyopathy is the most important cause of sudden cardiac death in people under the age of 35[14] and much work has gone into risk stratification. Until recently such investigations have not provided a high positive predictive accuracy, although the negative predictive accuracy of non-invasive investigation is reassuringly high.

Sudden cardiac death in hypertrophic cardiomyopathy is presumed to be arrhythmic and has provoked much electrophysiological interest. Whilst the factors involved in the pathogenesis of sudden cardiac death are complex, there is little doubt that the basic histological abnormality, myocardial disarray, provides a substrate capable of sustaining the lethal ventricular arrhythmias that are the presumptive final event in causing sudden cardiac death.[15,16] Attempts to identify individuals at risk of sudden cardiac death with a high degree of specificity using conventional electrophysiological stimulation techniques have by and large failed. A recently developed electrophysiological technique which attempts to quantify the degree of disarray offers considerable promise in this respect.[17]

## Difficulties in diagnosis

Hypertrophic cardiomyopathy is currently defined as an idiopathic heart muscle condition characterized by a hypertrophied and non-dilated left and/or right ventricle in the absence of any cardiac or systemic cause. These criteria have changed since the first descriptions in the 1960s, when clinical features of hyperdynamic systolic function and left ventricular outflow tract gradient were emphasized. It became apparent that only about 25 per cent of patients have resting outflow tract gradients, with a further 20 per cent having gradients after pharmacological provocation.[2] It also became evident that the magnitude of left ventricular hypertrophy and left ventricular outflow tract gradient did not correlate with patient symptom status.[4] The recognition of families with the characteristic histological abnormalities in the absence of hypertrophy suggests that the current diagnostic criteria are incomplete.[18]

The current definition seldom causes problems if classic features of the condition are present or if abnormalities are detected in first-degree relatives of patients undergoing evaluation. Difficulties may arise when other causes of left ventricular hypertrophy are present, such as in the highly trained athlete or the patient with mild hypertension and apparently disproportionate left ventricular hypertrophy.

Patients who present with classical symptoms of syncope, chest pain and dyspnoea do not present diagnostic difficulties. Symptomatic presentation may be at any age, although only 50 per cent of patients will present with symptoms,[2,4] the remainder having the diagnosis made as a result of family screening or routine physical, electrocardiographic or echocardiographic examination. Presentation in infancy/childhood may be at autopsy or with severe cardiac failure but is more usually during family screening studies.[19]

Fifty per cent of patients experience dyspnoea on exertion. This has been ascribed to high left atrial pressures consequent on left ventricular diastolic dysfunction. However, as with cardiac failure from other causes, there is no direct correlation between objective measures of exercise capacity and pulmonary capillary wedge pressures, suggesting that peripheral vascular mechanisms and subjective awareness are important determinants of exercise capacity.[20]

Chest pain is a symptom in 50 per cent of patients. This can either be typical angina pectoris with classical precipitants or atypical pain which can persist for hours without enzymatic evidence of myocardial damage.[21] The mechanism for such pain remains uncertain but the increased muscle mass will have greater oxygen demand with reduced coronary perfusion pressure in the presence of raised diastolic pressures.

Syncope is experienced in approximately 15 per cent of patients and is an ominous symptom with an increased risk of sudden death but is rarely related to documented conducting tissue disease, or to documented sustained arrhythmia. It often follows exertion and may be related to emotional stress.[22] Presentation in childhood or adolescence with syncope is an adverse feature, with such patients having at least a 6 per cent per annum risk of sudden cardiac death, this being significantly higher if adverse features such as syncope or a malignant family history are present.[23,24] This compares with the risk of sudden cardiac death in an adult population in a tertiary referral centre of 2.5 per cent per annum. Our experience does not confirm reports that the cause of syncope can be defined by electrophysiological investigation.[25] Frequently, the mechanism cannot be determined in the individual patient, but it is a bad prognostic feature and is strongly associated with the risk of sudden death, especially in the young.[26]

Atrial fibrillation is the commonest sustained arrhythmia seen and is present in approximately 5–10 per cent of patients at presentation and will develop in another 10 per cent over the next 5 years.[27] The establishment of atrial fibrillation was classically held to represent an important stage in the disease process, with universal functional deterioration and risk of systemic emboli, and was thought to carry a poor prognosis. The deterioration was explained on the basis of the uncontrolled ventricular response allowing little time for ventricular filling in ventricles with marked diastolic impairment. The relatively benign fate of a cohort of patients with hypertrophic cardiomyopathy and atrial fibrillation is well reported in a retrospective study of 52 patients from 1960 to 1985.[28] The acute onset of atrial fibrillation led to symptomatic deterioration in 89 per cent, but restoration of sinus rhythm (63 per cent) or control of ventricular rate with appropriate medical therapy (30 per cent) led to restoration of original NYHA functional class with no significant difference in mortality on long-term follow-up. This observation should be tempered by the fact that paroxysmal atrial fibrillation may initiate haemodynamic deterioration and sudden cardiac death before presentation to hospital.[29] Sustained ventricular tachycardia is rare in clinical practice.[30]

Physical examination may also be unrewarding, although there are subtle physical signs that can be elucidated. Patients may have a carotid pulse with a rapid upstroke consequent on rapid emptying of a ventricle with hyperdynamic systolic function. This may be obvious in younger patients but in elderly patients the emptying of a normal ventricle into rigid atherosclerotic major arteries can mimic a rapid upstroke. The venous pulse may show a dominant 'a' wave in the minority of patients with important right ventricular hypertrophy. A forceful left ventricular impulse may be detected, as may a palpable atrial contraction, which may or may not be associated with a significant atrial contribution to end-diastolic volume.

Auscultation will usually reveal normal first and second sounds. A loud fourth heart sound may be heard and is due to increased atrial systolic flow into a stiff, non-compliant left ventricle. The characteristic murmur of left ventricular outflow tract obstruction is only heard in the 25 per cent of patients who have a resting gradient. It is heard at the left sternal edge, starting after S1 and ending before A2, and radiating to the neck and the mitral area. It is increased in intensity by manoeuvres that decrease afterload or venous return (amyl nitrate, standing) and decreased in intensity by manoeuvres that increase afterload and venous return (squatting, phenylephrine). Mild mitral regurgitation may be difficult to separate from the murmur of left ventricular outflow tract obstruction but important mitral regurgitation will produce a murmur that radiates classically to the axilla. Mitral diastolic murmurs occur due to increased forward flow consequent on mitral regurgitation but more commonly are due to inflow turbulence. Rarely, right-sided ejection murmurs can be heard, denoting right ventricular outflow tract obstruction secondary to severe right ventricular hypertrophy.

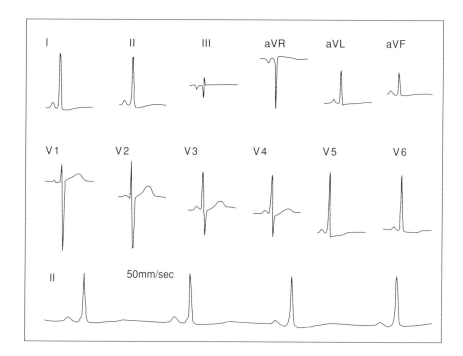

**Figure 16.1**
*Abnormal ECG showing left ventricular hypertrophy, T-wave abnormalities and a slurred upstroke to the QRS complex.*

## Investigations

### Electrocardiography

In keeping with the multiple morphological manifestations of hypertrophic cardiomyopathy, the electrocardiogram (ECG) may demonstrate multiple abnormalities.[31] There is no pattern diagnostic of hypertrophic cardiomyopathy and the best advice is to consider the diagnosis, particularly in young people, when presented with an abnormal ECG (Figure 16.1).

At presentation, 5–10 per cent of patients are in established atrial fibrillation, 20 per cent have left axis deviation and 5 per cent demonstrate complete right bundle branch block. The majority of patients will show an intraventricular conduction defect but true left bundle branch block is rare, although it may be seen after surgery and occasionally in the elderly. ST-segment depression, T-wave changes and voltage changes of left ventricular hypertrophy are the commonest abnormalities. Abnormal Q-waves may be present in the inferior leads or less commonly in the lateral or septal leads in about 20 per cent of patients.[2,32] Occasionally a short PR interval may be seen, together with a slurred upstroke to the QRS complex, although formal electrophysiological study rarely demonstrates an accessory pathway; however, such pathways have been described in hypertrophic cardiomyopathy. P-wave abnormalities of right or left atrial strain reflect the raised atrial pressures consequent on filling 'stiff' ventricles. Other subtle abnormalities such as J-point elevation, intraventricular conduction defects and T-wave abnormalities may be present in isolation or in combination with the abnormalities described above.

## Chest X-ray

The chest X-ray seldom demonstrates any pathognomonic features. Radiological features of left or right atrial or ventricular enlargement may be present, as may Kerley 'B' lines in the presence of chronically elevated left atrial pressures. Mitral valve calcification is not uncommon but aortic valve calcification should suggest aortic valvular stenosis rather than hypertrophic cardiomyopathy.

## Echocardiography

The development of M-mode echocardiography in the 1970s permitted the visualization of the interventricular septum and the posterior left ventricular wall at mitral valve level. These are the thickest and the thinnest myocardial segments respectively. M-mode echocardiography thus confirmed the earlier pathological descriptions of asymmetrical hypertrophy and led to the assertion that asymmetric septal hypertrophy (ASH) was the pathognomonic feature of the condition.[33] ASH is seen in 50–60 per cent of patients with hypertrophic cardiomyopathy, but is also found in other patient groups.[34] Cross-sectional (two-dimensional) echocardiography, currently the standard diagnostic technique, visualizes the entire heart and has shown that there is right

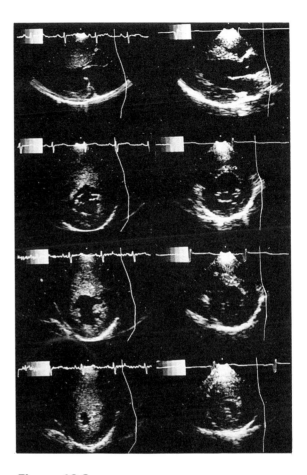

**Figure 16.2**

*Long-axis view and short-axis views taken at mitral valve papillary muscle and apex. The left-hand study demonstrates classical asymmetrical septal hypertrophy with maximal hypertrophy at the base of the septum. The right-hand study demonstrates hypertrophy maximal at the apex.*

ventricular hypertrophy in about a third of patients, and that left ventricular hypertrophy may be asymmetrical septal, symmetrical, or predominantly involve the distal ventricle[35–37] (Figure 16.2).

Colour Doppler flow mapping is a sensitive investigation for detecting left ventricular outflow tract turbulence and, when combined with continuous-wave Doppler studies, the peak velocity in the left ventricular outflow tract can be measured and, by using the modified Bernoulli equation, a value for the pressure gradient can be calculated which correlates well with those measured at cardiac catheterization.[38,39] When the outflow tract gradient is greater than 30 mm Hg then systolic anterior motion of the mitral valve is usually present. This is best demonstrated on M-mode recordings.[40,41] Associated echocardiographic findings include premature closure and fluttering of the aortic valve. Doppler evidence of mitral regurgitation, which can be severe, may also be present.

Cardiac catheterization and angiography is now seldom required for pressure measurements and assessment of left ventricular function, having been supplanted with modern echocardiographic techniques. Occasionally, invasive haemodynamic data may be helpful in refractory cases and particularly in attempting to assess the degree of mitral regurgitation. Coronary arteriography is still needed to evaluate chest pain, particularly in elder patients who may have coexistent atherosclerotic coronary artery disease.

Thus history, physical examination and simple non-invasive investigations may help to distinguish hypertrophic cardiomyopathy from other causes of left ventricular hypertrophy. The overlap with left ventricular hypertrophy secondary to athletic training is particularly significant, as hypertrophic cardiomyopathy is the most frequent cause of sudden cardiac death in young people participating in active sporting activities. Highly trained athletes demonstrate an upward shift of 3 mm in the bell-shaped distribution curve of left ventricular dimensions.[37] In such cases the overall context, including family history and symptomatology, are critical in making any final decision about diagnosis.

In establishing the diagnosis in children it should be noted that hypertrophy may develop during adolescent growth spurts.[42] Therefore it is wise to scan children every 5 years until puberty has been attained before finally committing to a diagnosis. Such progression of hypertrophy is not seen in adults.[43,44]

## Genetics

Simple genetic studies rapidly established that hypertrophic cardiomyopathy is usually familial and is transmitted in a pattern consistent with an autosomal dominant trait.[45] Retrospective clinical genetic studies suggested that approximately 55 per cent of cases were familial, with the remainder representing apparently sporadic new mutations. Detailed pedigree analysis and molecular genetic analysis suggests that an even greater percentage of cases are familial. Molecular genetic studies have demonstrated linkage of familial hypertrophic cardiomyopathy to the cardiac myosin heavy-chain genes on chromosome 14 in some but not all families, indicating genetic heterogeneity. Different mutations in the beta cardiac myosin heavy-chain mutation were initially identified in three affected families.[46,47] Subsequent work has extended the range of mutations documented in hypertrophic cardiomyopathy and correlated individual mutations with clinical outcome. Major structural abnormalities of the cardiac myosin heavy-chain genes are not a common cause of hypertrophic cardiomyopathy, and therefore molecular genetic techniques have been employed to identify point mutations affecting individual amino acids. In 12 of 25 families, seven different mutations of the beta cardiac myosin heavy-chain gene were identified.[6] These mutations are all mis-sense mutations involving single amino acid substitutions. In six of these mutations the charge of the substituted amino acid was altered, and this cohort of patients had a significantly shorter life expectancy compared to patients with the seventh mutation, which did not result in a change in the charge of the substituted amino acid. Patients with differing mutations did not have distinctive morphological or symptomatic manifestations of the condition.

## Difficulties in management of patients with refractory symptoms

Patients with hypertrophic cardiomyopathy require therapy for dyspnoea, angina pectoris and arrhythmias.

In the majority the natural history of the condition is one of slow progression of the symptoms with a high superimposed incidence of sudden death, which frequently occurs in those patients whose symptoms are mild, or who are asymptomatic.[48] Progression of symptoms seldom causes a limitation of lifestyle, although those who are severely symptomatic at the time of presentation have a poor prognosis from progressive impairment of left ventricular function. In addition, there is a further small subset (about 5 per cent) with a poor prognosis, who display progressive left ventricular wall thinning, possibly as a consequence of chronic subendocardial ischaemia, with deteriorating left ventricular systolic and/or diastolic function.[49] The former may experience a mild increase in end-diastolic dimensions but frank dilatation of the left ventricle is very rare.[44] Progressive impairment of diastolic function may lead to a picture resembling restrictive cardiomyopathy, with grossly enlarged atria and right heart failure with relatively preserved systolic function.

Dyspnoea is the commonest symptom in hypertrophic cardiomyopathy and is often attributed to the presence of a left ventricular outflow tract gradient. Braunwald's early clinical study, however, showed that there was no relationship between the presence or severity of a gradient and the patient's symptom status.[4] In Wigle's experience, however, the symptom status of those patients who have genuine obstruction to ventricular ejection (greater than 50 per cent of stroke volume in the ventricle at the onset of the gradient) is related to the severity of the gradient.[50] Many workers have demonstrated that pharmacological or surgical reduction of the outflow tract gradient in patients with obstruction does improve symptoms and exercise tolerance.[51] Rarely, dyspnoea may be associated with severe mitral regurgitation; mitral valve replacement is obviously appropriate in such patients. Careful angiographic and Doppler echocardiographic assessment of mitral regurgitation is necessary before proceeding to surgery; an elevated pulmonary capillary wedge pressure with a prominent 'v' wave may be seen in the absence of severe regurgitation, if the atria are themselves diseased and non-compliant.

Left ventricular hypertrophy, ischaemia, mitral regurgitation, obstruction to ventricular ejection and cellular disarray with associated fibrosis all contribute to impaired diastolic function and dyspnoea. It is seldom possible to identify a single cause of dyspnoea in any individual patient.

The mainstays of pharmacological therapy for dyspnoea are the beta-adrenergic blocking agents, of which greatest experience has been gained with propranolol and the calcium antagonists, notably verapamil.[7,8]

Propranolol slows the heart rate at rest and blunts the rate response to exercise, thereby reducing myocardial oxygen demand. By slowing the heart rate, propranolol prolongs diastole. It is also claimed to improve compliance, and may reduce left ventricular end-diastolic pressure. By virtue of its negative inotropism, propranolol can also reduce hyperdynamic systolic function and outflow tract gradients. There are no good controlled data on the effect of propranolol on mortality, although one non-randomized trial using very high doses of the drug showed good symptomatic control and no mortality over a 5-year period.[8] Our own experience suggests that while propranolol is a useful drug for the control of symptoms, it does not prevent sudden death.[2,48] Nevertheless, propranolol is usually well tolerated and its safety record is good.

Overall, the experience with calcium antagonists is less than with propranolol.[52] The effects of verapamil are similar to those of propranolol, although the mode of action is different. Like propranolol, verapamil slows the heart rate and exerts a negative inotropic effect. Its use is associated with increased exercise capacity, and with improved diastolic function (measured by radionuclide indices).[53] It can produce a significantly greater reduction in outflow tract gradient and left ventricular end-diastolic pressure than propranolol.[54] There is no evidence that verapamil can improve the prognosis of the condition, and indeed its use can be associated with serious complications.[55] It can suppress impulse formation in the sinus node and adversely affect conduction through the atrioventricular node. It has been associated with the development of complete heart block in patients with pre-existing, but unsuspected, conduction disease. The combination of conduction disturbance, negative inotropism and vasodilatory properties has caused pulmonary oedema and death in some patients. Use of nifedipine has been disappointing, primarily owing to its significant vasodilator properties. Diltiazem would appear to behave in a similar way to verapamil.

When choosing between them, propranolol is the safer drug, but patients with severe or refractory symptoms may not respond to propranolol. Though verapamil may be effective in this group, it is precisely these patients who are most at risk from its adverse effects. In such cases therapy with verapamil should be initiated in hospital.

Surgery offers another therapeutic option. The most common procedure is the removal of a segment of the upper anterior septum (myectomy), usually via a transaortic approach, although a transventricular approach has also been used. There is no doubt that myectomy can significantly improve symptoms in carefully selected patients, usually with basal septal hypertrophy, large resting gradients, true obstruction to left ventricular systole and symptoms refractory to medical therapy, but abolition of the outflow tract gradient is not necessarily the explanation of its success.[10,51] Surgery has a perioperative mortality of 5–10 per cent, even in the most experienced hands. The transventricular approach carries a higher risk of late death due to cardiac failure. A recent report of the use of intraoperative echocardiography to direct surgery suggests that the perioperative mortality can be reduced by echo-guided myectomy.[51] Mitral valve replacement has also been advocated in some patients. Good results have been obtained in the relatively small number of patients whose condition is complicated by severe mitral regurgitation.

Where possible, therapy should be chosen to treat specific symptoms. When dyspnoea is the dominant symptom in patients who show slow filling throughout diastole, prolongation of the filling time by slowing the heart rate, with either propranolol or verapamil, is appropriate. Conversely, those who show a 'restrictive' pattern of diastolic dysfunction, with rapid early filling, probably benefit from a relative tachycardia. In such patients negatively chronotropic agents should be avoided, while the role of beta-blockers with intrinsic sympathomimetic activity (ISA) should be investigated. In those patients who are dyspnoeic in relation to definite outflow tract obstruction (50 per cent or more of the left ventricular stroke volume within the ventricular cavity at the onset of the gradient), very high dose verapamil may be effective in reducing both the degree of obstruction and the symptoms. If this fails, myectomy may be worthwhile.

Angina may dominate the symptomatic presentation and is treated with beta-blockers or verapamil, although high doses may be required. Conventional coronary artery bypass grafting gives excellent results for obstructive coronary disease,[56] but myectomy may be required if hypertrophy and obstruction are thought to be responsible for myocardial ischaemia.

Sustained ventricular arrhythmias are rare in clinical practice.[30] The most common supraventricular arrhythmia is atrial fibrillation, which may be paroxysmal or established. Efforts should be made to restore sinus rhythm with DC cardioversion with or without the pharmacological background of amiodarone, but excellent symptomatic relief can be obtained with adequate control of ventricular rate with atrioventricular nodal blocking drugs or amiodarone. Atrial fibrillation carries a risk of embolization and such patients should be formally anticoagulated.

Intolerance or refractoriness to pharmacological therapy combined with the high morbidity from surgery has prompted consideration of alternative therapeutic approaches. Atrioventricular sequential pacing with a short programmed AV delay has been reported to be an effective treatment modality, with reductions in left ventricular outflow tract gradients, decreased filling pressures and improved treadmill exercise times, such improvement being maintained for up to 24 months.[11–13] The atrioventricular delay is deliberately shortened in order to ensure that the ventricle is always paced and hence always undergoes abnormal activation with a left bundle branch block pattern of activation on the surface electrocardiogram.

The precise pathophysiological mechanisms for improvement with pacing in this manner remain uncertain. The abnormal ventricular activation pattern consequent on ventricular stimulation at the right ventricular apex gives rise to paradoxical septal motion and may widen the left ventricular outflow tract and lessen Venturi forces, with consequent reduction in the gradient. Alternatively, the abnormal activation may reduce the total forces of left ventricular contraction, with consequent gradient reduction. Preliminary information suggests that DDD pacing may also improve diastolic filling of the left ventricle, and that this may help explain the subjective and objective improvements seen.[57]

Kappenberger has studied the effects of various pacing modes (AAI, VVI, VAT and DDD) in combination with a variety of atrioventricular delays in a small series of patients with hypertrophic cardiomyopathy and concludes that optimal haemodynamics occur when right ventricular stimulation is synchronized with atrial contraction such that the left ventricular apex is activated before the septum bulges (apical pre-excitation). This group has also followed patients with hypertrophic cardiomyopathy treated with permanent pacemaker implantation for up to 62 months and shown long-term symptomatic benefit, although the numbers are small.[13,58]

Fananapazir has studied the effects of DDD pacing in patients with hypertrophic cardiomyopathy and has shown significant reduction in outflow tract gradients, improvement in treadmill exercise times, improved NYHA functional class and improved symptomatology.[12] Interestingly, this group has also documented improvement in patients with hypertrophic cardiomyopathy without outflow tract gradients and sustained symptomatic improvement on discontinuing pacing. Pacing has also been associated with reductions in surface ECG voltages, suggesting a possible change in the mechanical function of the myocardium consequent on the abnormal activation sequence.[59,60]

The importance of chronotropic incompetence as a limiting factor in exercise capacity has only recently become apparent. Many patients who require pacing for sinus node disease also have important chronotropic incompetence. Such patients have been shown to benefit objectively and subjectively from DDDR pacing as compared to DDD pacing and the use of this mode is becoming more widespread.[61] A subgroup of patients with hypertrophic cardiomyopathy have been shown to be chronotropically incompetent at maximal and submaximal exercise using the above definitions and Wilkoff's formula for assessment of chronotropic incompetence at submaximal exercise.[62] Such patients have reduced exercise capacity as measured by $VO_2$max exercise testing when compared to patients with intact chronotropic response.[63] The variable of chronotropic incompetence has not been previously evaluated in assessing the effects of permanent pacemaker therapy in hypertrophic cardiomyopathy. It may well be that much improvement in symptomatic status can be gained by correction of chronotropic incompetence with rate-responsive pacing without recourse to non-physiological atrioventricular delay.

Permanent pacing would appear to offer an alternative to current therapeutic options but much work is needed to establish the precise mechanisms of benefit in order that patient selection can be optimized.

# Difficulties in risk assessment

One of the main aims in assessing patients with hypertrophic cardiomyopathy is the stratification of risk for sudden death. It rapidly became evident that certain families have a malignant pedigree with a high incidence of sudden cardiac death.[23] The recent genetic discoveries described above offer a potential basis to explain such families.

Young patients present a particular problem, with the highest incidence of sudden cardiac death. Syncope and a malignant family history of hypertrophic cardiomyopathy and sudden death are specific but relatively insensitive predictors of sudden death.[23,64] In older patients the presence of non-sustained ventricular tachycardia on Holter monitoring adds to risk stratification but is still only weakly predictive of subsequent sudden cardiac death.[27]

Gross anatomical morphology and symptomatic status do not predict future sudden cardiac death. The importance of the characteristic histological feature of hypertrophic cardiomyopathy, myocardial disarray,[15] would seem to be established. Myocyte disarray associated with an excess of loose connective tissue is quantitatively different in hypertrophic cardiomyopathy from the appearances seen in other forms of hypertrophy. The disorganized muscle bundles have a characteristic whorled pattern on light microscopy. Ultrastructural examination by electron microscopy has demonstrated that there is also disorganization of the myofibrils within individual cells (Figure 16.3).

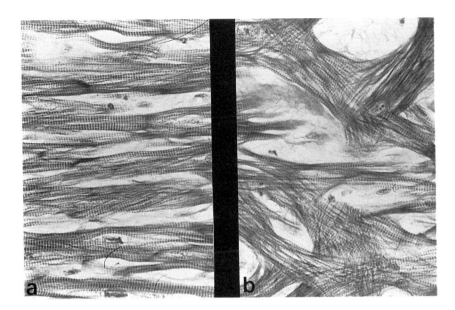

**Figure 16.3**
*(a) Normal myocardial cellular architecture. (b) Disordered myocardial architecture demonstrating myocardial disarray— the histological hallmark of hypertrophic cardiomyopathy.*

One of the clinical consequences of myocyte disarray is electrical instability of the heart, which may be relevant in the pathogenesis of sudden death. In addition, the cellular disorganization may contribute to the abnormalities of ventricular diastolic function.

The extent of disarray would seem to be associated with risk of sudden cardiac death. Patients with restrictive physiology, in whom examination of the explanted heart showed myocyte disarray in the absence of hypertrophy, have been described.[18] There is greater cellular disarray in the hearts of adolescents who die suddenly than in adults who die suddenly. Disarray is least in adults who die from other causes.[48,65] Until recently no quantitation of myocardial disarray or its effect on electrophysiological parameters of conduction has been available.

# Non-invasive risk stratification

## Holter monitoring

Non-sustained ventricular tachycardia is seen on Holter monitoring in approximately 25 per cent of patients with hypertrophic cardiomyopathy, and the presence of such episodes on Holter monitoring carries a seven-fold increase risk of sudden cardiac death.[27,66,67] Such arrhythmias appear to be clinically benign. Attacks are almost invariably asymptomatic, occurring at night or during periods of predominant vagal tone. The ventricular rate is usually relatively slow (mean heart rate 140 beats/min in one series of 400 episodes in 52 patients). Analysis of different episodes in the same patient shows multiple morphologies, suggesting multiple origins, in keeping with the diffuse histopathological nature of the disease. The presence of such arrhythmias is the best readily available marker of increased risk of sudden cardiac death in the adult patient. The negative predictive accuracy is high (97 per cent) but the positive predictive accuracy is low (23 per cent), reflecting the fact that the majority of patients with non-sustained ventricular tachycardia on Holter do not die during short-term follow-up. The arrhythmias may be suppressed and the risk of sudden cardiac death diminished with low-dose amiodarone therapy.[68]

## Abnormal exercise haemodynamics

A significant proportion of sudden deaths in hypertrophic cardiomyopathy occur during or immediately after a period of exertion.[69] Such sudden deaths may not be associated with arrhythmias. Exertional syncope is an important symptom and, as mentioned above, carries an increased risk of sudden cardiac death. Classically, exertional syncope in hypertrophic cardiomyopathy was thought to be due to true obstruction to left ventricular outflow in a manner akin to aortic stenosis. The occurrence of exertional syncope in patients without such gradients even with pharmacological provocation and the finding of exercise hypotension despite a normal increase in cardiac output has forced a revision of opinion.

One hundred and twenty-nine consecutive patients with hypertrophic cardiomyopthy were studied to evaluate the response of blood pressure to exercise.[70] Distinctly differing patterns of response were observed. The normal response to exercise, with a steady rise in blood pressure on exercise and a steady fall on recovery, was seen in 64 patients. Of the remaining patients, 5 showed a continuous fall in blood pressure from the commencement of exercise and 38 showed a dramatic fall from peak values whilst still exercising. A subgroup of 14 patients with exercise hypotension were further studied with invasive haemodynamic measurements. At peak exercise they showed similar cardiac index as compared to 14 controls with a normal blood pressure response but had a significantly lower systemic vascular resistance.

Patients with exercise hypotension had smaller left ventricular end-diastolic dimensions as assessed by echocardiography and had a significantly higher incidence of known risk factors, such as young age and an adverse family history, suggesting the possible importance of haemodynamic instability as a factor in initiating sudden cardiac death. Interestingly, the older patients described symptoms of fatigue, light-headedness and pre-syncope, causing them to discontinue exercise, whilst younger patients, who have a higher incidence of syncope, did not experience such warning symptoms. The failure of this 'early warning' system in the young may be an important determinant of exertional syncope and sudden death.

The abnormal drop in systemic vascular resistance during erect exercise is strongly associated with an inappropriate increase in forearm bloodflow during supine leg exercise. One hundred and three consecutive patients with hypertrophic cardiomyopathy were studied during symptom-limited supine bicycle exercise with forearm bloodflow measurement by plethysmography.[71] The normal response of reduction in forearm bloodflow as seen in 64 patients, as blood was preferentially channelled to the exercising musculature. No change or an increase in forearm bloodflow, suggesting inappropriate peripheral vasomotor control, was observed in 39 patients. Again, the abnormal population had echocardiographic evidence of smaller left ventricular end-diastolic dimensions. This latter group also showed an association with factors suggesting an adverse prognosis, providing further evidence of the possible importance of haemodynamic instability as a risk factor for sudden cardiac death. Further evidence to support this comes from case reports of syncopal episodes without cardiac arrhythmia. One of the authors (WJM) witnessed a syncopal episode in a 52-year-old woman with hypertrophic cardiomyopathy, syncope and frequent non-sustained ventricular tachycardia which occurred during Holter monitoring.[72] After complaining of palpitation and breathlessness the patient rested, but symptoms persisted with disappearance of her left ventricular outflow tract murmur and loss of consciousness. During this syncopal episode peripheral pulses were absent and signs of anoxia developed. Spontaneous recovery occurred. Analysis of the Holter revealed that loss of consciousness developed during sinus tachycardia (130 beats/min) in the absence of arrhythmias and evidence of syncope. The patient has subsequently undertaken exercise testing on a number of occasions with reproducible hypotension but no syncope, although she continues to experience syncope during 'normal' daily life.

## Supraventricular arrhythmias

Paroxysmal supraventricular tachycardia (including paroxysmal atrial fibrillation) may be seen in 30–50 per cent of patients during Holter recording.[73] When such arrhythmias are sustained for any length of time, important haemodynamic consequences may ensue. The acute onset of atrial fibrillation may be poorly tolerated haemodynamically, with rapid deterioration to ventricular fibrillation,[29] or be tolerated with minimal haemodynamic embarrassment.

The variable response to paroxysmal arrhythmias suggests that abnormal haemodynamic responses may be important determinants of outcome to such paroxysmal arrhythmias and may have an important role in the pathogenesis of sudden cardiac death.

The evaluation of blood pressure response to treadmill exercise simultaneously coupled with objective documentation of functional capacity by respiratory gas analysis and assessment of forearm bloodflow response to supine bicycle exercise form an important part of the non-invasive work-up of patients with hypertrophic cardiomyopathy at our institution.

## Electrophysiology

The information gained by the non-invasive tests described above fails to provide specific positive predictive accuracy about risk of sudden cardiac death. The arrhythmogenic substrate, myocardial disarray,[15] has attracted much attention from electrophysiologists in an attempt to determine a specific marker of risk for sudden cardiac death.

## Programmed stimulation

Conventional electrophysiological stimulation techniques attempt to induce arrhythmias for which a substrate, which may be latent, exists. Such studies, whilst demonstrating multiple electrophysiological abnormalities, have failed to provide a specific individual electrophysiological abnormality predictive of sudden death.

In a study of 155 consecutive patients (of whom 145 were placed at increased risk of sudden cardiac death on conventional criteria) undergoing invasive electrophysiological study, multiple electrophysiological abnormalities were documented.[74]

Asymptomatic abnormalities of sinus mode

function and His-Purkinje conduction were found in 66 and 30 per cent respectively. Accessory atrioventricular pathways were present in 5 per cent. Such pathways have been implicated in sudden cardiac death in patients with hypertrophic cardiomyopathy.[75] Atrial tachycardia could be induced in 10 per cent, of whom one-third had Holter evidence of the arrhythmia. Atrial fibrillation was inducible in 55 per cent of patients with documented paroxysmal atrial fibrillation compared to 7 per cent of patients with no previous atrial fibrillation.

A variety of responses to programmed ventricular stimulation were observed. Non-sustained ventricular tachycardia was induced in 14 per cent, sustained monomorphic ventricular tachycardia in 10 per cent and polymorphic ventricular tachycardia/ventricular fibrillation in 32 per cent. It was claimed that the induction of sustained ventricular arrhythmia (polymorphic ventricular tachycardia in the majority of the study patients) is an abnormal finding in hypertrophic cardiomyopathy that may provide a useful guide to therapy. The development of polymorphic ventricular tachycardia/ventricular fibrillation is usually regarded as a non-specific finding without clinical relevance in patients with coronary disease and would be induced in a significant number of normal controls at the levels of stimulation employed. The prognostic significance of the poorly tolerated polymorphic ventricular arrhythmias induced in the majority of patients undergoing conventional programmed stimulation remains uncertain,[76,77] and the induction of such arrhythmias is not used to guide therapy in our institution. Attempts to individually stratify the risk of ventricular fibrillation using programmed stimulation have been unsuccessful and the value of programmed ventricular stimulation must therefore be questioned, as the population

who require risk stratification are usually young and asymptomatic and the procedure is not without risk. Induced polymorphic ventricular arrhythmias may rapidly deteriorate to ventricular fibrillation from which prompt resuscitation is required.

## Electrogram fractionation

An alternative electrophysiological approach to risk stratification aims to record electrophysiological measurements which reflect the underlying myocardial disarray. It is based on the hypothesis that increased myocardial disarray leads to an increased number of possible conduction paths due to variations in fibre length and tortuosity. These different pathways would be expected to conduct with variable velocity on the basis of their physical properties.[78] Thus, non-homogeneous conduction may occur, with pathways recruited or blocked depending on the refractory state of the ventricle. Such dispersion of conduction may form one component of the substrate for re-entry and hence ventricular fibrillation.

The method is based on the analysis of the separate components of paced right ventricular electrograms recorded at multiple right ventricular sites. Such electrograms may contain components due to the individual conduction paths close to the electrodes. The electrograms are recorded during a computer-controlled pacing sequence, with an extra stimulus every third beat which has a gradually decreased coupling interval down to ventricular effective refractory period. With decreasing extra stimulus coupling interval, individual pathways may be blocked or recruited and the presence of such pathways may be inferred by studying the number of components within the recorded electrograms.

Thirty-seven consecutive patients with hypertrophic cardiomyopathy were studied.[17] The

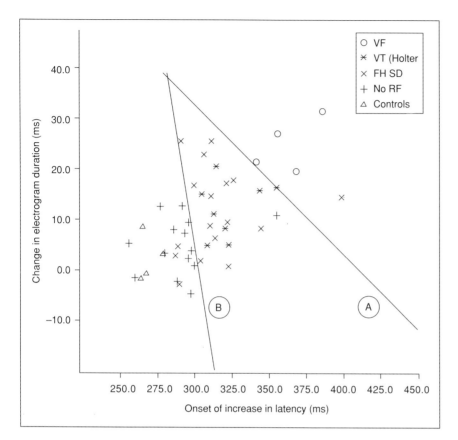

**Figure 16.4**
*Scatter plot of change in electrogram duration against S1–S2 at which latency starts to increase. The discriminant line A separates the patients with ventricular fibrillation (VF) from the remainder (p < 0.0001) and the line B separates the VF, ventricular tachycardia on Holter (VT) and family history of sudden cardiac death patients (FH SD) from low-risk patients (No RF) and controls (p < 10⁻⁶).*

study population included 4 patients who had sustained out-of-hospital cardiac arrest and were assumed or documented as having sustained ventricular fibrillation, 5 patients with non-sustained ventricular tachycardia on Holter, 15 patients with sudden death in a first-degree relative and 13 patients at low risk.

Analysis of the conduction curves generated centred on two variables: (1) the point at which latency began to increase; and (2) the width of the electrogram at ventricular effective refractory period. Normal controls showed an increase in electrogram width and increased latency at short coupling intervals. In contrast, patients who had sustained prior ventricular fibrillation showed early increase in latency, markedly increased electrogram width and increased numbers of transitions. A scatter plot of change of electrogram duration against S1–S2 coupling interval, at which latency increases, produced highly significant discrimination between the patients who had sustained cardiac arrest, who show a marked increase in electrogram width and early increase in latency, and controls and low-risk patients, who demonstrated late increase in latency and a small increase in electrogram width. Patients with familial sudden death and non-sustained ventricular tachycardia formed an intermediate group (Figure 16.4).

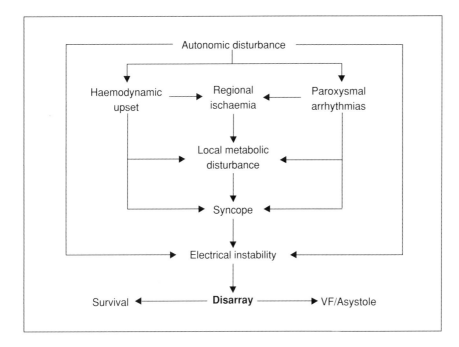

**Figure 16.5**
*Schematic diagram illustrating the interaction between triggering factors and underlying myocardial disarray in the pathogenesis of sudden death in hypertrophic cardiomyopathy.*

The technique requires prospective evaluation but offers for the first time an individual electrophysiological measure that may correlate with the extent of myocardial disarray and hence with the risk of sudden death.

## Difficulties in managing potential sudden cardiac death

### Mechanism of sudden cardiac death

The mechanism of sudden death in this group of patients is complex and is likely to reflect an interaction between numerous trigger factors such as abnormal haemodynamics, paroxysmal ventricular or supraventricular arrhythmias and abnormal autonomic control of the vasculature and an underlying myocardium with a histological substrate for lethal ventricular arrhythmias. The electrical stability of the underlying myocardium is determined by the extent and distribution of myocyte disarray (Figure 16.5). The technique described above, which attempts to quantify disordered conduction, may enable more individualized quantification of risk of sudden death. The majority of cases are thought to terminate in ventricular arrhythmias, although individual case reports have documented complete heart block, asystole, myocardial infarction and supraventricular tachycardia conducted rapidly to the ventricles via the atrioventricular node or by an accessory pathway, as antecedent events.[14,44,48]

Once patients have undergone risk stratification, therapy can be guided on an individualized basis. Conduction disease can be treated with a permanent endocardial pacemaker, left ventricular outflow tract obstruction can be dealt with by surgery or possibly dual chamber pacing with a short AV delay, and paroxysmal supraventricular arrhythmias can be treated with amiodarone. This approach may be successful in about 30 per cent of patients. In the remainder, features suggesting high risk may be present without clear evidence of the underlying mechanism. The management of adult patients with non-sustained ventricular tachycardia, a group with an annual mortality of 8 per cent, clearly falls into this category. Improved survival has been demonstrated with low-dose amiodarone over a number of years and it remains our policy to treat this group thus. Further refinement of the population at high risk may be possible with the use of the technique of electrogram fractionation.

Initially introduced as an anti-anginal agent, amiodarone has a wide spectrum of anti-arrhythmic effects and is a non-competitive sympathetic antagonist.[79] Unfortunately, its use in high doses is associated with a significant incidence of side-effects, ranging from the relatively trivial (corneal deposits) through the troublesome (sleep disturbance and photosensitization) to the life-threatening (pulmonary fibrosis). These adverse effects are generally seen with plasma amiodarone concentrations in excess of 2 mg/l.[80] Fortunately, there is now evidence that the benefit in hypertrophic cardiomyopathy can be obtained with plasma concentrations of <1.5 mg/l, when significant adverse effects are seldom seen.[81] Treatment with low-dose amiodarone significantly improves survival.[68] The mode of action of amiodarone at this low dose, particularly in the absence of sustained spontaneous arrhythmias, is speculative. Prevention of primary arrhythmias, particularly paroxysmal atrial fibrillation and raising the

threshold for ventricular fibrillation, and an effect on the control of peripheral blood flow may all be relevant.

Adult patients who are placed at high risk of sudden cardiac death by non-invasive and electrogram fractionation studies at our institution are placed on low-dose amiodarone.

Unfortunately there is no ideal algorithm for managing young patients. High-risk patients (with a history of out-of-hospital ventricular fibrillation, syncope or an unfavourable family history) need treatment with amiodarone, but they do not represent the majority at risk.[21,82] Those who are asymptomatic, have no arrhythmias on ambulatory monitoring and do not have an adverse family history will seldom receive therapy, although they are still at a significant risk (approximately 4 per cent per annum) of sudden death. The above high-risk group, together with those with marked hypertrophy, large resting gradients or a history of symptomatic arrhythmias, are advised to avoid competitive sport, but such advice often imposes unacceptable limitations on the lifestyle of a young, active patient population.[83]

There is a natural reluctance to commit young patients to an indefinite period of treatment with amiodarone, because of the potential side-effects. Nevertheless, we have seen encouraging results in an uncontrolled study using very low dose amiodarone (plasma concentrations of 0.5 mg/l) in the treatment of a group of high-risk children, with an expected annual mortality from sudden death of at least 8 per cent. There were no deaths over a 3-year period in a cohort of 15 patients.[22] This work needs to be confirmed with larger numbers and a longer period of follow-up.

The use of the automatic implantable cardioverter defibrillator (AICD) at this institution is reserved for those patients who have survived out of hospital ventricular fibrillation and those with refractory ventricular tachycardia. Such an approach is currently at the conservative end of the scale but the role of the AICD in patients with hypertrophic cardiomyopathy remains ill-defined at present. Amiodarone currently remains the mainstay of therapy in attempting to treat risk of sudden cardiac death but the advent of potentially identifiable individual risk together with improvements in implantable defibrillator technology render AICD implantation safer[84] and will maximize its cost-effectiveness.[85]

# If I had ...

If I was diagnosed as having hypertrophic cardiomyopathy I would wish to be evaluated at a major centre with experience in risk stratification and symptomatic management. If not already known, I would construct an extended family tree to document any premature sudden cardiac death which would place me at higher risk. I would be concerned if I was having syncopal episodes. I would have blood taken for molecular genetic studies in order to establish the presence of a mis-sense mutation. I would undergo a full echocardiographic study by an operator experienced in assessing hypertrophic cardiomyopathy to establish the anatomical extent of left ventricular hypertrophy and the extent of any mitral regurgitation, a Doppler assessment of left ventricular filling indices, and the calculation of a resting pressure gradient, if any. I would undergo 48-h Holter monitoring to document the presence of non-sustained ventricular tachycardia. I would undergo treadmill exercise testing with measurement of oxygen consumption and blood pressure to objectively measure functional capacity and document exercise hypotension. I would also undergo plethysmography to assess the forearm bloodflow response to exercise.

If any of the above investigations were abnormal I would undergo an electrophysiological fractionation study as described above. If this study suggested high risk of sudden cardiac death I would take low-dose amiodarone. If I had already sustained out-of-hospital ventricular fibrillation I would consider implantation of an AICD.

If symptomatic from dyspnoea and/or chest pain I would consider taking beta-blockers. If these agents were ineffective or poorly tolerated I would consider verapamil, although I would wish this therapy to be instituted in hospital. If drug therapy was ineffective and I had true obstruction to left ventricular outflow I would consider a myectomy. An alternative would be to consider implantation of a dual chamber permanent pacemaker although I would want to see more evidence that such devices are effective over a chronic period and that the device would be effective in my particular case.

If at high risk and/or symptomatic to the point of requiring drug therapy I would wish continued follow-up at a major centre.

# References

1 Teare RD, Asymmetrical hypertrophy of the heart in young adults, *Br Heart J* (1958) **20**:1–8.

2 McKenna WJ et al, Prognosis in hypertrophic cardiomyopathy. Role of age, and clinical, electrocardiographic and hemodynamic features, *Am J Cardiol* (1981) **47**:532–8.

3 Shapiro LM, Zezulka A, Hypertrophic cardiomyopathy: a common disease with a good prognosis: five year experience of a district general hospital, *Br Heart J* (1983) **50**:530–3.

4 Braunwald E et al, Idiopathic hypertrophic subaortic stenosis. I. Description of the disease based upon an analysis of 64 patients, *Circulation* (1964) **29**(suppl 4):111–19.

5 Jarcho JA et al, Mapping a gene for familial hypertrophic cardiomyopathy to chromosome 14qI, *N Engl J Med* (1989) **321**:1372–8.

6 Watkins H et al, Characteristics and prognostic implications of myosin missense mutations in familial hypertrophic cardiomyopathy, *N Engl J Med* (1992) **326**:1108–14.

7 Frank MJ et al, Long-term medical management of hypertrophic obstructive cardiomyopathy, *Am J Cardiol* (1978) **42**:993–1001.

8 Bonow RO et al, Effects of verapamil on left ventricular systolic function and diastolic filling in patients with hypertrophic cardiomyopathy, *Circulation* (1981) **64**:787–96.

9 Leon MB et al, Amiodarone in patients with hypertrophic cardiomyopathy and refractory cardiac symptoms: an alternative to current medical therapy, *Circulation* (1984) **70**(suppl 2):11–18 (abstr).

10 McIntosh C, Maron BJ, Current operative treatment of obstructive hypertrophic cardiomyopathy, *Circulation* (1988) **78**:487–95.

11 McDonald K et al, Functional assessment of patients treated with permanent dual chamber pacing as a primary treatment for hypertrophic cardiomyopathy, *Eur Heart J* (1988) **9**:893–8.

12 Fananapazir L et al, Impact of dual-chamber permanent pacing in patients with obstructive hypertrophic cardiomyopathy with symptoms refractory to verapamil and beta-adrenergic therapy, *Circulation* (1992) **85**:2149–61.

13 Jeanrenaud X, Goy J-J, Kappenberger L, Effects of dual-chamber pacing in hypertrophic obstructive cardiomyopathy, *Lancet* (1992) **339**:1318–23.

14 Maron BJ et al, Hypertrophic cardiomyopathy. Interrelations of clinical manifestations, pathophysiology and therapy (two parts), *N Engl J Med* (1987) **316**:780–9, 844–52.

15 Davies MJ, The current status of myocardial disarray in hypertrophic cardiomyopathy, *Br Heart J* (1984) **51**:361–3.

16 Nicod P, Polikar R, Peterson KL, Hypertrophic cardiomyopathy and sudden death, *N Engl J Med* (1988) **318**:1255–7.

17 Saumarez RC et al, Ventricular fibrillation in hypertrophic cardiomyopathy is associated with increased fractionation of paced right ventricular electrograms, *Circulation* (1992) **86**:467–74.

18 McKenna WJ, Nihoyannopoulos P, Davies MJ, Hypertrophic cardiomyopathy without hypertrophy: a description of 2 families with premature cardiac death and myocardial disarray in the absence of increased muscle mass, *Br Heart J* (1989) **61**:75.

19 Maron BJ et al, Hypertrophic cardiomyopathy in infants: clinical features and natural history, *Circulation* (1982) **65**:7–17.

20 Frenneaux MP et al, Abnormal blood pressure response during exercise in hypertrophic cardiomyopathy, *Circulation* (1990) **82**:1995–2002.

21 Cannon RO et al, Myocardial ischemia in hypertrophic cardiomyopathy: contribution of inadequate vasodilator reserve and elevated left ventricular filling pressures, *Circulation* (1985) **71**:234–43.

22 Loogen F et al, Clinical course and prognosis of patients with typical and atypical hypertrophic obstructive and with hypertrophic non-obstructive cardiomyopathy, *Eur Heart J* (1983) **4**(suppl F):145–53.

23  McKenna WJ et al, Arrhythmia and prognosis in infants, children and adolescents with hypertrophic cardiomyopathy, *J Am Coll Cardiol* (1988) **11**:147–53.

24  Maron BJ et al, 'Malignant' hypertrophic cardiomyopathy: identification of a subgroup of families with unusually frequent premature death, *Am J Cardiol* (1978) **41**:1133–40.

25  Kowey PR, Eisenberg R, Engel TR, Sustained arrhythmias in hypertrophic obstructive cardiomyopathy, *N Engl J Med* (1984) **310**:1566–9.

26  McKenna WJ, Deanfield JE, Hypertrophic cardiomyopathy: an important cause of sudden death, *Arch Dis Childhood* (1984) **59**:971–5.

27  McKenna WJ et al, Arrhythmia in hypertrophic cardiomyopathy: I. Influence on prognosis, *Br Heart J* (1981) **46**:168–72.

28  Robinson K et al, Atrial fibrillation in hypertrophic cardiomyopathy: a longitudinal study, *J Am Coll Cardiol* (1990) **15**:1279–85.

29  Stafford WJ et al, Cardiac arrest in an adolescent with atrial fibrillation and hypertrophic cardiomyopathy, *J Am Coll Cardiol* (1986) **7**:701–4.

30  Alfonso F, Frenneaux M, McKenna WJ, Clinical sustained monomorphic ventricular tachycardia in hypertrophic cardiomyopathy: association with left ventricular apical aneurysm, *Br Heart J* (1989) **61**:178–81.

31  Savage DD et al, Electrocardiographic findings in patients with obstructive and non obstructive hypertrophic cardiomyopathy, *Circulation* (1978) **58**:402–8.

32  Yamaguchi H et al, Hypertrophic cardiomyopathy with giant negative T waves (apical hypertrophy): ventriculographic and echocardiographic features in 30 patients, *Am J Cardiol* (1979) **44**:401–11.

33  Henry WL, Clark CE, Epstein SE, Asymmetric septal hypertrophy: echocardiographic identification of the pathognomonic anatomic abnormalities of IHSS, *Circulation* (1973) **47**:225–33.

34  Maron BJ, Epstein SE, Hypertrophic cardiomyopathy: recent observations regarding the specificity of three hallmarks of the disease: asymmetric septal hypertrophy, septal disorganisation and systolic anterior motion of the anterior mitral leaflet, *Am J Cardiol* (1980) **45**:141–54.

35  McKenna WJ et al, Echocardiographic measurement of right ventricular wall thickness in hypertrophic cardiomyopathy: relation to clinical and prognostic features, *J Am Coll Cardiol* (1988) **11**:147–53.

36  Maron BJ, Gottdiener JS, Epstein SE, Patterns and significance of distribution of left ventricular hypertrophy in hypertrophic cardiomyopathy: a wide angle, two dimensional echocardiographic study of 125 patients, *Am J Cardiol* (1981) **48**:418–28.

37  Shapiro LM, Kleinebenne A, McKenna WJ, The distribution of left ventricular hypertrophy in hypertrophic cardiomyopathy: comparison to athletes and hypertensives, *Eur Heart J* (1985) **6**:967–74.

38  Maron BJ et al, Dynamic subaortic obstruction in hypertrophic cardiomyopathy: analysis by pulsed Doppler echocardiography, *J Am Coll Cardiol* (1985) **6**:1–15.

39  Yock PG, Hatle L, Popp RL, Patterns and timing of Doppler-detected intracavitary and aortic flow in hypertrophic cardiomyopathy, *J Am Coll Cardiol* (1986) **8**:1047–58.

40  Gilbert BW et al, Hypertrophic cardiomyopathy: subclassification by M mode echocardiography, *Am J Cardiol* (1980) **45**:861–72.

41  Doi Y et al, M-mode echocardiography in hypertrophic cardiomyopathy: diagnostic criteria and prediction of obstruction, *Am J Cardiol* (1980) **45**:6–14.

42  Maron BJ et al, Development and progression of left ventricular hypertrophy in children with hypertrophic cardiomyopathy, *N Engl J Med* (1986) **315**:610–14.

43  Spirito P, Maron BJ, Absence of progression of left ventricular hypertrophy in hypertrophic cardiomyopathy, *J Am Col Cardiol* (1987) **9**:1013–17.

44  McKenna WJ, The natural history of hypertrophic cardiomyopathy. In: Brest AN, Shaver JA, eds. *Cardiovascular clinics* (F.A. Davis Company: Philadelphia 1988) 135–48.

45  Clark CE, Henry WL, Epstein SE, Familial prevalence and genetic transmission of idiopathic hypertrophic subaortic stenosis, *N Engl J Med* (1973) **289**:709–14.

46  Saez LJ et al, Human cardiac myosin heavy chain genes and their linkage in the genome, *Nucleic Acids Res* (1987) **15**:5443–9.

47  Geisterfer-Lowrance AAT et al, A molecular basis for familial hypertrophic cardiomyopathy: a beta cardiac myosin heavy chain missense mutation, *Cell* (1990) **62**:999–1006.

48  McKenna WJ, Goodwin JF, The natural history of hypertrophic cardiomyopathy. In: Harvey P, ed. *Current problems in cardiology*, Vol. VI (Year Book Medical Publishers: Chicago 1981) 5–26.

49  Spirito P et al, Occurrence and significance of progressive left ventricular wall thinning and relative cavity dilatation in patients with hypertrophic cardiomyopathy, *Am J Cardiol* (1987) **60**:123–9.

50  Wigle ED et al, Muscular (hypertrophic) subaortic stenosis (hypertrophic obstructive cardiomyopathy): the evidence for true obstruction to left ventricular outflow, *Postgrad Med J* (1986) **62**:531–6.

51  Maron BJ et al, Long-term clinical course and symptomatic status of patients after operation for hypertrophic subaortic stenosis, *Circulation* (1978) **57**:1205–13.

52  Lorell BH, Use of calcium channel blockers in hypertrophic cardiomyopathy, *Am J Med* (1985) **78**(suppl 2B):43–54.

53  Bonow RO et al, Effects of verapamil on left ventricular systolic function and diastolic filling in patients with hypertrophic cardiomyopathy, *Circulation* (1981) **64**:787–96.

54  Rosing DR et al, Verapamil therapy: a new approach to the pharmacologic treatment of hypertrophic cardiomyopathy. II. Effects on exercise capacity and symptomatic status, *Circulation* (1979) **60**:1208–13.

55  Epstein SE, Rosing DR, Verapamil: its potential for causing serious complications in patients with hypertrophic cardiomyopathy, *Circulation* (1981) **64**:437–41.

56  Cokkinos DV, Krajcer Z, Leachman RD, Coronary artery disease in hypertrophic cardiomyopathy, *Am J Cardiol* (1985) **55**:1437–8.

57  McDonald K et al, Dual chamber pacing improves left ventricular filling in patients with hypertrophic cardiomyopathy, *Eur Heart J* (1989) **10**(suppl):401 (abstr).

58  Kappenberger L et al, apical preexcitation reduces gradient in hypertrophic obstructive cardiomyopathy, *J Am Coll Cardiol* (1992) **19**:225A (abstr).

59  Cannon RO, Fananapazir L, Symptom and exercise benefit of synchronized atrial-ventricular pacing in nonobstructive hypertrophic cardiomyopathy, *Circulation* (1991) **84**(suppl):II-326(abstr).

60  McAreavey T, Epstein N, Fananapazir L, Electrotonic modulation of the QRS/T wave detected by signal-averaged ECG in patients with hypertrophic cardiomyopathy: relation of ECG findings to changes in outflow obstruction due to dual chamber pacing, *Circulation* (1991) **84**(suppl):II-145 (abstr).

61  Jutzy RV et al, Comparison of VVIR, DDD and DDDR pacing, *J Electrophysiol* (1989) **3**:194–201.

62  Wilkoff BL, Corey J, Blackburn G, A mathematical model of the cardiac chronotropic response to exercise, *J Electrophysiol* (1989) **3**:176–80.

63  Slade AKB et al, Chronotropic incompetence in hypertrophic cardiomyopathy and its association with impaired exercise capacity, *J Am Coll Cardiol* (1993) **21**:353A.

64  Fiddler GI et al, Idiopathic hypertrophic subaortic stenosis in the young, *Am J Cardiol* (1978) **42**:793–9.

65  McKenna WJ, Alfonso F, Arrhythmias in the cardiomyopathies and mitral valve prolapse. In: Zipes D, Rowlands D, eds. *Progress in cardiology* (Lea and Febiger: Philadelphia 1988) 59–75.

66  Maron BJ et al, Prognostic significance of 24 hour ambulatory electrocardiographic monitoring in patients with hypertrophic cardiomyopathy. A prospective study, *Am J Cardiol* (1981) **48**:252–7.

67  McKenna WJ, Sudden death in hypertrophic cardiomyopathy: identification of the 'high risk' patient. In: Brugada P, Wellens HJJ, eds. *Cardiac arrhythmias: where to go from here?* (Futura Publishing Co: Mount Kisco, New York 1987) 353–65.

68  McKenna WJ et al, Improved survival with amiodarone in patients with hypertrophic cardiomyopathy and ventricular tachycardia, *Br Heart J* (1985) **53**:412–16.

69  Maron BJ, Roberts WC, Epstein SE, Sudden death in hypertrophic cardiomyopathy: a profile of 78 patients, *Circulation* (1982) **65**:1388–94.

70  Frenneaux MP et al, Abnormal blood pressure response during exercise in hypertrophic cardiomyopathy, *Circulation* (1990) 82:1995–2002.

71  Counihan PJ et al, Abnormal vascular responses to supine exercise in hypertrophic cardiomyopathy, *Circulation* (1991) 84:686–96.

72  McKenna WJ, Harris L, Deanfield J, Syncope in hypertrophic cardiomyopathy, *Br Heart J* (1982) 47:177–9.

73  Savage DD et al, Prevalence of arrhythmia during 24 hour electrocardiographic monitoring and exercise testing in patients with obstructive and non obstructive hypertrophic cardiomyopathy, *Circulation* (1979) 59:866–75.

74  Fananapazir L et al, Electrophysiologic abnormalities in patients with hypertrophic cardiomyopathy: a consecutive analysis in 155 patients, *Circulation* (1989) 80:1259–68.

75  Krikler DM et al, Sudden death in hypertrophic cardiomyopathy: associated accessory atrioventricular pathways, *Br Heart J* (1980) 43:245–51.

76  Kuck K-H et al, Programmed electrical stimulation in hypertrophic cardiomyopathy. Results in patients with and without cardiac arrest or syncope, *Eur Heart J* (1989) 9:1777–85.

77  Fananapazir L et al, Prognostic determinants in hypertrophic cardiomyopathy: prospective evaluation of a therapeutic strategy based on clinical, Holter, hemodynamic and electrophysiological findings, *Circulation* (1992) 86:730–40.

78  Noble D, *The initiation of the heartbeat* (Oxford University Press: Oxford 1979).

79  Marcus F et al, Clinical pharmacology and therapeutic applications of the antiarrhythmic agent amiodarone, *Am Heart J* (1981) 101:480–93.

80  Harris L et al, Side effects of long-term amiodarone therapy, *Circulation* (1983) 67:45–51.

81  McKenna WJ et al, Amiodarone for long-term management of hypertrophic cardiomyopathy, *Am J Cardiol* (1984) 54:802–10.

82  McKenna WJ, Alfonso F, Arrhythmias in the cardiomyopathies and mitral valve prolapse. In: Zipes D, Rowlands D, eds. *Progress in cardiology* (Lea and Febiger: Philadelphia 1988) 59–75.

83  Maron BJ et al, Bethesda Conference No 16: 'Cardiovascular Abnormalities in the Athlete: Recommendations regarding eligibility for competition'. Task Force II: Hypertrophic cardiomyopathy and other myopericardial diseases; mitral valve prolapse, *J Am Coll Cardiol* (1985) 6:1215–17.

84  Lindemans FW, van Binsbergen E, Connolly D, European PCD™ Study: Patients with Transvene™ Lead systems. Clinical Evaluation Report, Bakken Research Centre, Maastricht 1991.

85  Anderson MH, Camm AJ, Implications for present and future applications of the implantable cardioverter-defibrillator resulting from the use of a simple model of cost efficacy, *Br Heart J* (1993) 69:83–92.

# 17

# Interventional cardiology in children

*Shakeel A Qureshi*

## Introduction

The pulmonary valve, whether or not as important haemodynamically as the other valves, has played a major part in the developments in paediatric cardiology. Over 40 years ago Brock[1] reported on the technique of closed surgical valvotomy for pulmonary valve stenosis. He later used the technique successfully for palliation of patients with tetralogy of Fallot. Since then it has become traditional that most patients requiring palliation or correction of congenital heart defects are treated surgically. However, within a few years of the publication of Brock's report, Rubio-Alvarez et al[2,3] described the technique of non-surgical pulmonary valvotomy using a catheter-mounted guidewire. Despite this innovation, no further progress was made in transcatheter techniques from the 1950s until the early 1980s, when experimental work with balloon dilation led to transcatheter treatment of pulmonary valve stenosis.[4] In between these dormant years, Rashkind and Miller tried to stimulate interest in transcatheter treatment when they reported the technique of balloon atrial septostomy[5] in 1966. It is in the last 10 years that transcatheter treatment has developed at an astonishing pace and interventional techniques have become established in the practice of paediatric cardiology. Some of these treatments have become universally accepted whilst others remain controversial and experimental.

The catheter-mounted balloons had to be collapsible, non-distensible envelopes of a predetermined size and geometry so that, when inflated, they exerted outward force against any structures that pressed against them. The inflation of the balloon thus produced a limited injury on the deforming structure, e.g. an arterial stenosis. Progress in the angioplasty equipment and in the use of the techniques in paediatric cardiology was delayed in part by the technical challenges in manufacturing small-sized and small-profile catheters and in part by the manufacturers' much larger interest in promoting the transcatheter techniques to adult cardiologists. During the same period, transcatheter embolization of vascular abnormalities gradually secured a place for itself in paediatric cardiology. A variety of devices were used, including plastic spheres,[6] microspheres and gelfoam particles,[7] tissue adhesives,[8] metal coils[9] and detachable balloons.[7,10] Just as the pulmonary valve was the 'guinea pig' for the development of surgical and non-surgical valvotomy techniques, the patent arterial duct has played a similar role in the hands of both the surgeons and the cardiologists. As long ago as 1967, Porstmann et al reported a transcatheter technique for the closure of the arterial duct.[11] Because of the large size of the equipment needing to be introduced through the femoral artery, this technique was applicable only to adolescents and adults. It was Rashkind who developed a device for closing the arterial duct by a transcatheter technique that could be used even in small children.[12]

There are two main types of transcatheter treatments that can be undertaken in the cardiac catheterization laboratory—valve and vessel dilation (valvoplasty and angioplasty) and vessel occlusion (embolization). In some congenital heart defects, such as pulmonary valve stenosis, these techniques have become accepted as the initial treatment of choice and have replaced surgery, whilst in others, such as aortic coarctation, their role is still under evaluation.

# Balloon valvoplasty and angioplasty

Balloon valvoplasty and angioplasty has been performed for pulmonary valve and pulmonary artery stenosis, aortic valve stenosis, aortic coarctation and postoperative aortic recoarctation. In addition, attempts have been made to relieve systemic and pulmonary venous stenoses, to treat subvalvar aortic stenosis and to palliate the tetralogy of Fallot.

## Pulmonary valve stenosis

Since the first report of balloon valvoplasty for congenital pulmonary valve stenosis by Kan et al,[4] extensive experience has been gained with this procedure worldwide. Since those early days, the technique has been refined partly with experience but mainly because of improved equipment. In modern practice, cardiac catheterization is no longer needed to make the diagnosis of pulmonary valve stenosis or to assess its severity, because Doppler echocardiography provides that information. Cardiac catheterization is only indicated to measure the size of the pulmonary valve

annulus and the right ventricular pressure prior to balloon dilation. At any age, a right ventricular systolic pressure in excess of 60 mm Hg and a transvalvar gradient greater than 35 mm Hg are accepted as the levels at which valvoplasty is performed. In neonates and small infants, in whom the systemic arterial pressure may only be in the region of 60–70 mm Hg, these indications have to be modified. In these a right ventricular pressure about about 60–70 per cent of the systemic arterial systolic pressure is an indication for valvoplasty.

A brief description of the technique of balloon pulmonary valvoplasty follows. Prior to the valvoplasty a right ventricular angiogram is performed in the lateral and, if available, antero-posterior projections, and the pulmonary valve annulus is measured in the lateral projection (Figure 17.1) using the external diameter of the catheter to correct for magnification. The valve is crossed using a guidewire, which is then positioned securely in the periphery of either pulmonary artery, preferably in one of the lower lobe pulmonary arteries. The balloon selected for the dilation is usually 20–30 per cent larger than the pulmonary valve annulus. The balloon catheter is introduced through the femoral vein and advanced over the guidewire. Modern very low profile valvoplasty (such as Tyshak balloon catheters, Numed Inc., Hopkinton, New York, USA, such as that shown in Figure 17.2) balloons can now be introduced through the introducer sheaths already inserted in the vessels, and this causes less trauma to the vessels than if the balloon were passed directly into the vessel over the wire. The balloon is sited with its centre portion at the level of the stenosed valve; it is then inflated with dilute contrast medium to the pressure recommended by the manufacturer. The inflation and deflation cycle has to be kept at less than 20 s for haemodynamic stability. With maximum inflation the indentation on the

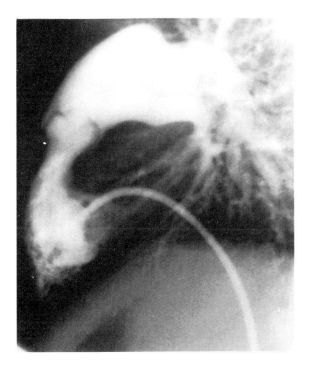

**Figure 17.1**
*A right ventricular angiogram in the lateral projection. The pulmonary valve is doming and stenotic. The pulmonary valve annulus is measured at the points of attachment of the valve leaflets.*

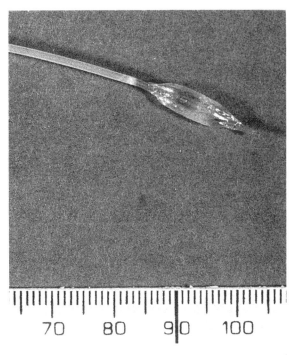

**Figure 17.2**
*A low-profile balloon valvoplasty catheter (Tyshak, Numed Inc., Hopkinton, New York). This example is one of a 5-mm-diameter balloon with a 4 Fr profile.*

balloon should disappear for an adequate valvoplasty to have been performed (Figure 17.3). If the balloon is correctly positioned, only one inflation is enough, but occasionally three or four may be required to ensure correct position of the balloon. The balloon catheter is removed, with the guidewire left in place; the diagnostic catheter is reintroduced over the wire, which is then removed and withdrawal pressures are recorded. After removal of the guidewire and the catheter from the pulmonary artery, no further attempt should be made to cross the dilated site. Usually, repeat right ventricular angiography is not performed because useful information may not be provided.

This procedure is technically much more difficult in the sick neonate with critical duct-dependent pulmonary valve stenosis. Several technical modifications may be needed. A right ventricular angiogram is performed prior to any attempts to cross the valve. A super-floppy steerable guidewire, which can be 0.014, 0.018 or 0.020 inch, is essential to negotiate the

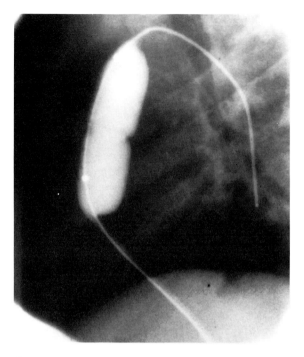 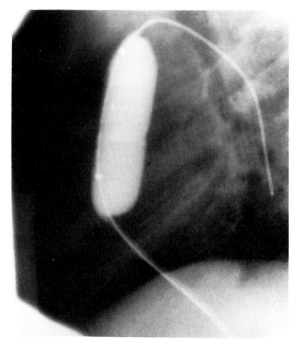

a                                                    b

**Figure 17.3**
*(a) A balloon with a residual indentation at the level of the stenotic pulmonary valve. (b) With increasing pressure, the indentation disappears, indicating a satisfactory valvotomy.*

severely stenosed valve safely. Sometimes, for further security, the tip of the guidewire can be placed in the descending aorta after passing it through the arterial duct. The balloon catheters need to be of the lowest profile for ease of passage across the valve and to minimize the trauma to the femoral vein. For maintaining haemodynamic stability in a patient with tight pin-hole orifice, balloon dilation may have to be performed with gradually increasing sizes of balloons. At the other extreme, in older children or adults with a larger valve annulus,

two balloons have to be used alongside each other through each femoral vein (Figure 17.4).

With this or a similar technique, several groups have reported considerable success in the relief of pulmonary valve stenosis.[13–18] In the VACA Registry, 784 patients had balloon dilation and the gradient was reduced from mean $71 \pm 33$ mm Hg to $28 \pm 21$ mm Hg.[18] The procedure was less effective in those patients with dysplastic valves with or without Noonan's syndrome. The complication rate was low, but was inversely related to age. Fontes et

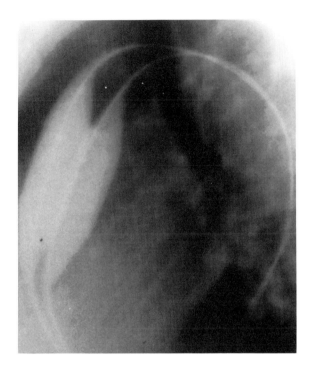

**Figure 17.4**
*Two 15-mm-diameter balloons maximally inflated across the pulmonary valve in an adult with pulmonary valve stenosis.*

al[17] reported the results of follow-up of 100 patients after balloon pulmonary valvoplasty. A significant reduction in the gradient occurred immediately after dilation, and this reduction was sustained at 12 months' follow-up. In a smaller series of 73 patients, we have obtained similar results.[19] The gradient was significantly reduced from a mean (±1 standard deviation) of $63 \pm 24$ mm Hg before to $29 \pm 22$ mm Hg after balloon dilation. In some patients in whom the first procedure is unsuccessful, or there is a late increase in the gradient, either a further balloon

procedure is required or, if the valve is dysplastic, surgery may be needed. Out of the original population, 12 per cent of our patients were referred for surgery. When successful, a sustained reduction in gradient is found both immediately and at review several months after the procedure. In the neonates, balloon dilation is successful in about 70 per cent of the cases,[20] and of these, two-thirds do not need further re-intervention. Several other workers have reported a similar experience. In age- and gradient-matched patients who had balloon dilation or surgery for pulmonary valve stenosis, the results were essentially similar but more severe and more frequent pulmonary regurgitation and lower gradients were noted after surgery and higher residual gradients and less pulmonary regurgitation after balloon dilation.[21,22] In the long term, 86 per cent of 46 patients had gradients less than 36 mm Hg at the latest follow-up and the gradients tended to be higher in those who had balloon dilation at under 2 years of age.[23] In those patients who develop restenosis, the use of larger balloons is effective in reducing the gradient and achieving satisfactory results.[24] These results stand comparison with those reported after surgery. Smolinsky et al[25] reported their results for 38 infants less than 1 year, who had closed pulmonary valvotomy between 1973 and 1989. Twenty-five of these were neonates. The operative mortality was 20 per cent in the neonates and 0 per cent for those between 1 month and 1 year. However, 45 per cent of the patients needed further surgery. In another series of 28 patients under the age of 3 months, the operative mortality from surgery was 25 per cent.[26]

In our experience, when the pulmonary stenosis is relieved by balloon dilation, although an early diastolic murmur may occasionally be heard, there is no significant pulmonary regurgitation or evidence of right ventricular volume overload on Doppler echocardiography. Individual failures occurred because of the use of too small a balloon or when the valve was dysplastic. Undue caution or problems with the original larger balloon profile led to the selection of balloons of the same diameter as, or a little smaller than, the pulmonary valve annulus. These problems are now avoidable because of the availability of lower profile balloon catheters. Occasionally it is impossible in older children or adults to attain the desired balloon size with one catheter. Two balloon catheters can then be introduced alongside each other, over separate guidewires, to achieve the desired size. A second reason for failure of balloon dilation is the dysplastic valve, a valve which is grossly thickened with space-occupying mucoid excrescences on the valve leaflets. This type of valve is not always suitable for balloon valvoplasty. Although some reduction in the gradient may be obtained, failure to achieve a good result should be treated by surgical excision or patch reconstruction of the pulmonary outflow.

The technique of balloon pulmonary valvoplasty is effective and safe not only in newborns, infants and children, but also in adults.[27] It is now the initial treatment of choice for most patients with pulmonary valve stenosis at all ages and, nowadays, no patient with pulmonary valve stenosis should be referred for surgery unless balloon dilation has failed.

## Aortic valve stenosis

Whilst there was no hesitation in clinicians accepting balloon pulmonary valvoplasty, the same view does not apply to congenital aortic valve stenosis. Indeed, some cardiologists and surgeons remain unconvinced about its value. All treatment for congenital aortic stenosis is palliative and, ultimately, aortic valve replacement will be required in the vast majority of the patients. Therefore, there are advantages for the patients if surgery can be delayed.

The basic principles in balloon aortic valvoplasty are similar to those in pulmonary valve stenosis. There are, however, some important differences in the technique. Although Lababidi reported good results of balloon aortic valvoplasty as long ago as 1983,[28,29] his modification of the technique, consisting of venting the left ventricle, by connecting the guidewire lumen of the balloon catheter to that of the venous catheter, was not universally accepted. Instead, it is preferable to leave a loop of the guidewire in the left ventricle to allow more stability of the balloon across the left ventricular outflow tract (Figure 17.5). Sometimes, despite this

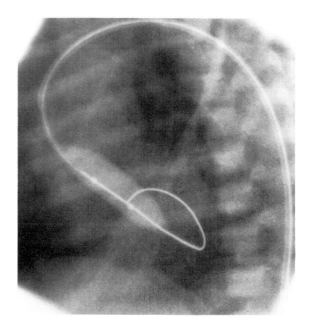

**Figure 17.5**
An inflated balloon across a stenotic aortic valve in an infant. Note the loop of the floppy wire in the left ventricular cavity.

loop, the balloon catheter is ejected out of the left ventricle. Balloon length longer than that commonly used should minimize this problem, although perhaps the only certain way of overcoming it is to use shaped balloons with properties for selective inflation of the distal half of the balloons initially and later complete inflation, such as the Innoue balloon catheters used in mitral valvoplasty. Another difference in technique is in the selection of the balloon size. This should be no larger than the aortic valve annulus measured at the junction of the valve leaflets with the aortic sinuses. Inflation and deflation needs to be even more rapid than in pulmonary valve stenosis.

The indications for balloon dilation in aortic stenosis are not as clear as in pulmonary stenosis. A transvalvar pressure gradient of 50–60 mm Hg at cardiac catheterization is generally considered a suitable level at which to intervene in patients older than 1 year. In younger patients and especially in neonates, the indications are much less clear. In these patients, left ventricular dysfunction can result in relatively low left ventricular pressures and transvalvar gradients despite severe aortic stenosis. Thus, treatment is indicated in symptomatic infants when the stenosis appears severe on cross-sectional echocardiography or angiography, and when no other anatomical cause for the myocardial dysfunction can be found. The major contraindication to the procedure is the presence of severe aortic regurgitation but balloon dilation is not necessarily ruled out by mild regurgitation.

Since the first report by Lababidi,[28] balloon dilation has been considered to be effective in reducing the gradient across the aortic valve. In a large series of patients reported from the VACA Registry, the pre-dilation gradient across the aortic valve was reduced from (mean ± standard deviation) $77 \pm 28$ mm Hg to $30 \pm 14$ mm Hg after balloon dilation, a reduction of about 60 per cent.[30] These results compare well with those achieved after surgical valvotomy.[31,32] Balloon dilation of the aortic valve has its own associated complications in children. These include death,[33] aortic regurgitation and femoral or iliac arterial injury or disruption.[34–36] Severe aortic regurgitation occurs infrequently, and is generally related to the use of oversized balloons. Whilst the results are acceptable in older children, balloon dilation is associated with increased risks and complications in neonates with critical aortic stenosis. However, in this age group, surgery also carries higher risks. Frequently, the main determinants of outcome are the size and function of the left ventricle and the presence of other left heart obstructions.[37,38] In fact, neither balloon dilation nor surgical valvotomy have been shown to be superior to each other.[39] In a comparison of the two types of treatments of neonatal critical aortic stenosis, Zeevi et al[39] demonstrated that the results of balloon dilation were similar to those after surgical valvotomy in their institution. In the past, poor balloon catheter technology resulted in higher incidence of failures of balloon dilation in the neonate, or of arterial damage. New, improved lower profile balloon catheters have increased the chances of a successful procedure and reduced the incidence of vascular damage.[40] In the literature, the mortality after surgery for critical aortic stenosis varies between about 18 and 64 per cent,[39,41,42] whether closed or open aortic valvotomy is performed. The number of patients with neonatal critical aortic stenosis who have undergone balloon dilation is small and, therefore, at present a meaningful comparison with surgery is not possible. However, in a report which pooled the results from the literature, the procedure-related mortality was 13 per cent,[43] but a further 26 per cent of patients died within 4 months of balloon dilation. Severe aortic regurgitation occurred in 7.7 per cent of patients, from cusp perforation or cusp avulsion. A higher percentage of neonates develop aortic restenosis, severe enough to warrant further balloon dilation or surgery, when compared with infants and older children. In contrast, in older infants and children, balloon dilation has not been associated with procedure-related mortality.[43] Aortic regurgitation occurred in 10–41 per cent of patients, but was severe in less than 5 per cent.

The application of balloon dilation has been limited by the complications associated with it, such as femoral arterial injury and cusp perforation or avulsion.[43] Once again, improved technology with the use of modern lower profile balloon catheters, super-floppy steerable guidewires and possible use of the antegrade approach via the femoral vein or retrograde umbilical arterial approach may reduce these complications and make the procedure more acceptable.

Although the long-term results of balloon dilation of the aortic valve are not available, it should be used as a palliative technique, which will usually delay the need for surgical treatment.

## Aortic coarctation and re-coarctation

Aortic coarctation has traditionally been treated by surgery. Various surgical techniques have been employed over the years. These have consisted of patch aortoplasty, resection of the coarctation combined with end-to-end anastomosis, subclavian flap aortoplasty and resection and extended aortoplasty. Various series over the years have reported good results with all these techniques, but complications have been noted also. The operative mortality for all

age groups was between 1.3 and 12 per cent.[44,45] In infants aged less than 1 year at the time of their repair, the operative mortality has varied between 5.1 and 17 per cent.[46–48] The late complications have included hypertension,[45] re-coarctation and aneurysm formation. An increased rate of these complications has been encountered in those patients who had their surgery in the neonatal period or early infancy. Late hypertension may occur in up to 17 per cent of the patients.[45,49] The rate of re-coarctation in infancy (less than 2 years at operation) was between 8.5 and 26 per cent.[46–50] The major risk factor for re-coarctation appears to be low weight at operation.[50] In one large series of neonates, who had resection of the coarctation and extended arch repair, the rate of re-coarctation was 12.5 per cent.[51] A more worrying complication is aneurysm formation. Unfortunately, this complication has not been sought systematically and therefore its reported incidence is usually an underestimate. Malan et al[49] found only two (1.7 per cent) patients with aneurysms in their large series but, unfortunately, the method of detection of aneurysms was by a chest X-ray, a method which is completely unreliable. However, Mendelsohn et al[52] reported a prevalence of aneurysms of 23 per cent after patch aortoplasty in their small series. Even more worrying was the fact that in five out of the six patients, an increase in the size of the aneurysm was noted over a 3–5-year period. False aneurysms such as those that occur after Dacron patch aortoplasty may leak and cause haemoptysis.[53] It seems clear from the literature that all of the current surgical techniques for the repair of aortic coarctation are associated with a significant incidence of all of these complications.

It is against this background of the surgical literature that the results of balloon dilation for native coarctation should be compared.

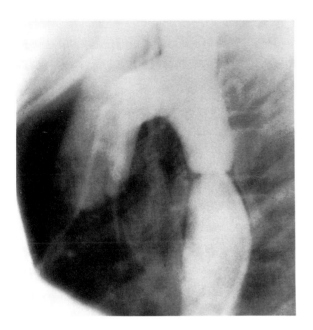

**Figure 17.6**
*An arch aortogram showing a localized coarctation of the aorta.*

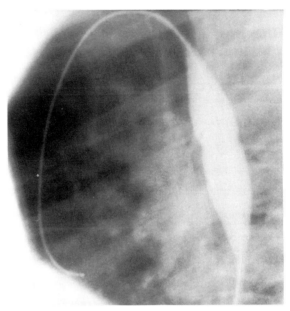

**Figure 17.7**
*The inflated balloon should be no larger than the descending aorta at the level of the diaphragm. Note the indentation on the balloon caused by the coarctation.*

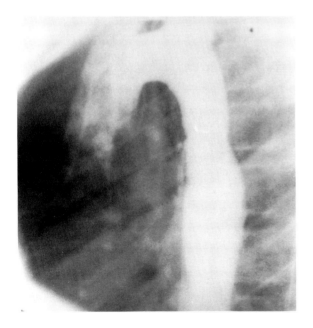

**Figure 17.8**
*Aortogram showing a satisfactory result of balloon dilation of the coarctation.*

Balloon dilation of aortic coarctation was first reported clinically in 1982.[54] Since then its use has waxed and waned. The technique is little different from other angioplasties. After a haemodynamic assessment and diagnostic aortogram have been performed, the required-size balloon catheter is introduced over a guidewire retrogradely via the femoral artery and positioned at the site of the coarctation. The balloon is inflated and deflated in a 15-s cycle, withdrawn and replaced by a catheter through which an aortogram is repeated. The size of the balloon is usually similar to the diameter of the aorta at the level of the diaphragm and certainly no larger (Figures 17.6, 17.7 and 17.8). Early studies of dilation of surgically excised coarctation segment showed that this treatment was feasible,[55,56] but the mechanism of relief of the stenosis is intimal and medial tearing. Good results have been obtained in older children, adolescents and adults.[57,58] These series have included a similar number of patients. In one series, the mean gradient across the coarctation was reduced from $67 \pm 20$ mm Hg to $9 \pm 11$ mm Hg.[58] Re-coarctation occurred in 7.7–13 per cent of the patients and aneurysm formation in 8.7–13 per cent of the patients who had repeat catheterization.[57–59] The most data available are from the VACA Registry report.[60] In this multi-centre report on 140 patients aged between 3 days and 29 years, the immediate haemodynamic results were good. There was, however, one death (a mortality rate of 0.7 per cent) and eight (5.7 per cent) aneurysms were reported. These data suggest that dilation of native coarctations can be performed effectively and safely, but do not establish superiority of this technique over the various surgical techniques. In neonates and infants, the story is even less clear. In 20 neonates and infants, who were less than 1 year old when they had balloon dilation, the gradient was reduced from a mean of $40 \pm 12$ mm Hg to $11 \pm 8$ mm Hg.[61] None of the patients needed immediate surgery. During a short follow-up of a mean of 12 months, no aneurysms were seen but re-coarctation occurred in 31 per cent of patients, some of whom had surgery and others further dilation. This reflects the problem in neonates, which is further highlighted by Redington et al, who reported on dilation of coarctation in 10 consecutive neonates.[62] Two patients with severe isthmus hypoplasia had no change in the gradient, whilst one patient had a technical failure. Thus, good immediate haemodynamic results were obtained in seven patients. In five of these, severe re-coarctation developed between 5 and 12 weeks after dilation. These

authors strongly recommended that balloon dilation should not be performed in neonates with aortic coarctation. However, it seems likely that balloon dilation is effective in aortic coarctation once the arterial duct has closed, but not when it is still patent.

Compared with native coarctation, balloon dilation has become the treatment of choice for postoperative aortic re-coarctation.[63,64] This complication of surgery used to be treated traditionally by reoperation, but in most centres it is now treated by balloon dilation. The technique is the same as that used in balloon dilation of native coarctation. The selection of the balloon size is also similar. In the past, the results have been presented in an inconsistent manner and, at times, decisions and policies have been determined more on emotional grounds than facts. Contribution to the debate is made by variable definitions of successful balloon angioplasty. If strict definitions of a good result are adhered to, as in a recently reported series,[63] then a clearer picture emerges. In this series, a good late haemodynamic result was defined as systemic blood pressure within the normal range for age and absolute residual gradient across the restenosis of less than 20 mm Hg. Fifty-eight per cent of the patients had a sustained good late haemodynamic result and further surgery was needed in only 19 per cent of the patients, the remainder being treated conservatively. Two (8 per cent) patients developed aneurysms after balloon angioplasty, one of these requiring surgery for progressive increase in size of the aneurysm. Aortic arch hypoplasia was the best predictor of a poor late haemodynamic result and the results were influenced by balloon/aortic diameter ratio at the level of the diaphragm. The major concern with this treatment, as in native coarctation, is the development of aneurysms at the site of the angioplasty (Figure 17.9). This complication is

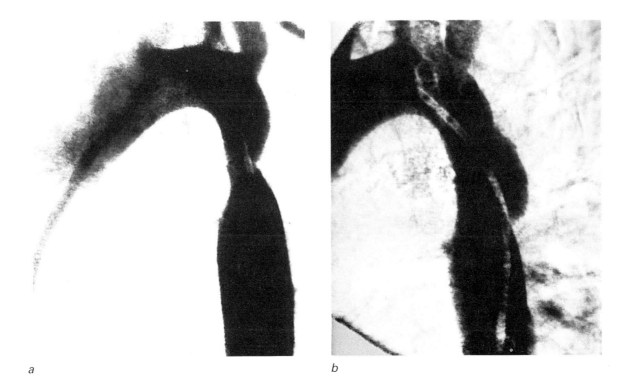

a

b

**Figure 17.9**
Arch aortogram showing a severe coarctation (a)
in a 12-year-old boy. Immediately after balloon
dilation an extensive aneurysm has formed (b).

inherent in the technique of angioplasty and it is difficult to see how it can be avoided. Only time will reveal the significance of this, but to balance it, we have to be aware that various surgical treatments of coarctation are also associated with late aneurysm formation.[65] In the VACA Registry,[64] the results in 200 patients, with an age range of 1 month to 26 years, relief of the pressure gradient was achieved regardless of the type of previous surgery. Overall, 75 per cent of the patients

had good results (defined by a residual pressure gradient of <20 mm Hg). However, there was an important mortality rate of 2.5 per cent (5/200) related to the procedure. All the deaths occurred within 36 h of the procedure, and of major concern is one death due to acute aortic rupture. Death from balloon dilation of aortic re-coarctation has been reported by others also.[66] Other acute complications included small aortic tears, neurological complications (1.5 per cent) and femoral artery injury (9 per cent). From the literature review, it appears as if the only chronic complication of concern, aneurysm formation, has an incidence of about 7 per cent.[67] However, because of the lack of systematic follow-up evaluation, the exact incidence of aneurysm formation remains unknown. Thus, from the available information and until the long-term results are known, balloon dilation is preferable to surgery for aortic re-coarctation, as it does offer satisfactory palliation.

## Balloon dilation of other defects

The value of balloon dilation of other defects is being defined slowly. In the tetralogy of Fallot, dilation of the right ventricular outflow tract has been proposed as an alternative method of palliation to a Blalock–Taussig shunt in those patients, under the age of 1 year, who are considered unsuitable for primary repair.[68–70] The technique is similar to that used in dilation of pulmonary valve stenosis, but usually multiple inflations in different positions across the outflow tract are needed to ensure adequate dilation. Also, the balloon is generally approximately 50 per cent larger than the pulmonary valve annulus. Satisfactory palliation is achieved in over two-thirds of the patients and some of the patients may need repeat balloon dilation. This method will clearly be applicable in those units which have adopted a policy of palliative surgery for tetralogy of Fallot in the first year of life. It has the advantage of avoiding the complications associated with shunt surgery, such as shunt stenosis or occlusion, or shunt-related distortion or stenosis of branch pulmonary arteries. It has to be recognized, however, that whilst the majority of the patients will derive benefit from dilation, some will need early surgery because of inadequate improvement in oxygenation.[70] Other lesions in which balloon dilation has been used with limited success include discrete subaortic stenosis,[71] postoperative systemic and pulmonary venous stenoses[72,73] and congenital or post-surgical branch pulmonary artery stenoses.[74] Of all the clinical situations where balloon dilation is used, pulmonary arteries are the most difficult, with unpredictable results and significant complications. Although the technique is similar to that used in other lesions, the selected balloon is usually four times the stenosis diameter. For the tough lesions, balloons which tolerate high inflation pressures (up to 18 atmospheres) are recommended. Relief of the stenosis is usually accompanied by significant arterial wall damage. Recent results suggest that the technique is successful in about 60 per cent of cases, has a mortality rate of 1 per cent and that there is aneurysm formation in 3 per cent.[75] However, a major problem exists in the interpretation of results reported in the literature, which is made difficult by soft and variable criteria used to define success. Some of these criteria include: an increase in diameter to >50 per cent of the pre-dilation diameter of the pulmonary artery; an increase in blood flow in the affected lung of >20 per cent, and a decrease of >20 per cent in the ratio of systolic pressures in the right ventricle to the aorta.[76] It can be seen that misleading success of the procedure may be reported without normalization of the right ventricular or proximal pulmonary artery pressure. It has occasionally been seen in clinical practice that the pulmonary artery stenosis seems to dilate well, but as soon as the balloon is deflated, it returns to its previous configuration. In pulmonary artery or pulmonary or systemic venous stenoses, evidence is now becoming available that stent implantation may be a better non-surgical technique, and this will be dealt with later in the chapter.

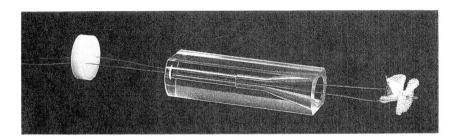

**Figure 17.10**
*The Rashkind double-umbrella occluder ready for attachment to a delivery catheter for closure of the arterial duct.*

# Transcatheter occlusion/embolization

## Patent arterial duct

In most centres in the UK and Europe, patent arterial duct is the commonest vessel to be occluded by transcatheter occlusion techniques. There are two techniques most commonly used. The oldest is the one described by Porstmann et al in 1967, in which an ivalon plug is placed in the arterial duct retrogradely via the femoral artery.[11] The size of the introducing catheter for the ivalon plug limits the use of this technique to adolescents and adults. Much more widely used is the technique of implantation of a double-umbrella device reported by Rashkind and Cuaso in 1979.[77] The device consists of a small metal double-umbrella frame with a single 12-mm or 17-mm polyurethane disc attached to the distal umbrella, which will be sited at the aortic end of the duct. A similar disc is attached to the proximal metal frame and both frames or umbrellas are joined in the middle by a hinge. The proximal umbrella has a small metal eye attached to it at the centre (Figure 17.10), by which it is attached via a kuckle on to the delivery wire. The whole device is loaded inside a pod at the distal end of the delivery catheter. With this method, arterial ducts can now be closed in children weighing as little as 6–7 kg.

The technique consists of positioning of an arterial catheter, via the femoral artery, in the distal aortic arch for the purposes of aortography to delineate the duct anatomy and the landmarks (Figure 17.11). A venous catheter placed in the pulmonary artery is then manipulated through the arterial duct into the

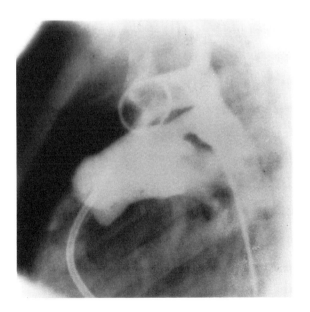

**Figure 17.11**
*An arch aortogram in the lateral projection showing a large patent arterial duct opacifying the pulmonary artery.*

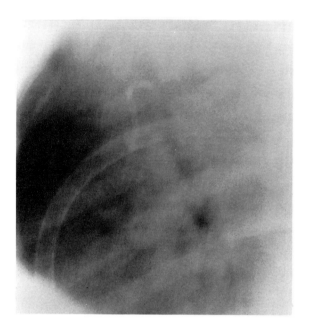

**Figure 17.12**
*A 11 French Mullins trans-septal sheath has been placed via the femoral vein across the arterial duct a short distance into the descending aorta. Through this sheath a 17-mm double-umbrella device can be implanted across the duct.*

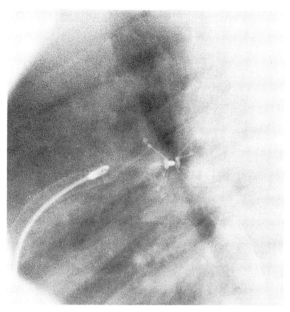

**Figure 17.13**
*Once the position of the umbrella is satisfactory, it can be released from the delivery catheter.*

descending aorta. Using an exchange 0.035-inch guidewire, this catheter is withdrawn and replaced by either an 8 Fr or 11 Fr Mullins trans-septal sheath with its dilator (depending on the size of the arterial duct at its narrowest point). The dilator is withdrawn once the distal end of the sheath has been positioned in the descending aorta a few centimetres from the aortic end of the duct (Figure 17.12). For arterial ducts less than 3 mm in diameter at the narrowest point, a 12-mm umbrella is used, and for ducts larger than this, the 17-mm umbrella device is implanted. With the sheath in position, the umbrella device is pushed carefully out of the sheath until only the distal

umbrella is fully open. The sheath and the device delivery catheter are slowly withdrawn until the hinge point of the umbrellas is at the level of the pulmonary artery end of the duct. The distal umbrella is now engaged in the aortic end of the duct. At this point, the sheath is slowly withdrawn until the proximal umbrella is fully open. Aortography is repeated to ensure correct positioning of the umbrellas, before the release mechanism is actuated (Figure 17.13). The technique has been described in much more detail elsewhere.[78]

Most centres use the double-umbrella device rather than the ivalon plug technique for the closure of the arterial duct. The results have

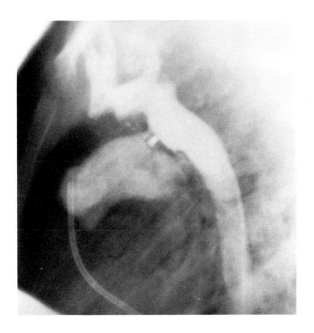

**Figure 17.14**
*An aortogram in the lateral projection showing
significant residual leak past a 17-mm umbrella
device correctly positioned across the arterial
duct.*

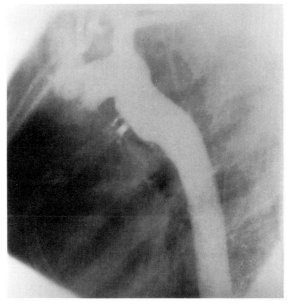

**Figure 17.15**
*An aortogram in the lateral projection showing
complete occlusion of the arterial duct after
implantation of another umbrella device
alongside the first umbrella. The patient is the
same as in Figure 17.14.*

been widely reported over the last few years and
are remarkably similar in all the centres. In a
series of 190 patients in whom the umbrella
device was attempted, the rate of residual shunting was 34 per cent at 1 year, 19 per cent at 2
years and 11 per cent at 40 months.[79] In another
series of 200 patients, complete occlusion of the
duct occurred in 89 per cent of the patients. In
a report of a large series from the European
Registry, 686 patients were entered into the
study and Kaplan–Meier analysis showed
complete occlusion rates of 83 per cent at 1
year.[80] In those patients with significant residual
shunting (Figure 17.14), two umbrella devices
can be implanted alongside each other (Figure

17.15) and this should reduce the incidence of
residual shunts considerably, with actuarial rates
of occlusion rising to 95 per cent at 30 months.[80]
Complications are uncommon.[78,80] Inadvertent
embolization of the device to the pulmonary
artery branches (Figure 17.16) or the descending aorta, haemolysis and endocarditis are the
main complications.[78–80] The devices that have
been inadvertently embolized can be retrieved by
retrieval baskets by transcatheter means (Figure
17.17), thus avoiding surgery. These results
compare favourably with those after surgical
ligation, and those reported worldwide support
the continued use of this technique to close the
patent arterial duct.

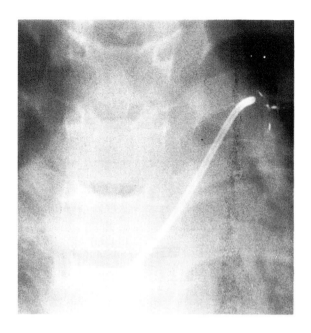

**Figure 17.16**
*The 12-mm umbrella device has embolized to the proximal left pulmonary artery (anteroposterior projection).*

# Atrial and ventricular septal defects

Various other devices are currently under evaluation for closure of atrial and ventricular septal defects. The reason for this is that, quite early on, it became apparent that the double-umbrella device used to close the arterial duct was unsuitable for other defects. The device, which is currently under evaluation in the USA, is also a double-umbrella device, with hinges in the mid-portion of each umbrella arm (i.e. Lock Clamshell Occluder). It is available in diameters ranging between 17 mm and 40 mm. It has been used to close both atrial and ventricular septal defects.[81–83] Other devices are also being investigated. These include the Sideris buttoned double-disc device, which has been used in closure of atrial septal defects.[84] For all of these devices, patient selection seems to be the most important determinant of success of the procedure. For effective closure,

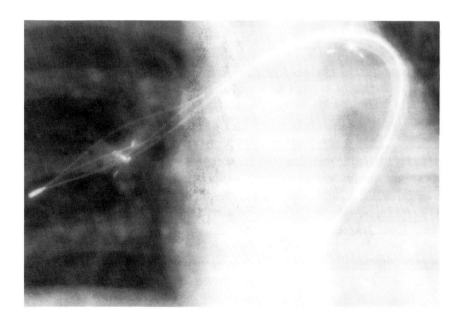

**Figure 17.17**
*Cine frame in the anteroposterior projection shows a 12-mm umbrella device embolized to the right pulmonary artery. The device is being retrieved by a Dotter basket introduced alongside the device through a 11 Fr trans-septal sheath.*

the atrial septal defect must have a complete rim of atrial septum and be far away from the atrioventricular valves and pulmonary veins and, for the fenestrated atrial septal defects, the openings must be close enough for the device to close all the holes when it is implanted through one of them.[82] Deployment and positioning of the device is facilitated by transoesophageal echocardiography. In a multicentre trial in the USA, this device was placed in 400 patients ranging in age between 21 days and 78 years.[85] Implantation was successful in 393 (98 per cent) of the patients and there were complications in 28 (7 per cent) patients. Device embolization was the most frequent complication, necessitating removal by transcatheter means or by surgery. At 1-month follow-up evaluation by Doppler echocardiography, there were small residual leaks in 33 per cent of the patients.

The same device has been used to close muscular or postoperative residual ventricular septal defects or post-myocardial infarction ventricular septal defects.[83] In the UK, the clamshell device has not been available thus far, and so the Rashkind duct umbrella device has been used in some of these clinical situations.[86] At present none of these devices are commercially available. Not all the questions have been answered with regard to the closure of atrial and ventricular septal defects by these devices, and their durability, and there is a long way to go before all the answers do become available.

## Embolization by coils or detachable balloons

Occlusion techniques using materials such as detachable balloons or stainless steel coils via catheters have been employed in closing abnormal vessels such as arteriovenous fistulas, aortopulmonary collateral arteries, or patent Blalock–Taussig shunts.[87,88] On occasions the complexity of the defect may necessitate the simultaneous use of coils and balloons in the same vessel.[89] The commonest indication for transcatheter embolization in congenital heart disease is the presence of aortopulmonary collateral arteries in patients with pulmonary atresia and ventricular septal defect. The other indications are residual patent Blalock–Taussig shunts after previous surgical ligation, congenital coronary artery fistulas and pulmonary arteriovenous malformations. The technique of embolization is similar, but different types of equipment may be needed for different types of vessels, especially taking account of tortuosity of the vessels. The vessel to be embolized is selectively catheterized by a non-tapered guiding catheter and angiography performed to define the landmarks and to determine the position where the occluding device is to be placed. A trial occlusion is often needed with a flow-directed balloon angiographic catheter to assess the effect of temporary occlusion of the vessel on the systemic arterial oxygen saturation. If there is no deterioration, then an appropriate-diameter coil or detachable balloon is selected. In paediatric cardiology practice, stainless steel or platinum coils are generally used, but, rarely, detachable balloons may be needed. The procedure and the equipment have been described in detail in the literature.[89] The coils selected are generally about 20 per cent larger than the artery to be embolized, in order to minimize the possibility of inadvertent embolization to the wrong site. Technical progress has been made with the coils. Currently, a few different types of controlled-delivery coils are under evaluation. These need small guiding catheters (usually 5–6 Fr) for implantation and the coils can be withdrawn, if the position of the coil is not secure, almost at the last second whilst the last

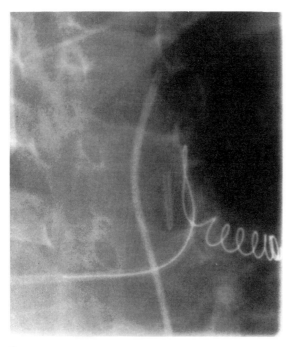

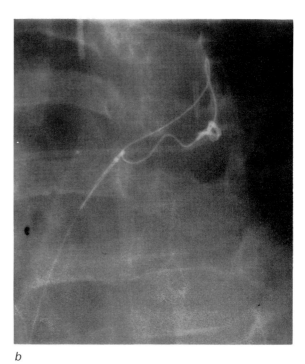

a

b

**Figure 17.18**
*A stainless steel coil inadvertently embolized into the left pulmonary artery during attempted occlusion of left Blalock–Taussig shunt. Part of the coil is still inside the guiding catheter (a) and it cannot be removed safely. With the use of a snaring catheter the coil protruding outside the catheter can be safely trapped and removed (b).*

few millimetres are still inside the guiding catheter. This makes the procedure even safer than previously. Despite this, if a coil is embolized inadvertently, it can be retrieved by transcatheter means with retrieval baskets or snaring catheters (Figure 17.18). Some authors have even used the Rashkind double-umbrella device for occluding a residual patent Blalock–Taussig shunt.[90]

# Miscellaneous techniques

## Laser valvotomy in pulmonary valve atresia

The last two years have seen the development of non-surgical catheter treatments for other complex congenital heart defects which have implications for the future. Surgical treatment

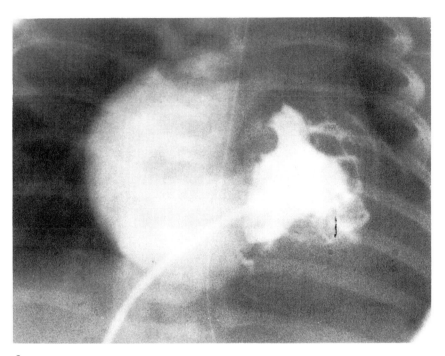

a

**Figure 17.19**
A right ventricular angiogram in a 2-day-old neonate in the anteroposterior (a) and lateral (b) projections. These show valvar pulmonary atresia, with small cavity right ventricle. In (a), moderate tricuspid regurgitation is seen.

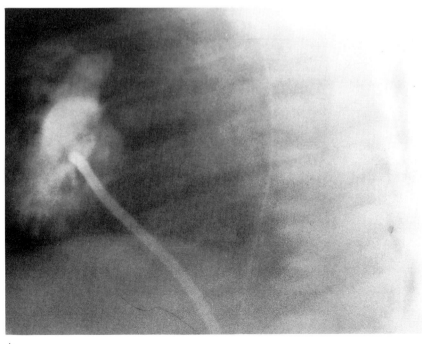

b

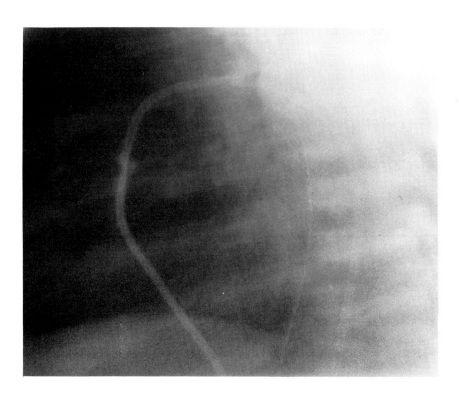

**Figure 17.20**
The venous catheter is passed into the right ventricle and is positioned just below and in contact with the pulmonary valve. The arterial catheter has been passed retrogradely from the aorta through the arterial duct and positioned just above and in contact with the pulmonary valve. This positioning of catheters is essential for defining landmarks prior to laser or radiofrequency valvotomy.

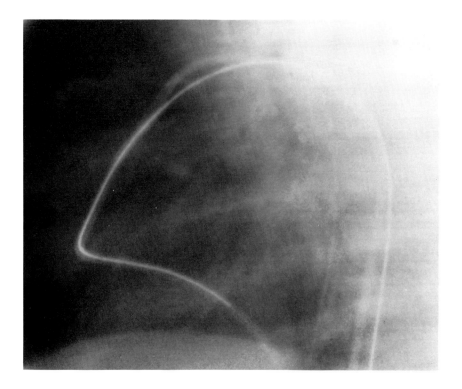

**Figure 17.21**
The laser wire has been passed from the right ventricle through the pulmonary valve and the arterial duct and into the descending aorta.

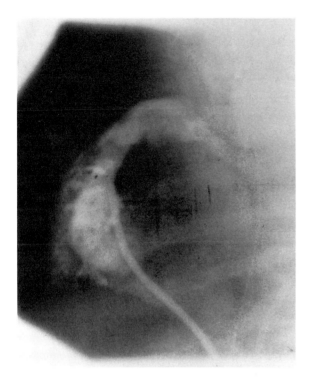

**Figure 17.22**
*Right ventricular angiogram in the lateral projection showing a satisfactory way through a patent pulmonary valve after laser-assisted balloon valvotomy.*

for pulmonary valve atresia with intact ventricular septum is usually performed in two or three stages, consisting of Blalock–Taussig shunt, pulmonary valvotomy or right ventricular outflow tract patch, and final complete repair with closure of the shunt. Laser-assisted pulmonary valvotomy has been proposed as an alternative to surgery for pulmonary valve atresia (Figure 17.19) and has produced acceptable results, especially when it is considered that the learning experience is included in the reporting of the results.[91–93] The technique

consists of positioning a venous catheter just under the pulmonary valve and an arterial catheter, passed through the arterial duct or through a previously constructed shunt, just above the pulmonary valve (Figure 17.20). Once the position and the landmarks have been clearly defined, the laser generator is switched on and energy of about 5 W is delivered for 5 s or until the wire has crossed the pulmonary valve. The wire is usually passed antegradely (Figure 17.21), but occasionally a retrograde approach may have to be considered. Following this, balloon dilation is performed by the conventional methods as for the pulmonary valve in order to remove the obstruction as fully as possible (Figure 17.22). Laser technology is not essential, because we have found that delivery of heat to the tip of the guidewire by radiofrequency energy is equally effective in perforating the atretic pulmonary valve.[93] Can this technique preserve or promote biventricular circulation? The answer is not yet available but the technique has exciting potential.

## Stents in congenital heart disease

Failure of balloon dilation to achieve effective dilation in rigid lesions or those that recoil, or restenose late, after an acceptable initial result stimulated the use of endovascular stents in paediatric cardiology. This was particularly the case in branch pulmonary artery stenoses, whether naturally occurring or post-surgical. Stent implantation has been one of the most important advances in the non-surgical treatment of congenital heart defects in the last few years. The two most frequently used stent types are those that are mounted on a balloon, and those that are self-expanding. Benson et al[94] reported on stent implantation in pigs with experimentally created pulmonary artery stenoses and O'Laughlin et al[95] reported

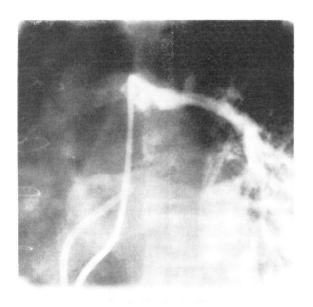

**Figure 17.23**
A left pulmonary angiogram in a long axial
oblique projection in a 6-year-old child. This
shows a severe long segment left pulmonary
artery stenosis discovered after correction of the
tetralogy of Fallot.

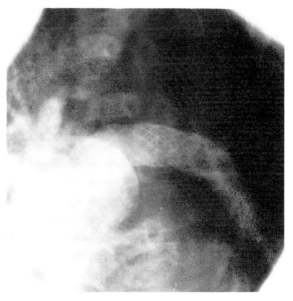

**Figure 17.25**
Left pulmonary angiogram now shows adequate
relief of the stenosed left pulmonary artery after
the implantation of two balloon-expandable
stents.

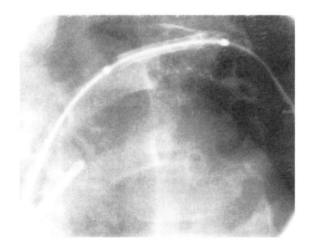

**Figure 17.24**
One balloon-expandable stent already has been
placed across the stenosed left pulmonary artery.
To cover the entire length of the stenotic
segment, another stent is about to be deployed.

encouraging short-term results in 23 patients,
who had 36 stents implanted in stenosed
pulmonary arteries. The technique consists of
haemodynamic and angiographic assessment of
the pulmonary artery stenosis (Figure 17.23).
Usually the lesion is crossed with a 0.035-inch
heavy-duty guidewire, and then a 11 Fr trans-
septal sheath is manoeuvred up to or past the
stenosis. On occasions, prior balloon dilation
of the stenosis with a 6-, 8- or 10-mm balloon
is needed to facilitate the passage and positioning of this sheath. The stent (mounted on a
high-inflation pressure balloon) is then passed

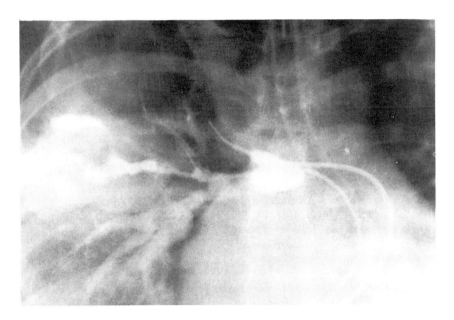

**Figure 17.26**
*Right pulmonary angiogram in the anteroposterior projection in a 22-
year-old girl with multiple peripheral pulmonary artery stenoses. There is
a tear in one of the branches of the right upper lobe pulmonary artery.
Contrast has spilled into the lung parenchyma. A balloon has been
inflated in the proximal right pulmonary artery to control the bleeding,
and subsequently the torn pulmonary artery was successfully occluded
with coils.*

through the sheath and positioned at the appropriate site, and the balloon is inflated to deploy the stent (Figures 17.24 and 17.25). Complications have included tears in the pulmonary artery (Figure 17.26), misplacement of the stent (Figure 17.27), necessitating surgical removal, transient pulmonary oedema, and even death.[95,96] Obstruction of the systemic venous pathways after the Mustard or Senning operations or pulmonary venous obstruction are also amenable to dilation by stents.[95,97] Clearly, in these clinical situations the ideal age for stent implantation is at the time when the

patient has achieved full growth potential. If the stents are implanted earlier than this, they will need to be re-dilated at a later date. An innovative use of stents has been reported by Gibbs et al[98] recently. Stents were implanted to maintain the arterial duct open in two neonates with duct-dependent pulmonary atresia. The technique is certainly much more demanding and there is a strong possibility of misplacement of the stent in the occasionally tortuous duct. This approach is likely to be controversial, as the results will need a comparison with currently available surgical treatments.

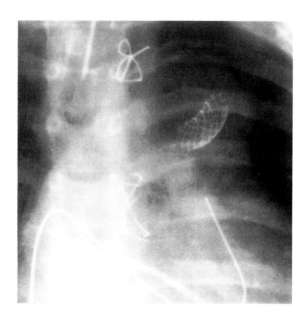

**Figure 17.27**
*Cine frame in the anteroposterior projection of a balloon-expandable stent which had been deployed in the left pulmonary artery. On removal of the balloon, the stent was displaced into the proximal aneurysmal main pulmonary artery. This child had had correction of the tetralogy of Fallot, but was found to have left pulmonary artery stenosis and an aneurysm of the right ventricular outflow tract.*

However, a similar approach of stenting open the arterial duct in the hypoplastic left syndrome as an adjunct to a later cardiac transplantation has much more to offer in the future and is currently under evaluation in a few centres.

There is not much doubt that the development of interventional techniques in congenital heart disease at a remarkable pace has revolutionized paediatric cardiology practice over the last 10 years. When the revolution will end, we know not!

# If my child had ...

If my child was born with moderate or severe pulmonary valve stenosis, there is not much doubt in my mind that I would want balloon dilation to be performed in the first instance, even if the valve appeared dysplastic. This is because in neonates all stenotic pulmonary valves may appear dysplastic, but sustained and good relief of the gradient can be obtained in the majority. If he had mild pulmonary stenosis, with gradient <36 mm Hg, then I would want conservative policy pursued, because there is no evidence of benefit. Even if restenosis occurred, I would want balloon dilation to be repeated. If this did not produce a good gradient relief, then I would prefer a surgical valvotomy.

The decisions are more difficult for aortic stenosis. If my child presented in the neonatal period with severe aortic stenosis and a poor left ventricle, then either the surgical or balloon dilation approach produces a similar outcome and so I would support balloon dilation. In older children, I would recommend balloon dilation in the first instance, and in case of failure of this or if there was more than moderate aortic regurgitation present, I would prefer surgery. If the valve did not seem suitable for surgical valvotomy, then surgery should consist of pulmonary autograft replacement of the aortic valve and implantation of an aortic homograft in the pulmonary position.

If my child presented as a neonate with severe duct-dependent aortic coarctation, I have no doubt that I would prefer surgery to be the first line of treatment. A good subclavian flap aortoplasty seems preferable to other techniques and I would not want the surgeon to use any patches, if at all possible. In an older child with coarctation, I would recommend balloon dilation if there was no important hypoplasia of the transverse aortic arch and there was a discrete coarctation. If the child had had previous surgery and had developed a re-coarctation, I would not hesitate to recommend balloon dilation as the treatment of choice and only if this failed despite the use of an appropriate-sized balloon would I allow the surgeons to reoperate. The only other situation when I may want a surgeon's help would arise if an aneurysm formed immediately at the end of the balloon dilation. If it did not, then I would want regular magnetic resonance scans as part of the follow-up evaluation.

If my child was found to have a patent arterial duct, then I would pick an experienced operator to perform implantation of an umbrella device, as the results with this technique are as good as surgery. In case of a residual leak, I would prefer my child to have another device implanted in order to achieve complete occlusion.

For defects such as aortopulmonary collateral arteries, congenital coronary artery fistulas and Blalock–Taussig shunts with residual leaks after surgical ligation, I would have no hesitation in recommending closure of these with transcatheter techniques. I would prefer my child to have these vessels embolized by transcatheter techniques in a unit where the operators were very experienced and where a wide range of embolization devices were available. Nowadays, with the availability of different sizes and diameters of controlled-release coils, I would prefer these to be used than detachable balloons. These techniques will avoid surgery in congenital coronary fistulas and residual leaks in shunts, but complement it in aortopulmonary collaterals.

Pulmonary valve atresia and intact ventricular septum is associated with high risks with any treatment. I would hope that this diagnosis could be made prenatally for termination of pregnancy to have been a better and more realistic option. After birth, transcatheter laser or radiofrequency-assisted valvotomy, although experimental, still achieves the same aims as surgery, but with perhaps lower risks. A more difficult problem, as far as treatment is concerned, is branch pulmonary artery stenosis, more commonly as a result of previous surgery. I would do my utmost to stop the surgeons dealing with this, as stent implantation has much more to offer, deals with the stenosis more effectively and again avoids reoperation.

If my child was found to have an atrial or ventricular septal defect with a significant left-to-right shunt, I would have no hesitation in asking a good paediatric cardiac surgeon to close these surgically rather than allowing transcatheter umbrella closure to be performed. At present, the devices are not freely available and are under investigation in a limited number of centres in the USA, and there is no experience as yet in the UK.

# References

1 Brock RC, Pulmonary valvulotomy for the relief of congenital pulmonary stenosis, *Br Med J* (1948) **1**:1121–6.

2 Rubio-Alvarez V, Limon Lason R, Treatment of pulmonary valvular stenosis and tricuspid stenosis with a modified cardiac catheter. In: *Proceedings of 1st National Conference on Cardiovascular Disease*, Washington DC, 1950.

3 Rubio-Alvarez V, Limon RL, Soni J, Valvulotomias intracardiacas por medio de un cateter, *Arch Inst Cardiol Mexico* (1953) **23**:183–92.

4 Kan JS et al, Percutaneous balloon valvuloplasty: a new method for treating congenital pulmonary valve stenosis, *N Engl J Med* (1982) **307**:540–2.

5 Rashkind WJ, Miller WW, Creation of an atrial septal defect without thoracotomy: palliative approach to complete transposition of the great arteries, *JAMA* (1966) **196**:991–2.

6 Luessenhop AJ et al, Clinical evaluation of artificial embolization in the management of large cerebral arteriovenous malformations, *J Neurosurg* (1965) **23**:400–17.

7 Reidy JF et al, Embolization procedures in congenital heart disease, *Br Heart J* (1985) **54**:184–92.

8 Zuberbuhler JR et al, Tissue adhesive closure of aortic-pulmonary communications, *Am Heart J* (1974) **88**:41–6.

9 Gianturco C, Anderson JH, Wallace S, Mechanical devices for arterial occlusion, *Am J Roentgenol* (1975) **124**:428–35.

10 White RI Jr et al, Therapeutic embolization with detachable balloons, *Radiology* (1978) **126**:521–3.

11 Porstmann W, Wierny L, Warnke H, Der vershluss des ductus arteriosus persistens ohne thorakotomie, *Thoraxchirurgie* (1967) **15**:199–203.

12 Rashkind WJ, Interventional cardiac catheterization in congenital heart disease, *Int J Cardiol* (1985) **7**:1–11.

13 Tynan M et al, Percutaneous balloon pulmonary valvuloplasty, *Br Heart J* (1985) **53**:520–4.

14 Lababidi Z, Wu J, Percutaneous balloon pulmonary valvuloplasty, *Am J Cardiol* (1983) **52**:560–2.

15 Rocchini AP et al, Percutaneous balloon valvuloplasty for the treatment of pulmonary valvular stenosis in children, *J Am Coll Cardiol* (1984) **3**:1005–12.

16 Sullivan ID et al, Percutaneous balloon valvuloplasty for pulmonary valve stenosis in infants and children, *Br Heart J* (1985) **54**:435–41.

17 Fontes VT et al, Pulmonary valvoplasty—experience of 100 cases, *Int J Cardiol* (1988) **21**:335–42.

18 Stanger P et al, Balloon pulmonary valvuloplasty: results of the Valvuloplasty and Angioplasty of Congenital Anomalies Registry, *Am J Cardiol* (1990) **65**:775–83.

19 Tynan M et al, Balloon pulmonary valvoplasty. In: Hombach V, Koch M, Camm AJ, eds. *Interventional techniques in cardiovascular medicine* (Kluwer Academic Publishers: Dordrecht 1991) 187–93.

20 Ladusans EJ et al, Balloon dilation of critical stenosis of the pulmonary valve in neonates, *Br Heart J* (1990) **63**:362–7.

21 O'Connor BK et al, Intermediate-term outcome after pulmonary balloon valvuloplasty: comparison with a matched surgical control group, *J Am Coll Cardiol* (1992) **20**:169–73.

22 Vogel M et al, Brock transventricular pulmonary valvotomy in patients with pulmonary stenosis: long-term results, *Pediatr Cardiol* (1990) **11**:191–4.

23 McCrindle BW, Kan JS, Long-term results after balloon pulmonary valvuloplasty, *Circulation* (1991) **83**:1915–22.

24 Ali Khan MA et al, Results of repeat percutaneous balloon valvuloplasty for pulmonary valvar restenosis, *Am Heart J* (1990) **120**:878–81.

25  Smolinsky et al, Surgical closed pulmonary valvotomy for critical pulmonary stenosis: implications for the balloon valvuloplasty era, *Thorax* (1992) **47**:179–83.

26  Caspi J et al, Management of neonatal critical pulmonic stenosis in the balloon valvotomy era, *Ann Thorac Surg* (1990) **49**:273–8.

27  Pepine CJ, Gessner IH, Feldman RL, Percutaneous balloon valvuloplasty for pulmonic valve stenosis in an adult, *Am J Cardiol* (1982) **50**:1442–5.

28  Lababidi Z, Aortic balloon valvuloplasty, *Am Heart J* (1983) **106**:751–2.

29  Lababidi Z, Wu J, Walls JT, Percutaneous balloon aortic valvuloplasty: results in 23 patients, *Am J Cardiol* (1984) **53**:194–7.

30  Rocchini AP et al, Balloon aortic valvuloplasty: results of the Valvuloplasty and Angioplasty of Congenital Anomalies Registry, *Am J Cardiol* (1990) **65**:784–9.

31  Jones M, Barnhart GR, Morrow AG, Late results after operations for left ventricular outflow obstruction, *Am J Cardiol* (1982) **50**:569–79.

32  Messmer BJ, Hofstetter R, von Bernuth G, Surgery for critical congenital aortic stenosis during the first three months of life, *Eur J Cardiothorac Surg* (1991) **5**:378–82.

33  Waller BF, Girod DA, Dillon JC, Transverse aortic wall tears in infants after balloon angioplasty for aortic valve stenosis: relation of aortic wall damage to diameter of inflated angioplasty balloon and aortic lumen in seven necropsy cases, *J Am Coll Cardiol* (1984) **4**:1235–41.

34  O'Connor BK et al, Intermediate-term effectiveness of balloon valvuloplasty for congenital aortic stenosis. A prospective follow-up study, *Circulation* (1991) **84**:732–8.

35  Witsenburg M et al, Short- and midterm results of balloon valvuloplasty for valvular aortic stenosis in children, *Am J Cardiol* (1992) **69**:945–50.

36  Cikrit DF et al, Complete external iliac artery disruption after percutaneous aortic valvuloplasty in two young children: successful repair with hypogastric artery transposition, *Surgery* (1991) **109**:623–6.

37  Leung MP et al, Critical aortic stenosis in early infancy. Anatomic and echocardiographic substrates of successful open valvotomy, *J Thorac Cardiovasc Surg* (1991) **101**:526–35.

38  Rhodes LA et al, Predictors of survival in neonates with critical aortic stenosis, *Circulation* (1991) **84**:2325–535.

39  Zeevi B et al, Neonatal critical aortic stenosis: a comparison of surgical and balloon dilation therapy, *Circulation* (1989) **80**:831–9.

40  Beekman RH, Rocchini AP, Andes A, Balloon valvuloplasty for critical aortic stenosis in the newborn: influence of new catheter technology, *J Am Coll Cardiol* (1991) **17**:1172–6.

41  Messmer BJ, Hofstetter R, von Bernuth G, Surgery for critical congenital aortic stenosis during the first three months of life, *Eur J Cardiothorac Surg* (1991) **5**:378–82.

42  Pelech AN et al, Critical aortic stenosis: survival and management, *J Thorac Cardiovasc Surg* (1987) **94**:510–17.

43  Roth SJ, Keane JF, Balloon aortic valvuloplasty, *Prog Pediatr Cardiol* (1992) **1**:3–16.

44  Amato JJ, Galdieri RJ, Cotroneo JV, Role of extended aortoplasty related to the definition of coarctation of the aorta, *Ann Thorac Surg* (1991) **52**:615–20.

45  Bobby JJ et al, Operative survival and 40 year follow up of surgical repair of aortic coarctation, *Br Heart J* (1991) **65**:271–6.

46  Shrivastava CP et al, The early and long-term results of surgery for coarctation of the aorta in the 1st year of life, *Eur J Cardiothorac Surg* (1991) **5**:61–6.

47  Messmer BJ et al, Surgical correction of coarctation in early infancy: does surgical technique influence the result? *Ann Thorac Surg* (1991) **52**:594–600.

48  Dietl CA et al, Risk of recoarctation in neonates and infants after repair with patch aortoplasty, subclavian flap, and the combined resection-flap procedure, *J Thorac Cardiovasc Surg* (1992) **103**:724–31.

49  Malan JE, Benatar A, Levin SE, Long-term follow-up of coarctation of the aorta repaired by patch angioplasty, *Int J Cardiol* (1991) **30**:23–32.

50  Brouwer MH et al, Repair of aortic coarctation in infants, *J Thorac Cardiovasc Surg* (1991) **101**:1093–8.

51  Lacour-Gayet F et al, Hypoplastic transverse arch and coarctation in neonates. Surgical

reconstruction of the aortic arch: a study of sixty-six patients, *J Thorac Cardiovasc Surg* (1990) **100**:808–16.

52 Mendelsohn AM et al, Rapid progression of aortic aneurysms after patch aortoplasty repair of coarctation of the aorta, *J Am Coll Cardiol* (1992) **20**:381–5.

53 Holdright DR, Kilner PJ, Somerville J, Haemoptysis from false aneurysm: near fatal complication of repair of coarctation of the aorta using a Dacron patch, *Int J Cardiol* (1991) **32**:406–8.

54 Singer MI, Rowen M, Dorsey TJ, Transluminal aortic balloon angioplasty for coarctation of the aorta in the newborn, *Am Heart J* (1982) **103**:131–2.

55 Lock JE et al, Balloon dilation of excised aortic coarctation, *Radiology* (1982) **143**:688–91.

56 Sos T et al, Percutaneous transluminal dilation of coarctation of thoracic aorta post-mortem, *Lancet* (1979) ii:970.

57 Tyagi S et al, Balloon angioplasty of native coarctation of the aorta in adolescents and young adults, *Am Heart J* (1992) **123**:674–80.

58 Fawzy ME et al, Balloon coarctation angioplasty in adolescents and adults: early and intermediate results, *Am Heart J* (1992) **124**:167–71.

59 Fontes VF et al, It is valid to dilate native aortic coarctation with a balloon catheter, *Int J Cardiol* (1990) **27**:311–16.

60 Tynan M et al, Balloon angioplasty for the treatment of native coarctation: results of Valvuloplasty and Angioplasty of Congenital Anomalies Registry, *Am J Cardiol* (1990) **65**:790–2.

61 Rao PS, Chopra PS, Role of balloon angioplasty in the treatment of aortic coarctation, *Ann Thorac Surg* (1991) **52**:621–31.

62 Redington AN et al, Primary balloon dilation of coarctation of the aorta in neonates, *Br Heart J* (1990) **64**:277–81.

63 Anjos R et al, Determinants of hemodynamic results of balloon dilation of aortic recoarctation, *Am J Cardiol* (1992) **69**:665–71.

64 Hellenbrand WE et al, Balloon angioplasty for aortic recoarctation: results of Valvuloplasty and Angioplasty of Congenital Anomalies Registry, *Am J Cardiol* (1990) **65**:793–7.

65 Martin MM et al, Aortic aneurysms after subclavian angioplasty repair of coarctation of the aorta, *Am J Cardiol* (1988) **61**:951–3.

66 Balaji S, Oommen R, Rees PG, Fatal aortic rupture during balloon dilation of recoarctation, *Br Heart J* (1991) **65**:100–1.

67 Rocchini AP, Balloon angioplasty of postoperative aortic recoarctation, *Prog Pediatr Cardiol* (1992) **1**:28–34.

68 Qureshi SA et al, Balloon dilation of the pulmonary valve in the first year of life in patients with tetralogy of Fallot: a preliminary study, *Br Heart J* (1988) **60**:232–5.

69 Rao PS et al, Balloon pulmonary valvuloplasty in the management of cyanotic congenital heart defects, *Cathet Cardiovasc Diagn* (1992) **25**:16–24.

70 Sreeram N et al, Results of balloon pulmonary valvuloplasty as a palliative procedure in tetralogy of Fallot, *J Am Coll Cardiol* (1991) **18**:159–65.

71 Suarez de Lezo J et al, Immediate and follow-up results of transluminal balloon dilation for discrete subaortic stenosis, *J Am Coll Cardiol* (1991) **18**:1309–15.

72 Benson LN, Yeatman L, Laks H, Balloon dilation for superior vena caval obstruction after the Senning procedure, *Cathet Cardiovasc Diagn* (1985) **11**:63–8.

73 Cooper SG et al, Balloon dilation of pulmonary venous pathway obstruction after Mustard repair for transposition of the great arteries, *J Am Coll Cardiol* (1989) **14**:194–8.

74 Perry SB, Keane JF, Lock JE, Interventional catheterization in pediatric congenital and acquired heart disease, *Am J Cardiol* (1988) **61**:109–17.

75 Rothman A et al, Early results and follow-up of balloon angioplasty for branch pulmonary artery stenoses, *J Am Coll Cardiol* (1990) **15**:1109–17.

76 Rothman A, Balloon angioplasty of pulmonary artery stenosis, *Prog Pediatr Cardiol* (1992) **1**:17–27.

77 Rashkind WJ, Cuaso CC, Transcatheter closure of patent ductus arteriosus: successful use in a 3.5 kilogram infant, *Pediatr Cardiol* (1979) **1**:3–8.

78 Mullins CE, Transcatheter closure of patent ductus arteriosus, *Prog Pediatr Cardiol* (1992) **1**:55–62.

79  Hosking CK et al, Transcatheter occlusion of the persistently patent ductus arteriosus, *Circulation* (1991) **84**:2313–17.

80  Report of the European Registry, Transcatheter occlusion of patent arterial duct, *Lancet* (1992) **340**:1062–6.

81  Lock JE et al, Transcatheter closure of atrial septal defects: experimental studies, *Circulation* (1989) **79**:1091–9.

82  Rome JJ, Transcatheter closure of atrial septal defects, *Prog Pediatr Cardiol* (1992) **1**:63–71.

83  Bridges ND, Lock JE, Transcatheter closure of ventricular septal defects. *Prog Pediatr Cardiol* (1992) **1**:72–7.

84  Sideris EB et al, Transvenous atrial septal defect occlusion by the buttoned device, *Am J Cardiol* (1990) **66**:1524–6.

85  Latson LA et al, Transcatheter closure of atrial septal defect—early results of multicenter trial of the Bard clamshell occluder, *Circulation* (1991) **84**(Suppl):II-544.

86  Redington AN, Rigby ML, Novel uses of the Rashkind ductal umbrella in adults and children with congenital heart disease, *Br Heart J* (1993) **69**:47–51.

87  Reidy JF et al, Embolization procedures in congenital heart disease, *Br Heart J* (1985) **54**:184–92.

88  Fuhrman BP et al, Coil embolization of congenital thoracic vascular anomalies in infants and children, *Circulation* (1984) **70**:285–9.

89  Reidy JF et al, Transcatheter embolization in the treatment of coronary artery fistulas, *J Am Coll Cardiol* (1991) **18**:187–92.

90  Houde C, Zahn EM, Benson LN, Transcatheter closure of Blalock–Taussig shunts with a modified Rashkind umbrella delivery system, *Br Heart J* (1993) **69**:56–8.

91  Qureshi SA et al, Transcatheter laser-assisted balloon pulmonary valve dilation in pulmonic valve atresia, *Am J Cardiol* (1991) **67**:428–31.

92  Parsons JM, Rees MR, Gibbs JL, Percutaneous laser valvotomy with balloon dilation of the pulmonary valve as primary treatment for pulmonary atresia, *Br Heart J* (1991) **66**:36–8.

93  Tynan M et al, Laser treatment in congenital heart disease, *Curr Opinion Ped* (1992) **4**:839–41.

94  Benson LN et al, Percutaneous implantation of a balloon-expandable endoprosthesis for pulmonary artery stenosis: an experimental study, *J Am Coll Cardiol* (1991) **18**:1303–8.

95  O'Laughlin MP et al, Use of endovascular stents in congenital heart disease, *Circulation* (1991) **83**:1923–39.

96  Mulcahy D, Sigwart U, Somerville J, Successful stenting of a life threatening pulmonary arterial stenosis, *Br Heart J* (1991) **66**:463–5.

97  Chatelain P, Meier B, Friedli B, Stenting of superior vena cava and inferior vena cava for symptomatic narrowing after repeated atrial surgery for D-transposition of the great vessels, *Br Heart J* (1991) **66**:466–8.

98  Gibbs JL et al, Stenting the arterial duct: a new approach to palliation for pulmonary atresia, *Br Heart J* (1992) **67**:240–5.

# 18

## Endocarditis

*Celia M Oakley*

Some diseases are new or obscure. Some have known causes, others not and many still have no cure. Infective endocarditis is none of these. It is a classic disease and well known to all doctors. It was described more than a century ago and has been curable for more than 50 years. Yet the diagnosis is still missed, the disease poorly treated and the outcome too often death or disability.

## *Definitions*

Infective endocarditis is a microbial infection of the endothelial lining of the heart (or of the vascular endothelium in infection of aortic coarctation or patent ductus arteriosus).

Non-infective endocarditis occurs in rheumatic fever and in other auto-immune diseases such as systemic lupus erythematosus (Libman Sacks endocarditis). Sterile thrombotic (marantic) endocarditis is characteristically associated with adenocarcinoma. Secondary infection of originally sterile endocarditis may occur but is rare. This chapter deals only with infective endocarditis.

The term bacterial endocarditis has been dropped because any micro-organisms apart from viruses may infect the endocardium. Similarly, the terms acute, subacute and chronic (lente) used to be applied arbitrarily according to the duration of the illness between onset and death in the pre-antibiotic era. Virulent pyogenic organisms such as *Staphylococcus aureus* and *Streptococcus pneumoniae* were thought to infect previously normal valves, and used to cause death within 1 or 2 months. Subacute and chronic endocarditis were caused by less virulent organisms, typically viridans streptococci, which infected previously abnormal valves, with a duration of illness which occasionally lasted 1 or 2 years. Infection by coxiella can last years or rarely even decades untreated, without killing the patient.

The modern classification is usually into native valve and prosthetic valve endocarditis.

## *Changes*

The demography of infective endocarditis has changed dramatically since Osler's description of it in 1885. It was then usually associated with obvious sepsis such as pneumonia, surgery, trauma or the puerperium. Since the virtual disappearance of endocarditis complicating overt sepsis and the reduction in rheumatic and syphilitic heart disease, the most common underlying conditions now are calcified aortic valves (congenitally bicuspid or degenerated tricuspid) or mitral valves with 'wear and tear' prolapse, congenital heart disease and the normal valves of intravenous drug abusers. Infection on prosthetic valves accounts for up to 30 per cent of cases seen in most regional centres. The increasing numbers of elderly in

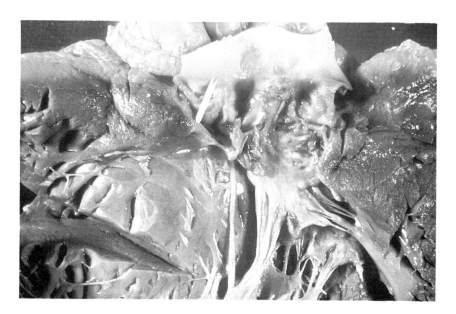

**Figure 18.1**
*Untreated fatal infective endocarditis. Vegetations have destroyed the aortic valve and infection has been seeded onto the mitral valve, which shows ruptured chordae. Planar vegetations are seen on the aortic wall.*

the population, more often now with their own teeth, seeking, deserving and getting diagnosis and treatment, account for the high proportion of patients with degenerative valve disease. At the other end of the age spectrum, the success of surgeons in palliating complex congenital cardiac malformations accounts for an increasing number of infections in the young.

Nosocomial endocarditis has increased with the increase in procedures, particularly patients with newly placed prosthetic valves (early prosthetic valve endocarditis), patches or conduits. Central venous lines and pulmonary artery catheters predispose to infective endocarditis in seriously ill medical and surgical patients but the disease is remarkably uncommon in immunocompromised bone marrow transplant and chronic haemodialysis patients. This is almost certainly because bloodstream infections are so frequent that

they are promptly sought and treated in these vulnerable patients. Underlying heart disease has frequently been absent in patients with nosocomially acquired endocarditis.

The incidence of the disease is not really known but has been estimated as 2 cases per 100 000 population per year in the UK. The incidence is higher in men than in women because of the higher prevalence of aortic valve disease in men and the decline in the incidence of rheumatic heart disease, which was more common in women.[1]

## Pathogenesis

The pathognomonic lesion of infective endocarditis is the vegetation. Damaged endothelium provides a nidus for infection. Endothelial damage is particularly likely to be caused by high-velocity jets, as in flow from a high- to a low-pressure chamber in aortic or mitral regurgitation, aortic stenosis or small ventricular septal defect. High-pressure streams are associated with low-pressure sinks, and bacterial deposition occurs in these low-pressure areas through the Venturi effect. Damaged endothelium is thrombogenic so that the bacteria are rapidly covered in platelet fibrin aggregates, the characteristic vegetations of the disease. These develop downstream to the jet: on the atrial surface of the mitral valve, on the right ventricular side of a ventricular septal defect, distal to a coarctation or on the venous end of an arteriovenous fistula.

Within the cardiac vegetation, micro-organisms are protected from host defence mechanisms by a dense covering of fibrin within which they initially multiply rapidly until they reach maximal density, after which they become metabolically inactive and are no longer easily killed by antibiotics, which are most effective against rapidly dividing bacteria.

That is why antibiotics have to be given in high dosage and for a long time compared with ordinary infections.

Untreated infective endocarditis is always fatal (Figure 18.1). With antibiotic treatment it should always be curable but the mortality seems only to have fallen from a presumptive 100 per cent down to an estimated 30 per cent and to have stuck there.

## Symptoms

Symptoms usually start within 2 weeks or earlier of the inciting bacteraemia when this is known, but diagnosis often takes very much longer due to patient delay (usually short), doctor delay (commonly measured in weeks, occasionally in months) and then failure to make the diagnosis promptly in hospital.[2] Fever is present in almost all patients except after antibiotic therapy or in the elderly and debilitated. Virulent organisms such as

| **Signs of infection** | | **Signs of a heart disorder** |
|---|---|---|
| Fever | and | Murmur |
| Chills | | Changing cardiac signs |
| Night sweats | | |
| Malaise | | |
| Weight loss | | |
| Anaemia | | |
| Splenomegaly | | |
| **Immunological activation** | | **Embolism** |
| Nephritis | | Focal neurological lesion |
| Vasculitis | | Stroke |
| Rheumatoid factor positive | | Psychiatric |
| | | Retinal |
| | | Limb |
| | | Skin etc. |

Symptoms and signs. The classic triad. Now a quartet.

- **Isolated tricuspid endocarditis**
  Addicts
  Non-addicts

- **With congenital heart disease and left-to-right shunt e.g. ventricular septal defect**
  Pleuritic pain
  Embolic pneumonia
  Lung abscesses

*Staphylococcus aureus* may cause high fevers and rigors but in most patients the fevers are low grade and remittent. Chills and night sweats are characteristics of endocarditis with, eventually, malaise, fatigue, anorexia and weight loss.

Nearly all patients have cardiac murmurs but they may not be prominent and may be attributed to the fever itself. The exception is tricuspid valve endocarditis, which usually does not give rise to murmurs because the right ventricular pressure is low and regurgitation is not associated with a high-velocity jet. In patients with *Staphylococcus aureus* infection, valve destruction can be amazingly rapid, with severe aortic or mitral regurgitation developing within hours of a normal examination. The development of new murmurs or changes in murmurs may be missed because of lack of auscultatory skills in this modern age. Elderly patients may simply present with worsening of chronic congestive heart failure.

Rarely, vegetations may grow so large that they cause obstruction of valves. Large vegetations are particularly characteristic of fungal infection but may also be seen with *Haemophilus parainfluenzae*. Myocardial infarction may result from coronary embolism or occlusion of a coronary ostium from a vegetation on an aortic prosthesis. Embolic myocardial abscesses may cause conduction disturbances, particularly in aortic valve endocarditis, or pericarditis may be septic from direct extension of infection or sterile in association with aseptic coronary embolism. Generalized myocardial depression can develop

- **Abscess**
  Continuing fever
  Continuing raised C-reactive protein
  New conduction defect on ECG
  Pericarditis
      CT scan of brain        White cell scan
  CT scan of spleen

- **Embolism**
  Pulse loss
  Neurological deficit
      CT scan of brain
  CT scan of spleen

- **Mycotic aneurysm**
  Focal pain or petechiae
      DSA

*Recognition of complications.*

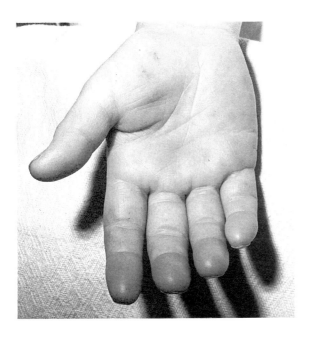

**Figure 18.2**
*Osler's nodes on the thenar eminence of a patient with staphylococcal prosthetic valve endocarditis.*

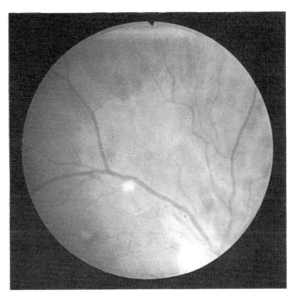

**Figure 18.3**
*Multiple Roth spots in the retina. They have a white centre and a red surround.*

unexpectedly.[3] It may be missed, picked up on echo or be the cause of cardiac arrest but it is reversible. Splenomegaly is uncommon in patients with a short history and tends to be associated with more indolent and prolonged infection.

Skin lesions are a useful clue to the diagnosis, with petechiae being most common and found on conjunctivae, buccal mucosa, neck and extremities. They are associated with local vasculitis or microemboli. New splinter haemorrhages have similar origin and may appear in crops. One or two splinter haemorrhages are not infrequent in patients on admission to hospital, often old, black and towards the nail tip. These are due to previous trauma. Important splinter

haemorrhages are new, red and close to the nail base. Osler's nodes (Figure 18.2), Janeway lesions and Roth spots (Figure 18.3) should all be sought but are relatively rare.

Clubbing like splenomegaly takes time to develop and is a difficult physical sign unless gross. Arthralgia and myalgias are common.

Systemic embolism may occur early or late, and cerebral embolism or rupture of an intra-cerebral mycotic aneurysm is a major cause of death. Cerebral and splenic emboli may be silent but are commonly found if sought by CT scanning, a useful ancillary to a difficult diagnosis.

Major embolism to a limb artery suggests fungal endocarditis. The embolus should be

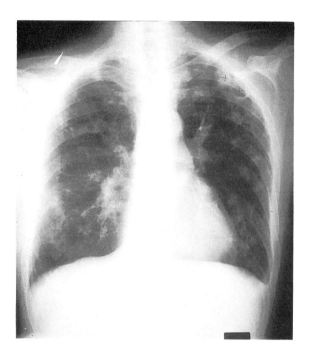

**Figure 18.4**
*Embolic pneumonia in a patient with tricuspid endocarditis. Multiple abscess cavities and infarctions are seen. The heart is not enlarged.*

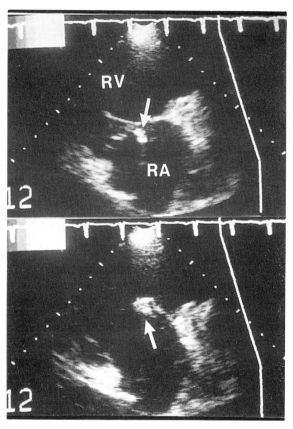

**Figure 18.5**
*Vegetation shown on the tricuspid valve protruding into the right atrium (RA) in systole (top) and flopping towards the right ventricle (RV) in diastole (lower frame).*

removed promptly to restore bloodflow and for examination, which may reveal fungal hyphae, *Coxiella* or even that the patient has a left atrial myxoma.

Patients with right-sided endocarditis may present with an atypical (embolic) pneumonia (Figure 18.4) or with pulmonary embolism and infarction. Narcotic addicts with tricuspid endocarditis (Figure 18.5) may also have left-sided valve involvement. Isolated tricuspid endocarditis is occasionally seen in infants following umbilical infection, in infants or children following skin infection and in previously healthy adults.

Neurological manifestations of endocarditis are frequent, most often due to emboli. Psychiatric presentations are sometimes seen but more often hemiplegia or cranial nerve palsies or occasionally a multi-infarction presentation suggestive of multiple sclerosis or cerebral or subarachnoid haemorrhage resulting from rupture of mycotic aneurysms. Meningitis is rare but an aseptic meningitis may result from occult cerebral infarction or purulent meningitis in patients with acute pyogenic infection. Careful and repeated neurological examinations often reveal transient or minor abnormalities.

Mycotic aneurysms result from infected emboli occurring before treatment has sterilized the vegetations and may not become clinically manifest until after the patient has completed successful treatment. Again, they can arise anywhere: in the facial artery, mimicking toothache, in the splenic artery, giving rise to an acute abdomen on rupture, or in a limb artery, when they may present with a pulsatile mass. Complaint of severe focal pain or a shower of emboli to a single limb should raise the possibility.

Impairment of kidney or liver function plus anaemia and loss of weight may all be present by the time a patient recurrently treated with antibiotics reaches the hospital. The antibiotics have delayed the diagnosis, modified the features of the disease and extended the patient's life, but made it more likely that the patient is referred not to a cardiologist, but to a non-cardiac specialist. The advent of major embolism or cardiac failure may then come as a surprise when the still infected valve eventually gives way, often in association with extensive paravalvular infection and abscess formation, making the surgeon's life difficult and greatly reducing the patient's chance of survival, cure and future health and fitness.

The combination of late onset of proper treatment and inadequate use of surgical rescue undoubtedly accounts for the continuing high mortality and morbidity of the disease. Early suspicion of a serious underlying disorder is often allayed by a patient's prompt early response to antibiotics and, each time he relapses, another 'course' is given. Early hospital suspicion of the diagnosis is often allayed

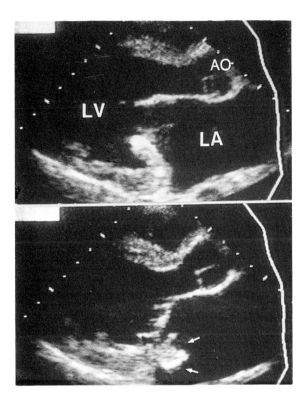

**Figure 18.6**
*Long-axis echocardiographic view of the mitral valve showing a large mobile vegetation on the posterior leaflet of the mitral valve. In diastole (top) it appears within the ventricle (LV) and in systole (lower) it prolapses into the atrium (LA). The vegetation is arrowed.*

by negative blood cultures caused by the previous antibiotics and too often by a 'negative' echocardiographic report.

## Echocardiography

Echocardiography is of tremendous value in the diagnosis of endocarditis (Figure 18.6), in following the response to treatment and in the

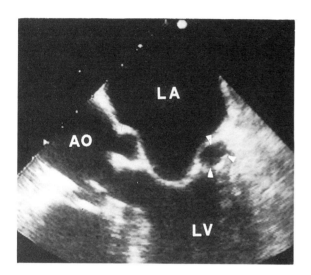

**Figure 18.7**
Transoesophageal view to show a mitral
paravalvular abscess (arrowed). Ao = aorta.

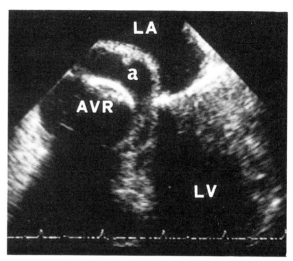

**Figure 18.8**
Transoesophageal view of a patient with an
infected aortic prosthesis (AVR) and a large
abscess cavity (a) in the left posterior sinus of
valsalva which bulges towards the left atrium
(LA).

recognition of complications but it requires
skill and it helps if the operator is alerted to
the possibility. Particularly useful in poor echo
subjects, transoesophageal echocardiography
provides a reliable unobstructed near view of
the heart (Figures 18.7 and 18.8) but, even
with the high definition of transoesophageal
views, errors may be made. Both the exuber-
ant reaction to rheumatism seen particularly in
patients with rheumatic valve disease from the
African continent and myxomatous degeneration with expanded 'cotton wool bud' appearance of ruptured mitral chordae may
masquerade as infection. Conversely, vegetations may be planar (Figure 18.1) rather than

pedunculated and so not move independently
of the valve structures. Furthermore, new
vegetations may embolize. Echocardiograms
have to be viewed, discussed and repeated. This
is easy for the cardiologist. The non-cardiolo-
gist, having suspected endocarditis, may well
be content with a report but he should chase
it up.

## Laboratory findings

The problem of persistently negative blood
cultures has declined, probably because of
better and specialized blood culture media and

holding the cultures for longer periods in suspected cases. The use of serological techniques in patients infected by cell-dependent organisms such as *Coxiella* and *Chlamydia* has further increased the proportion of positive diagnoses. Previous antibiotic therapy is still the commonest cause for negative blood cultures. Fastidious bacteria which fail to grow are the second commonest cause. These are usually streptococci and sensitive to a penicillin plus aminoglycoside combination. Unusual organisms are usually sought these days. Fungal infection by *Candida* and *Aspergillus* is never primary but occurs in chronically ill patients with indwelling lines, often having parenteral feeding and frequent courses of antibiotics, as well, of course, as in patients with prosthetic heart valves.

A high C-reactive protein and raised sedimentation rate are nearly always present, though non-specific. Serum albumin may be low in patients with very high C-reactive protein.

Circulating immune complexes due to a polyclonal gammopathy are typical, particularly in late diagnosed cases, giving rise to latex and rheumatoid factor positivity. Low serum complement levels are found in patients with renal involvement.

The anaemia of chronic infection usually develops. Mechanical haemolysis occurs rarely in patients with infected native valves but much more often in prosthetic valve endocarditis with a new paraprosthetic leak. The effects of mechanical haemolysis are exaggerated by poor marrow response in these patients. Anaemia, neutropenia or thrombocytopenia or all three may be a complication of high penicillin dosage. This is often confused with penicillin sensitivity, which it is not. It indicates only a need to lower the dosage and does not preclude future use of penicillin.

Penicillin sensitivity is associated with recurrence of fever, often with eosinophilia and usually a skin rash.

The urine is normal in early cases but evidence of renal involvement is nearly always present later in endocarditis. Haematuria may be due to infarction from embolism but focal crescentic glomerulonephritis of immunological origin is indicated by the presence also of protein and casts. Rarely, a more diffuse glomerulonephritis develops and gives rise to renal failure which may even be the presenting feature of the illness. If a renal biopsy is carried out, the pathologist can make the diagnosis from the pathognomonic finding of crescents plus 'lumpy-bumpy' deposition of immunoglobulin on the basement membrane shown by immunofluorescent staining.

Blood cultures should be included in the routine primary investigation of any patient with a pyrexia of unknown origin. When positive blood cultures are obtained in the absence of suggestive clinical features of endocarditis the significance depends on absence of other cause such as pneumonia, the identity of the micro-organism and the detection of susceptible heart disease or vegetations on echo plus clinical reappraisal. Bacteraemia is constant in endocarditis so that all culture bottles will usually be positive unless the bacterial concentration in the blood is very low. That is why multiple cultures are taken.

A diagnosis of 'septicaemia' cannot easily be made in a patient with valvular or congenital heart disease but when the time and source of the bacterial entry is known, the antibiotic course can be appropriately short.

The differential diagnosis in atypical cases includes collagen vascular diseases, reticuloses and other neoplasms, and protracted infections, including tuberculosis, viral infections and AIDS.

| | |
|---|---|
| • Proliferative glomerulonephritis | 'Active' urinary sediment blood and casts<br>Proteinuria |
| • Skin | Vasculitic rash<br>Purpura<br>Janeway lesions |
| • Retina | Roth spots |
| • Pericardium | Sterile effusion |
| • Blood | Hypocomplementaemia<br>Polyclonal rise in immunoglobulins, positive rheumatoid factor |

*Immunological phenomena.*

# Treatment

Correct choice of an appropriate antimicrobial regime is crucial to the successful treatment of infective endocarditis. Treatment is started before receipt of laboratory information on the blood cultures when the clinical probability is high.

No patient with collagen vascular disease, sarcoidosis or reticulosis was ever harmed by antibiotics but patients with endocarditis whose bacteria are multiplying most rapidly early in the illness may be greatly harmed by treatment delays, which can result in mycotic aneurysm, stroke or severe damage to the infected heart valve.

Initial therapy is empirical and targeted against the most likely organism in the clinical setting. Subacute presentation suggests infection with streptococci. Therapeutic regimes should be active against streptococci and aimed at the most resistant organisms, enterococci. That is why high-dose intravenous penicillin coupled with gentamicin is chosen.[4] In the setting of acute onset with rigors, skin sepsis or previous surgery, *Staphylococcus aureus* is targeted, incorporating a penicillinase-resistant penicillin, flucloxicillin. In patients with prosthetic valves, *Staphylococcus epidermidis* is likely to be a nosocomial organism even in patients up to a year after operation and to be resistant to all beta-lactam antibiotics.[5] Vancomycin should be used in such patients.

Older patients have a higher chance of an enterococcus or of *Staphylococcus epidermidis*. Patients who have suffered occupational or surgical skin trauma may also be infected by this organism, which should not be dismissed as a contaminant. Patients who have had recent cardiac surgery are likely to have a staphylococcal, fungal or opportunist organism such as a diphtheroid. Fungal infection must be thought about in other surgical patients, particularly those who have had intravenous lines. Intravenous drug abusers usually have staphylococci but may have multiple organisms.

| | |
|---|---|
| • Medical | Mainly streptococci |
| • Medical elderly | More enterococci |
| | More *Staphylococcus epidermidis* |
| • Addicts | Mainly staphylococci |
| | Some multiple infections |
| | Fungi |
| • Surgical | Mainly Staphylococci, coagulase positive |
| | and |
| | *Staphylococcus epidermidis* |
| | also |
| | Fungi |

*Classification of patients for choice of antibiotics,*

Once the infecting organism has been isolated from blood culture, both minimum inhibitory concentrations (MIC) and minimum bactericidal concentrations (MBC) are determined. The MIC is the minimum concentration of antibiotic which inhibits growth in vitro. The MBC is the minimum concentration which achieves a 99.9 per cent decrease in numbers of bacteria at 24 h. Agents for which the MBC is equal to (or within a dilution of) the MIC are considered bactericidal. If the difference between MIC and MBC is equal to or greater than 16 dilutions, the agent is considered to be bacteriostatic. Optimal therapy of endocarditis requires bactericidal therapy. Combination therapy is frequently necessary or desirable to achieve or to enhance bactericidal activity. The serum bactericidal titre or killing level is the greatest dilution of the patient's serum that kills a standard inoculum of the patient's organism. Its use is controversial, partly because of variations in performance of the test. A bactericidal titre of one in eight or

greater has traditionally been felt to represent adequate therapy. Tolerance is the situation in which a particular organism shows a substantial difference between MIC and MBC for an antibiotic which is normally bactericidal and usually represents a slower than expected rate of kill of organisms. Enterococci are always tolerant to the action of cell wall active agents such as penicillin, and the combination of a cell wall active agent plus an aminoglycoside is usually needed for cure. Many strains of staphylococci are tolerant to cell wall active agents. Some streptococci may be tolerant to penicillin. Endocarditis due to tolerant streptococci may respond more slowly than that due to non-tolerant strains and require longer treatment if penicillin alone is used, so combination therapy is chosen to provide enhanced bactericidal activity and to decrease the likelihood of the emergence of resistance and to shorten the necessary course of treatment.[6]

Guidelines for the treatment of streptococcal and staphylococcal endocarditis have been

Treatment regimes.

- **Fully penicillin-sensitive streptococci**
  (MIC < 0.1 µg/l)
  Penicillin 12 mega U/24 h i.v. given 6-hourly
  +
  Gentamicin 1 mg/kg per 24 h i.v. given 12-hourly (monitoring peak and trough levels) for 4 weeks, or for 2 weeks followed by amoxycillin 1.5 g 8-hourly plus probenecid

  *Penicillin-allergic patients*
  Vancomycin 30 mg/kg per 24 h infused i.v. 12-hourly over 1 h (monitoring peak and trough levels) for 2 weeks

- **Relatively resistant streptococci**
  (MIC >0.1 and <0.5 µg/ml)
  Penicillin 20 mega U/24 h i.v. for 4 weeks + gentamicin 1 mg/kg per 24 h i.v. for first 2 weeks

- **Enterococci (other than *Strep. bovis*)**
  (MIC >0.5 µg/ml)
  Penicillin 20 mega U/24 h i.v. for 6 weeks, or amoxycillin 12 g/24 h i.v. given 6-hourly for 6 weeks, or ampicillin + gentamicin 1 mg/kg per 24 h i.v.

  *Penicillin-allergic patients*
  Vancomycin for 6 weeks + gentamicin for 2 weeks

- **Fully sensitive staphylococci**
  Flucloxacillin 12 g/24 h i.v. given 6-hourly for 4–6 weeks + gentamicin 1 mg/kg per 24 h for first 2 weeks

  *Penicillin-allergic patients*
  Vancomycin for 4 to 6 weeks + gentamicin for 2 weeks

- **Resistant staphylococci**
  Vancomycin for 6 weeks + rifampicin 300 mg 8-hourly orally + gentamicin for first 2 weeks

- **HACEK organisms**
  Amoxycillin or ampicillin 12 g/24 h i.v. given 6-hourly for 4 weeks + gentamicin 2 mg/kg per 24 h i.v. for 4 weeks

- **Pseudomonas**
  Piperacillin 18 g/24 h i.v. given 4-hourly + ceftazidime 6 g/24 h i.v. given 8-hourly

NB: All regimes variable according to response and presence of a prosthetic valve.

published by the Working Group on Antibacterial Chemotherapy and are well known.[7] Most serious infections require parenteral therapy to ensure complete bioavailability. Although oral therapy has been used successfully, absorption from the gut may be unreliable, peak serum levels are usually lower and there may be poor compliance with a self-administered regime. Fluroquinalones, rifampicin and fusidic acid are well absorbed from the gut and may be valuable as oral treatment but, in general, intravenous treatment is recommended through a central line by bolus injection (except for vancomycin) with the line filled with heparin in between. This line should not be used for withdrawing blood.

The duration of therapy varies with the infecting organism, the duration of illness, the rapidity of response and the presence or not of prosthetic material. The minimum duration is 2 weeks of intravenous therapy but 6 weeks is necessary for enterococcal infection and for most prosthetic valve infections.

Treatment must be rigorously monitored. Serum levels of aminoglycosides should be followed by measuring peak levels half an hour after intravenous injection or 1 h after intramuscular injection, and trough levels immediately before the next dose, aiming at peaks of <5 mg/l and troughs of <1 mg/l when gentamicin is used synergistically with penicillin. Renal function must be followed, as creatinine clearance tends to fall progressively in patients receiving aminoglycosides. Complete blood counts are needed because some drugs cause haemolytic anaemia, neutropenia or thrombocytopenia. Liver enzymes should be measured as markers of hepatotoxicity.

Once the infecting organism has been recovered from blood culture and sensitivities determined, the initial regime can be altered to provide the most effective therapy with the least toxicity and cost. If cultures are negative but the clinical response is good, therapy should be continued. If no pathogen is recovered and there is no response to treatment, the possibility of unusual organisms should be considered, particularly *Coxiella* and *Chlamydia*. Fungal endocarditis should be sought in patients with prosthetic valves and in intravenous drug abusers, especially if large vegetations are seen on echo or there have been emboli. Fastidious Gram-negative organisms (so-called HACEK organisms) account for up to 10 per cent of infections, and empirical treatment towards these with ampicillin and gentamicin should be considered in such patients.

Failure to respond despite a sensitive organism may be due to local or metastatic abscess formation, while recurrence of fever after an initially satisfactory response suggests the development of antibiotic sensitivity.

## Indications for surgical intervention

The most urgent indication for surgical intervention is the development of severe valvar regurgitation. Other indications include failure to respond either because of localized abscess formation in a patient with a susceptible organism or because of a resistant organism such as a slime-producing *Staphylococcus epidermidis*. Most patients with early prosthetic valve endocarditis need the valve to be replaced urgently, although in some patients who have refused operation or been regarded as too frail to sustain repeat operation, the infection has been cured medically. Despite this, the principle is urgent reoperation for patients with early prosthetic valve endocarditis caused by a nosocomial organism. Patients with infection caused by *Coxiella* (Q fever) or *Chlamydia* usually respond clinically to treatment with

---

> Acute valve failure
> Increasing valvar regurgitation
> Failure to respond: resistant organism or paravalvular abscess
> Recurrent embolism
> Prosthetic valve dysfunction: leaking or obstructed

*Indications for surgery: early surgery when medical treatment is failing.*

---

tetracyclines or rifampicin but the organism is not eradicated. Treatment has therefore to be semi-permanent, particularly as *Coxiella* often lodges in the liver and even valve replacement will then not be curative.

## Prosthetic valve endocarditis

This may be caused either by organisms which gain entry at the time of operation or shortly after it, often in association with sternotomy infection (early prosthetic valve endocarditis), or later on by the same organisms which infect native valves (late prosthetic valve endocarditis). Nosocomial staphylococci remain unduly common for the first year after valve implantation, indicating that these organisms may lie dormant for long periods because of perioperative antibiotic treatment. Fungal infection may appear late because of lack of constitutional reaction on the part of the host until embolization of the fungal vegetations brings the problem to light. These emboli are often large and multiple but may be small and give rise to curious complaints in an otherwise seemingly well patient.

Mechanical prosthetic valve endocarditis does not lead to any change in the valve opening and closing sounds unless there is interference with moving parts by vegetation or thrombus. No new murmurs are heard until a paraprosthetic abscess ruptures, with the development of regurgitation, or a large vegetation becomes obstructive. Echocardiographic recognition of vegetations on mechanical valves may be difficult because of the extreme echogenicity of the prosthetic material but this can be overcome by the transoesophageal approach (Figure 18.8). Even then, the complex structure of prostheses may make vegetations hard to visualize. This is less of a problem with bioprostheses. Infection of mechanical prostheses is necessarily paravalvular, though vegetations and thrombi may extend over the valve. Infection of bioprostheses may be both paravalvular and involve the valve cusps. There seems to be little difference in incidence of infection between mechanical and bioprosthetic valves or in curability, and there is no justification for the choice of a tissue valve to replace an infected mechanical valve unless the patient's prognosis is felt to be shorter than that of the prosthesis by virtue of age or other disease.

Prosthetic valve endocarditis can be cured with antibiotic treatment when the infecting organism is sensitive but treatment should be extended for a longer period of time, aiming for at least 2 weeks after the temperature has become normal, all signs of infection have gone and C-reactive protein has been normal.[8]

## Penicillin sensitivity

Many patients give a history of sensitivity to penicillin but if a careful history is taken it often becomes apparent that this was not the case. Unless the history is of anaphylaxis or a convincing rash, the patient should be given penicillin with preceding hydrocortisone and standby adrenaline. The reason for this is that penicillin is still the most effective, safest and least costly of the antibiotics that we have. Desensitization is difficult and usually unsatisfactory. Skin testing for penicillin sensitivity is worthless (often falsely positive).

The most common time for development of true penicillin sensitivity is in the third week of treatment as shown by recrudescence of fever, a sharp rise in C-reactive protein in the blood and often an eosinophilia. Withdrawal of antibiotics results in resolution of all these features. The decision may be made to stop treatment altogether or to substitute rifampicin plus erythromycin for the final week.

## Conclusion

In spite of advances in medical technology, the diagnosis of endocarditis still depends primarily on clinical suspicion. Consideration of this diagnosis should be given to any patient with unexplained fever and a multisystem illness. The clinical manifestations are diverse, almost unlimited, involving any organ system. The classic criteria for diagnosis include fever, cardiac murmurs, anaemia, splenomegaly and embolic phenomena but clinicians miss the cardiac origin of the disease because the syndrome is generally incomplete and because the cardiac abnormality is missed or underestimated.

## Prevention

The rationale on which attempts at prevention of endocarditis are based is quite clear:

- Infective endocarditis follows bacteraemia.
- Bacteraemias are known to follow procedures such as dental extraction.
- These organisms can cause infective endocarditis.
- Antibiotics can prevent bacteraemia after dental extraction and other bacteraemias after known interventions.
- Antibiotics should be given to patients with susceptible cardiac disease before procedures known to cause bacteraemia.

On the basis of this impeccable logic it is standard procedure to recommend antibiotic prophylaxis before dental and other procedures known to carry a high risk of causing bacteraemia. Although bacteraemia has been amply demonstrated after tooth extraction, as well as the efficacy of amoxycillin in preventing this, the efficacy of antibiotic prophylaxis in the prevention of infective endocarditis has not been shown. The reasons are that very few cases of endocarditis are caused by unprotected tooth extraction, and spontaneous low-grade bacteraemias with oral organisms are frequent occurrences. These spontaneous bacteraemias, although lower grade than after dental extraction, represent a far greater cumulative risk to patients with predisposing heart disease than a rare dental procedure. Cases of 'failed' prophylaxis are collected, but who knows whether these are not cases of successful prophylaxis before the dental procedure with subsequent spontaneous bacteraemia causing infection within the requisite time frame? This is in any case unknown but probably less than 2 weeks rather than up to 3 months. Efforts have been made to assess the efficacy of dental prophylaxis.[9] It seems clear

Recommendations for
endocarditis
prophylaxis.

(1) *Dental Extractions, Scaling, or Periodontal Surgery under local or no anaesthesia*

(a) For patients not allergic to penicillin and not given penicillin more than once in the previous month:
*Amoxycillin*
Adults: 3 g single oral dose taken under supervision 1 hour before dental procedure
Children 5–10 years: half adult dose
Children under 5 years: quarter adult dose

(b) For patients allergic to penicillin:
*Clindamycin*
Adults: 600 mg single oral dose taken under supervision 1 hour before dental procedure
Children 5–10 years: half adult dose
Children under 5 years: quarter adult dose
*Under general anaesthesia*

(c) For patients not allergic to penicillin and not given penicillin more than once in the previous month:
*Amoxycillin Intravenously or Intramuscularly*
Adults: 1 g intravenously or 1 g in 2.5% lignocaine hydrochloride intramuscularly at the time of induction plus 500 mg by mouth 6 hours later
Children 5–10 years: half adult dose
Children under 5 years: quarter adult dose
or
*Amoxycillin orally*
Adults 3 g oral dose 4 hours before anaesthesia followed by a further 3 g by mouth as soon as possible after the operation
Children 5–10 years: half adult dose
Children under 5 years: quarter adult dose
or
*Amoxycillin and probenecid orally*
Adults: amoxycillin 3 g together with probenecid 1 g orally 4 hours before operation

*Special risk patients who should be referred to hospital:*
(I) Patients with prosthetic valves who are to have a general anaesthetic
(II) Patients who are to have a general anaesthetic *and* who are allergic to penicillin or who have had a penicillin more than once in the previous month
(III) Patients who have had a previous attack of endocarditis
Recommendations for these patients are:

(d) For patients not allergic to penicillin and who have not had penicillin more than once in the previous month:
Adults: 1 g amoxycillin intravenously or 1 g amoxycillin in 2.5 ml 1% lignocaine hydrochloride intramuscularly plus 120 mg gentamicin intravenously or intramuscularly at the time of induction: then 500 mg amoxycillin orally 6 h later

Children 5–10 years: amoxycillin half adult dose; gentamicin 2 mg/kg body weight

Children under 5 years: amoxycillin, quarter adult dose; gentamicin 2 mg/kg body weight

(e) For patients allergic to penicillin or who have had a penicillin more than once in the previous month:

    (I)    Adults: vancomycin 1 g by slow intravenous infusion over at least 100 min followed by gentamicin 120 mg intravenously at the time of induction or 15 min before the surgical procedure

Children under 10 years: vancomycin 20 mg/kg by intravenous infusion followed by gentamicin 2 mg/kg intravenously

or

    (II)    Adults: telcoplanin 400 mg intravenously plus gentamicin 120 mg intravenously at the time of induction or 15 min before the surgical procedure

Children under 14 years: telcoplanin 6 mg/kg intravenously plus gentamicin 2 mg/kg intravenously

or

    (III)    Adults: clindamycin 300 mg by intravenous infusion over at least 10 min at the time of induction or 15 min before the surgical procedure, followed by 150 mg orally or 150 mg by intravenous infusion over at least 10 min 6 hours later

Children 5–10 years: half adult dose

Children under 5 years: quarter adult dose

(2) *Surgery or Instrumentation of Upper Respiratory Tract*
Recommended cover is for 1(a) to 1(e)(III), but postoperative antibiotics may have to be given intramuscularly or intravenously if swallowing is painful.

(3) *Genitourinary Surgery or Instrumentation*
For patients with sterile urine the suggested cover is directed against faecal streptococci and is as for 1(d), 1(e)(I), or 1(e)(II) above*. If the urine is infected prophylaxis should also cover the pathogens involved.

(4) *Obstetric and Gynaecological Procedures*
Cover is suggested for patients with prosthetic valves or patients who have had a previous attack of endocarditis and is as for 1(d), 1(e)(I), or 1(e)(II) above because of the risk from faecal streptococci*.

(5) *Gastrointestinal Procedures*
Cover is suggested for patients with prosthetic valves or patients who have had a previous attack of endocarditis and is as for 1(d), 1(e)(I), or 1(e)(II) above because of the risk from faecal streptococci*.

*Clindamycin regimens are not suitable for this purpose.

that it is probably effective, although not many cases are prevented because not very many cases follow dental procedures anyway. This does not mean that dental prophylaxis should be abandoned but emphasizes the importance of optimal oral hygiene for patients with susceptible heart disease in order to minimize the frequency and intensity of the low-grade spontaneous bacteraemias which are probably responsible for most cases.

Relatively few cases of endocarditis originate from the gastrointestinal tract distal to the oral cavity. Gram-negative organisms are rarely responsible but enteric streptococci may cause endocarditis after diagnostic procedures involving the gut or an infected genitourinary tract and so suitable prophylaxis is recommended.

Recommendations for prophylaxis from the UK,[10] the European Society of Cardiology and the American Heart Association have recently come together with only minor differences. In the UK amoxycillin 3 g taken as a single oral dose 1 h before the dental procedure is recommended. Clindamycin 600 mg also given as a single oral dose 1 h before the procedure is recommended for penicillin-allergic patients. Gentamicin is added for in-hospital gastrointestinal or genitourinary procedures for patients at especially high risk. Vancomycin infusion is recommended for such patients who are allergic to penicillin.

The full guidelines are available free from the British Heart Foundation, printed on cards for issue to patients.

## If I had ...

I expect that I would diagnose it really early! But joking apart, I hope that my general practi-
tioner would get blood cultures or refer me to hospital without delay and before starting antibiotics. I hope that my GP would recognize my underlying heart condition and refer me to a cardiologist. If he did not do so, I hope that the junior doctor on the firm on take would listen to my heart, ask for an echo study and suggest to her chief that I be referred to the cardiologist, and I hope that her chief would listen. I hope that intravenous penicillin and gentamicin would be started immediately after taking the blood cultures on suspicion of the diagnosis, that a friendly microbiologist would be involved and the cardiac surgeon informed. I would hope that cardiac surgery was performed in my hospital; otherwise I would be fearful that indications for surgical intervention would not be recognized simply because of lack of experience of benefit from surgery in previous patients like me. If not, I would hope that my physician would inform a cardiologist and cardiac surgeon from the nearby major cardiac surgical centre and keep them informed of my progress. I would expect a careful all-over examination every day looking for new skin lesions, pulse loss or any deterioration in function of my valve and for this to be complemented by regular echocardiographic studies. I would not expect to develop labyrinthine problems from excessive gentamicin dosage and I would expect clear directions about how to prevent and how to detect a possible further attack.

## Acknowledgement

I am grateful to my colleague Dr Petros Nihoyannopoulos for the echocardiographic figures.

# References

1   Bayliss R et al, Incidence, mortality and prevention of infective endocarditis, *J R Coll Physicians* (1985) **20**:15–20.

2   Nihoyannopoulos P et al, Duration of symptoms and the effects of a more aggressive surgical policy: factors affecting prognosis of infective endocarditis, *Eur Heart J* (1985) **6**:380–90.

3   Hackett D et al, Myocardial depression and nephrotic syndrome in strep sanguis endocarditis, *Q J Med* (1985) **57**:867–73.

4   Oakley CM Infective endocarditis, *Med Int* (1989) **70**:2928–34.

5   Westaby et al, Surgical treatment of infective endocarditis with special reference to prosthetic valve endocarditis, *Br Med J* (1983) **287**:320–3.

6   Oakley CM, Treatment of infective endocarditis, *Prescribers J* (1990) **30**:152–65.

7   British Society of Antimicrobial Chemotherapy, Antibiotic Treatment of Streptococcal and Staphylococcal Endocarditis. Report of the Working Party, *Lancet* (1985) **ii**:815–17.

8   Oakley CM, Treatment of prosthetic valve endocarditis, *J Antimicrob Chemother* (1987) **20**(suppl A): 181–6.

9   Van Der Meer JTM et al, Efficacy of antibiotic prophylaxis for prevention of native valve endocarditis, *Lancet* (1992) **339**:135–8.

10  British Society for Antimicrobial Chemotherapy, Antibiotic Prophylaxis of Infective Endocarditis. Recommendations from the Endocarditis Working Party, *Lancet* (1990) **335**:88–9.

# Further reading

Kaye D, ed. *Infective endocarditis* 2nd edn (Raven Press: New York 1992).

# Index